MODERN PERSPECTIVES IN PSYCHIATRY
Edited by John G. Howells

9

MODERN PERSPECTIVES IN THE PSYCHIATRY OF MIDDLE AGE

MODERN PERSPECTIVES IN PSYCHIATRY

Edited by John G. Howells

Modern Perspectives in the Psychiatry of Middle Age

Edited by

JOHN G. HOWELLS
M.D., F.R.C.Psych., D.P.M.
Director, the Institute of Family Psychiatry
The Ipswich Hospital
England

BRUNNER/MAZEL, Publishers • New York

EDITOR'S PREFACE

As old age recedes, so middle age lengthens. Yet books devoted to the psychiatry of this long period of adult experience are rare. Both the intrinsic requirememts of the subject and its novelty demand a place for it in the Modern Perspectives Series. Middle age is taken here to be the phase of life experience following young adulthood and preceding old age—between 40 and 65 years approximately.

This volume deals with its subject as with all others in the series; it selects the growing points in the field for description by acknowledged experts. The approach is clinical with the right balance of theoretical and research input. Contributors are international and write from Australia, Canada, England, Scotland and the U.S.A.

This is the ninth volume in the Modern Perspectives Series, by now an international encyclopaedia of psychiatry. Thus there must be subjects in the previous volumes that touch the theme here. Readers are referred to the cumulative index at the end of Volume Five. Particular attention is drawn to the following previously published topics:

In Volume Three, Modern Perspectives in International Child Psychiatry, are found the following: Chapter 4, Mother-Child Relationship; Chapter 5, Fathering; Chapter 10, Culture and Child Rearing; Chapter 21, Dysfunctions of Parenting.

In Volume Five, Modern Perspectives in Psycho-Obstetrics, are found the following: Chapter 2, Psychosomatic Infertility in the Male and Female; Chapter 3, Pseudocyesis; Chapter 4, The Couvade Syndrome; Chapter 5, The Psychology of Human Sexual Behavior; Chapter 7, Childbirth is a Family Experience; Chapter 9, The Control of Conception; Chapter 10, Termination of Pregnancy; Chapter 20, Emotional and Psychotic Illness Following Childbirth; Chapter 21, Lactation—Its Psychologic Components.

In Volume Seven, Modern Perspectives in the Psychiatric Aspects of Surgery, will be found the following: Chapter 3, The Psychopathology of Cancer; Chapter 4, The Accident-Prone Syndrome; Chapter 5, Delay in Surgery: Patients' Motivations; Chapter 7, Mental Changes as Indicators of

Brain Tumors; Chapter 19, The Psychological and Social Sequelae of Mastectomy; Chapter 20, Psychiatric Aspects of Hysterectomy; Chapter 23, Psychiatric Aspects of Cosmetic Surgery; Chapter 34, Psychological Care of the Dying Child and His Relatives.

In Volume Eight, Modern Perspectives in the Psychiatry of Infancy, are found the following: Chapter 8, Disadvantaged Infants as Parents; Chapter 15, Upbringing in the Super-Rich; Chapter 16, Intergenerational Exchange: Transference of Attitudes Down the Generations; Chapter 19, Mourning for Young Children; Chapter 29, Foster Care.

With each succeeding volume, my work as editor, due to the enthusiasm and responsiveness of the contributors, appears to become easier. My editorial assistant, Mrs. Livia Osborn, has fashioned and guided the work after its conception and completes the volume with yet another extensive name and subject index.

CONTENTS

vii

CLINICAL ISSUES

BASIC THEORY

1

THE DEVELOPMENTAL PSYCHOLOGY OF MIDDLE AGE

DAVID A. CHIRIBOGA, PH.D.

Associate Professor of Psychology in Residence
Human Development and Aging Program
University of California, San Francisco

"It was the the the best of times, it was the worst of times . . . "
Charles Dickens, A *Tale of Two Cities*

INTRODUCTION

The purpose of this chapter is to pull together some of the often divergent theoretical and empirical perspectives on the psychology of middle age. We will begin with the question whether the term "development" can be applied with justification to the study of the middle years. Some psychologists believe that only when age and behavior show a strong and orderly relationship can the term development be used. Such an age-related orderliness is most prevalent in studies of children and the aged (5) and much less obvious in studies of middle life. The argument against a developmental psychology of the later years was presented most cogently by Flavell (39), who suggested over ten years ago that to substantiate itself a psychology of the middle years must demonstrate the major changes, the directionality, and the cross-individual commonality typical of development in childhood and adolescence. For Flavell, change in adulthood seemed minor and the result of more or less random circumstances.

A decade later, we have begun to accumulate the kind of information about middle age which does in fact demonstrate that major changes do occur, that the changes manifest direction, and that individuals within this phase of the life course share certain psychological characteristics. We still

3

know very little about middle age, and what we do know is often gleaned from studies which only coincidentally have included the middle years. The growing body of literature does suggest, however, that middle age not only may be a justified topic of developmental inquiry, but also is a pivotal phase of the life course.

How, then, does one proceed with a developmental inquiry into middle age? There are several issues to be dealt with. One issue is how to identify the age boundaries of the period. In most research, some arbitrary age range is selected, usually from age 40 to 65 or 69, but occasionally dropping down to 35 or extending up to 70. The use of chronological age as a definer of the life course has become suspect, however, as researchers learn more about the factors which underlie apparent age effects (see, for example, Wohlwill (113), and Neugarten (84). Two such factors are social class and cultural background. Thus, Neugarten and Peterson (89) found upper-middle-class respondents to report 40 to be the "prime of life" and middle age to start at 50. In contrast, those from the lower class saw the prime age to be in the 30s and middle age to start at 40. In a similar fashion, Bengtson, Kasschau, and Ragan (9) found Mexican-Americans to perceive a more accelerated aging progress than black Americans, who in turn perceived a more accelerated progress than did representatives of the dominant culture.

Group differences in perceptions of the timing or pace of the life course may be reflecting differences in the salience of social and biological cues of the aging process. Bühler (14) presents a simple model which illustrates this point. Imagine, if you will, a graph representing the biological curve of life for some individual. Typically it will rise rapidly during childhood and adolescence, maintain a long plateau, and then begin to show decrement in the 40s and 50s. A biographical (or psychosocial) curve might show a similar rise and plateau, but a later and less rapid decline. Such a model helps to explain the influence of at least socioeconomic status on timing: Those with physically demanding occupations may notice a decline in performance earlier than those whose jobs are less linked to the biological curve.

Ultimately, of course, the onset of middle age is a very individual matter. For some, middle age may begin the day your son beats you at tennis or your daughter announces her engagement. For others, grey hair or a balding pate, stroke, or other physical change may herald the transition. For most, the onset of middle age is prompted by a combination of such factors, and it becomes clear that the use of rigid age boundaries for middle age, while convenient, is in fact nothing more than that: a convenience.

Regardless of the age boundaries chosen, some investigators make another more or less arbitrary classification: They may decide to treat middle age as one undifferentiated period, or they may impose subdivisions on the period. The placement and duration of these subdivisions of middle age reflect the concerns of the investigator. Levinson (65), for example, was interested in the regular alternation, across the life course, of cross-era transitions and development of "life structures" compatible with each of four eras, or seasons: childhood and adolescence, young adulthood, middle adulthood, and late adulthood. His classification includes a mid-life transition which lasts from roughly age 40 to 45; a middle adult phase which is subdivided into entrance, age 50 transition, and culmination; and a late adult transition from approximately age 60 to 65. Frenkel-Brunswik (41) employed a much simpler classification system. She was interested in changes in accomplishments and productivity over the life course. Much as Neugarten (83) subdivided old age into the "young old" (ages 55-74) and the "old old" (ages 75 and above) stages, Frenkel-Brunswik distinguished two periods which are relevant to mid-life. One, the culmination phase, begins in the late 20s and extends to the late 40s. The second begins in the late 40s and lasts until the early 60s. The former period is probably the most eventful one of the life course, as will be discussed later in this chapter, and a time of peak productivity. The latter period is one marked by the growing presence of social and biological losses; productivity is maintained, but at some cost.

Another question faced by investigators of middle age is whether evaluation of the period should be done in the context of earlier and later periods, whether middle age should be treated separately. While the latter approach is perhaps the simplest and most economical, it may foster an artificial sense of uniqueness and difference. Many developmental psychologists therefore counsel against separate evaluations of people at some particular life stage, especially if the characteristics of the phase are little understood (6, 84). To the extent that the major changes in middle age reflect gradual shifts in behavior or functioning that begin before this life phase, the full explication of these changes can be enhanced by life span rather than phase-specific studies.

Even when the researcher has grappled with the issues outlined above, problems remain. After laboring over an investigation, and following all the usual methodological guidelines for proper research, it is often frustrating to realize the limitations to generalization which are imposed upon life span research. Two major limitations to generalization which are endemic in such research are those imposed by historical and cohort effects (99). Elder's (32, 33) study of children of the Great Depression in America demonstrates that being born only a few years before or after critical periods of historical change may lead to marked differences in adult development. Cohort effects may be even more influential. As described by Neugarten (83), those who now can be categorized as middle-aged are far better educated, more politically active, healthier, and better nourished than those of any previous cohort in American history. She predicts that successive cohorts of the middle-aged will continue to improve in these qualities.

In the face of all the obstacles imposed on research on middle age, or indeed on any age, it may appear surprising to the reader that any systematic body of knowledge has been generated. In fact, there is a great deal that is known about middle age, although our knowledge still is only a fraction of what should be known before theory, research, and service delivery can be integrated effectively. In the following sections, no attempt is made to review all that is known about middle age from a developmental perspective. Instead, some of the more representative findings and theories will be addressed. The first section discusses three theoretical models which have been of seminal value for studies of middle age: those of C. G. Jung, R. J. Havighurst, and E. H. Erikson. The selection of these three is not meant to demean the work of current theorists such as Fiske (38), Gould (42), Levinson (65), Neugarten (82), or Schaie (98), but merely to indicate the continuing heuristic value of the earlier works. Several topics of particular relevance to a developmental psychology of the middle years are then presented, and the chapter ends with some comments about the dualism inherent in the status of being middle-aged.

THREE THEORETICAL PERSPECTIVES ON MIDDLE AGE

From a historical point of view, the theories of Jung, Havighurst, and Erikson have exerted a pervasive influence on the psychology of later life. Jung (60) divided psychological development into two phases, with the second commencing around the age of 40. Up until age 40, most people are preoccupied with meeting obligations which revolve around bearing and raising a family and establishing one's place in society. Meeting these obligations imposes constraints on the developing personality such that men often focus on the instrumental and achievement-oriented facets of personality, while women focus on the more expressive and nurturant.

As the demands of the family lessen, people are freed to balance their personality by giving expression to its suppressed aspects. They acccomplish this "union of opposites" by paying greater heed to the inner world, and bringing parts of this world to consciousness (58). This confrontation with the inner world may be a threatening experience, since it involves giving up the image of youth and recognizing the finitude of life. The transition to an inner orientation is therefore often associated with a period of "storm and stress" (59) and is one people often attempt to elude, preferring to retain the no longer appropriate life-style of the first half of life (60). Unfortunately, this balancing out is not only a possibility afforded by the growing freedom from obligations and social demands, but also a requirement for successful adjustment during the middle years. "What youth found and must find outside, the man of life's afternoon must find within himself" (58, p. 114). One of the major causes of neurosis among people in the second half of life results from the perseveration of an inappropriate life-style (60).

If the individual successfully completes the transition to an inner orientation, he or she can continue to function with undiminished motivation and effectiveness. Acquiring a mature sense of responsibility for oneself also involves developing a feeling of responsibility to the community, and the balanced person in the mid-life is often a leader. At the same time, however, an inner world awareness sensitizes one to the beginnings of the aging process. Acceptance of diminishing capacity and increasing losses is a first step towards coping with the problems in the later years (58).

Havighurst (48) also presents a model of development which suggests that successful resolution of the challenges posed in particular phases of the life course leads to both personal adjustment and the ability to play a highly effective and influential role in society. For Havighurst, each phase of life is associated with a specific set of "developmental tasks" to be dealt with. For middle age, these tasks are to:

Achieve adult civic and social responsiblity;
Establish and maintain an economic standard of living;
Assist teenage children to become responsible and happy adults;
Develop adult leisure-time activities;
Relate to one's spouse as a person;
Accept and adjust to the physiological changes of middle age;
Adjust to aging parents.

A perusal of the literature on later life during the 32 years since Havighurst (48) first published his model demonstrates its continuing validity. Some tasks, such as adjustment to aging parents, have only recently begun to receive empirical attention. Others, such as the use of leisure, are still awaiting attention. In contrast, the theoretical model of Erikson has prompted much direct research application. For Erikson (36), personality develops across a series of epigenetic stages that occur from childhood through old age. Each stage incorporates a central conflict which demands attention if growth is to occur. Although his theory does not emphasize the later aspects of life, being primarily a treatise on childhood and adolescence, two of the eight stages fall within the second half of life. In very general terms, these two involve guiding the succeeding generation, and establishing an enduring sense of personal worth. According to Erikson (35), the central crisis of the middle years is one of generativity versus rejectivity. By generativity is meant a commitment to care for others and a willingness to guide and counsel. Since caretaking tends in some measure to be selective (i.e., one cannot care for everyone), an inherent component of generativity is rejectivity: the exclusion of some or all people from one's concern. For example, middle-agers may be concerned only with their own children or grandchildren, or with the grooming of specific social heirs with whom they have formed a mentor relationship.

One grave danger of the middle years is to become overly concerned with the self, to the exclusion of all, or almost all, others. The extremes of rejectivity lead to feelings of stagnation, which may manifest itself in destructive impulses directed towards one's children, social heirs, or the larger social community (while young men fight wars, it is often the middle-aged who start them). This form of alienation, with the world defined as one very small "me" and a vast array of "theys," may be a source of problems in the next and last stage of life, where the central conflict is described by Erikson (36) as one of integrity versus despair. At this stage the individual must either accept his or her life as having been productive and meaningful or be left with feelings of disgust and despair.

In several important ways, the above three theories share a similar perspective on middle age. All employ life course models of development, although they differ on the timing, duration, and number of phases included within the life course. All make use of some version of the concept of developmental task: Jung and Erikson prefer a single omnibus task per phase, while Havighurst resorts to several more specific and concrete tasks. All assume that personal adjustment depends a great deal on how well the task or tasks of each phase are worked out. All allow some flexibility in the timing of passage through each phase. And, finally, all suggest that middle-aged people may assume a position of responsibility and guidance vis-à-vis social others. That these similarities may be grounded in the actual psychosocial characteristics of the middle-aged is suggested in much of the research reviewed in the following section.

SELECTED TOPICS IN THE PSYCHOLOGY OF MIDDLE AGE

The topics in this section are, as noted in the Introduction, only a sampling of those which have been studied in the field of middle age. Two of the topics, those concerned with stability over time and with the prediction of mental health, look at the middle-aged in terms of their characteristics in the past. The third examines the characteristics of the middle-aged in the present.

Stability or Change: A Continuing Dialogue

Nearly all research on adult personality and behavior has addressed itself directly or indirectly to the question of stability over time. One school of thought emphasizes the stability of personality. As William James once stated, by the age of 30 an individual's "character has set like plaster and will never soften again" (55, p. 121). On the opposing side are those who suggest that life in modern societies promotes discontinuity. Lifton (66), for example, sees the pace and fragmentation of modern life to result in what he calls "Protean Man," an individual with a chameleon-like ability to change his persona in midstream. A more moderate position, and one which reflects the thinking of many developmental researchers, is voiced by Margaret Clark:

> A person is not a pile of stone, no matter how artfully arranged, laid down in concrete early in life. . . . Personality is rather an ongoing process of interaction between the sociocultural world and the internal life of the individual—a process that continues throughout the life-cycle (26, p. 63).

Research evidence for or against stability is inconclusive, even though the results consistently point in the direction of greater stability. In part, the lack of definitive answer is due to the state of the art in lifespan studies: There are few studies which cover the period from childhood or adolescence to middle age (or, for that matter, even shorter periods of time); the same instruments are rarely used across studies; and social scientists sometimes resort to highly inferential strategies in order to impute stability or change. To illustrate this latter point, in some research involving children and adults, different measures are employed at different times in order to measure the same underlying characteristic (see, for example, McKee and Turner (78), Kagan and Moss (61)). Other researchers will infer "genotypic" continuity if personality characterisitics measured at one point in time predict different personality characteristics at another time (67, 74). The main cause of the continuing lack of closure in stability research, however, may be that we have simply been asking the wrong questions. It is probably not a matter of whether there is any evidence of stability, because there usually is. At issue is *how much* stability is required before we can comfortably say that a given behavior or personality/characteristic is stable over time, and what are the preconditions for change.

Even though researchers may have been asking the wrong questions, their results are impressive. In longitudinal research spanning from ten to 50 years, the majority of studies which have examined psychological characteristics in mid-life have found evidence in support of stability (see, for example Block (10); Costa and McCrae (27); Fozard and Thomas (40); Grombach (43); Haan and Day (46); Schaie and Parham (100); Sears (102)). At the very least, the results suggest that there are underlying consistencies in how people approach life, and direct attention towards the need to identify those conditions which lay the groundwork for both stability and change (105).

Antecedents of Mental Health at Mid-life

For health practitioners, particularly those working in the area of prevention, the relationship of early experiences to later mental health is of more than passing interest. Here we will discuss the effect of childhood stress upon mental health during middle age, and whether psychosocial characteristics in youth are related to later health.

Childhood stress has been demonstrated in several studies to exert an influence on adult functioning, and the influence is not necessarily a negative one. The research of Elder on the Great Depression of 1929 provides one example of this type of research. Elder (32, 33) found that boys who had been exposed for longer periods of time to deprivation experiences related to the Depression exhibited lower levels of adaptation in adult life. In another study which used longitudinal data extending from early childhood to middle age, Macfarlane (75) found that discrete episodes of stress during childhood had little more than a temporary influence on mental health. In fact, she reports that many of the adults classified as mature had experienced severe stress as children. Chronically unhappy childhoods or long-term problems seemed to be more effective predictors of mental health in middle age. Macfarlane concludes that it is not the presence of stresses alone that creates later problems, but the duration and context of the stress condition.

Vaillant (110) also reports that while stressful life events may have caused some immediate disturbances during childhood for his all-male sample, these stresses did not necessarily affect mental health in middle age. Like Macfarlane, he found some evidence that early stresses may create a growth-enhancing climate that results in a more mature personality during the middle years. On the other hand, if children experienced multiple stress events, or continuing conditions of deprivation and neglect, mental health in later life was likely to be below average. A similar finding was reported by Lowenthal et al. (73).

Attempts to predict mental health in middle age on the basis of early social and psychosocial characteristics has yielded mixed results. Vaillant and McArthur (111) report little association between mental health during adolescence and health during mid-life. Several characteristics of young adulthood did predict subsequent health, however; these characteristics included the capacity to maintain a happy marriage, occupational success, and the maturity of defenses (110).

Oden (91) used another approach in predicting health. She classified middle-aged members of the original Terman sample of gifted children according to success in their occupations. The most successful middle-agers had been better adjusted as children, had come from more advantaged homes, and were less likely to come from broken homes; they were more likely to be rated by teachers and parents as persevering, goal-directed, self-motivated, and future-oriented. When the respondents were approximately age 30, the successful group was distinguished by their high achievement level; ratings by significant others at ages 30 and 40 indicated them to be more goal-directed and confident. It is perhaps not too surprising that at age 50 the most successful respondents were also the better adjusted.

In a sophisticated attack on the problem of early prediction, Livson and Peskin (68) compared data drawn from early and later adolescence with mental health status at age 40. Among both men and women, the personality factors derived from Q-sort ratings of intensive interviews conducted during adolescence predicted health at 40. Although there was considerable variation both by sex and by early and later adolescence concerning which factors predicted best, Intellectual Competence (a factor composed of five ratings: values intellectual matters, wide interests, appears intelligent, verbally fluent, and interesting) was associated, for both sexes and both periods of adolescence, with later health. For men, and to a somewhat lesser extent for women, the results could be interpreted to mean that healthy adolescents become healthy middle-agers (68).

Psychological and Behavioral Characteristics of the Middle-aged

After reviewing a decade of personality research on middle age and aging, Neugarten (82) concluded that little had been accomplished except for the creation of numerous untested models of development and some complex analytic designs. She uttered a plea for more attention to the description of behavior and functioning in later life. This section reviews some of the major areas in which developmental psychologists have conducted descriptive research.

Cognitive performance

Research on cognitive status has generally established that there are minimal to moderate decrements in performance during the middle years, followed by more severe decrements in the later years. Much of the attention has focused on crystallized intelligence, measured by general verbal tests like WAIS Vocabulary and Information, and fluid intelligence, measured by often nonverbal, integrative performance tests like WAIS Block Design, Picture Arrangement, and Digit Symbol. Crystallized intelligence shows little if any decline during the middle years, particularly when factors such as education, cohort, sex, and health are controlled (11, 12, 98). Fluid intelligence is likely to show a significant decline as early as the 40s (11, 12, 31).

Research on learning and memory suggests that there is mild but progressive decline in performance after the 20s (3, 28, 53). By middle age, the decline is clearly evident in test performance even though not excessive: The middle-aged still are closer in their performance levels to young adults than to those 65 and older (2, 28). Much of the problem middle-age respondents have with learning and memory tests appears to center on how they organize the material, and on decreasing use of mediating strategies to encode material for more effective storage (3, 28, 53, 94). In short, there are progressive problems with both the acquisition and retrieval of information.

Not all the research findings point unequivocally in the direction of decline in the middle years, however. Particularly in the area of intelligence there have been suggestions that characteristics of the individual are of primary importance in determining the presence or absence of decline. For example, longitudinal studies of superior adults often report stability or improvement in test performance during the middle years (62, 90, 102). In one of the more carefully executed life span studies on cognition, as well as one of the most criticized (51), Schaie (98) and his colleagues have examined change over a 14-year period on the Primary Mental Abilities Test. Little evidence for cognitive decline was found until well past middle age—as long as health was maintained. In subsequent analyses, Schaie (98) experimented with the results produced with different analytic designs. Repeated measurement design results suggested that decline generally does not occur until after the 50s, although an independent random sample design indicated some decline in mid-life for two of the five subtests of the PMA: Reasoning and Word Fluency. Schaie (98) also reports that cohort differences were more substantial than age differences, while demographic factors such as income, education, and occupational status influenced scores on the PMA but did not eliminate the age effect.

Themes of power and mastery

In a surprising number of studies, the middle-aged have been found to exhibit qualities of power and mastery. The Spanish philosopher Ortega y Gasset (92) labels them the "dominant generation" and maintains that people in this phase of life are the natural leaders in the various activities they participate in. While such a view might be suspected to be reflective only of a rather small and elite portion of the middle-aged, it is in fact a view shared by people of other ages: The middle-aged are viewed as the most intellectually capable and powerful age group (15, 16, 96).

Ortega y Gasset is not the only theorist to be impressed by the middle-aged. Based on his life span studies of cognition, Schaie (98) is in the process of developing a stage theory of cognitive development. His stage of "responsibility" falls within the middle years, and is depicted as a stage where people have assumed responsibilities for fairly complex "microsystems" within the home and at work. For those who assume greater responsibilities, Schaie postulates an "executive" stage which also falls within the middle years. Tenure in the executive stage may be more durable than in the responsible stage, according to Schaie (98), since its occupants represent an elite group whose cognitive performance (as noted in a previous section of this chapter) should continue at a high level well past the average age of decline.

Neugarten (86) has also found men and women in mid-life to occupy a pivotal relationship to other age groups. Drawing on the findings from an admittedly elite population (they were chosen from Who's Who in America and American Men of Science, and similar sources), the middle-aged are portrayed as the most powerful and influential age group. A major theme which arose from her in-depth interviews was the feeling that middle age was prime time, a period when the individual could get things done and feel competent in almost any situation. These individuals manifested a sense of competence and self-knowledge that allowed an active mastery of life's problems. Moreover, they were highly skilled in using others, when necessary, to accomplish tasks.

Somewhat masked by the sense of dynamism and accomplishment, however, was an undercurrent of alarm. These respondents were becoming aware in a very personal way about the reality of death, and some spoke of restructuring time in terms of amount left rather than amount lived. Time had become a precious commodity, to be used carefully and wisely. Subtle—and sometimes not so subtle—cues of biological decline were resulting in an increased awareness of bodily condition: "body monitoring" (19, 86).

The strong sense of purpose and mastery found by Neugarten may have been influenced by the social class of her respondents. There are, however, similar studies drawn from lower-middle-class populations. In one such study, Chiriboga and Thurnher[25] found mastery themes again to be present, but there were marked sex differences. Among those 40 to 55, the men could be characterized by a concern with instrumental activity and by their sense of control and confidence. The women appeared to lack confidence and were more troubled and dependent. However, those respondents who were slightly further along in middle age, and who were postparental, showed an interesting shift. The men seemed to have distanced themselves from the manipulative and assertive stance of early middle age, and were moving in the direction of emotional sensitivity and interest in interpersonal relations. The women, on the other hand, were moving in the opposite direction—towards assertiveness, mastery, and self-confidence.

In a similar study of non-elite men and women in middle age and over, Neugarten and associates (87) found a heightened ability to organize and synthesize information among the middle-aged which seems to be the hallmark of most studies of this "executive" age group. However, changes in intrapsychic functioning were evident in the 40s and 50s: an increasing orientation to the inner world, and a growing distancing from the environment which Neugarten and associates (87) characterized as a form of psychological disengagement. There were no signs of social disengagement, either in terms of social activities or what Havighurst (47) has called "social competence," among the middle-aged members of the sample.

Sex differences in mastery styles comparable to those reported by Chiriboga and Thurnher were also found. The men in the middle years were more involved in an active and aggressive mastery of the social environment, but findings from the older men indicated a shift towards a more nurturant, sensual and affiliative orientation (88). In contrast, women moved from a more submissive and nurturant orientation to one more accepting of aggressive and self-centered activity. In pursuing these findings in other samples, Gutmann (44) has found cross-cultural evidence that, among men, there is a shift from passive mastery styles in young adulthood to active mastery in middle age and a recurrence of passive mastery in later life. Although his investigation of age differences in women is less complete, Gutmann reports some cross-cultural corroboration for the initial finding of a change from a dependent and passive style to one of more active mastery.

Masculinity and femininity: Coming to balance

In the changes of mastery style reported above, the men were adopting styles that are more associated with the traditional female role, and the women were adopting styles more associated with the male role. In short, the findings suggest that there may be a balancing out of the suppressed aspects of one's personality in middle age, as suggested by Jung (60). A number of other studies support the notion of a balance being reached (i.e., Terman and Oden (104); Cameron (17); Monge (80). For example, in one study of men and women aged 18 to 79, the respondents were asked what age groups they would most associate with masculinity and femininity; the middle-aged were seen both as the most masculine and as the most feminine (17). Gutmann (45) speculates that this movement towards balance in mid-life may be prompted by changes in the family.

Early in the family cycle, the tasks of raising and providing for children necessitate divisions of labor. The male, in adopting active and instrumental roles, suppresses his needs for nurturance and dependency. The female, adopting the more socio-expressive roles, suppresses her assertive and aggressive inclinations. As the children assume adult responsibilities, the parents are freed to strike a more appropriate balance between the masculine and feminine sides of their personality.

Crisis and Transition in Mid-life

There is a remarkable consensus of opinion among both researchers and theoreticians that entrance into middle age is frequently accompanied by storm and stress (14, 34, 41, 42, 59, 65, 95). There is, of course, undoubtedly a considerable range of variation in how people react to the changes they face in mid-life. Whether the period is stormy or not, however, the personal transition into middle age can be a dramatic period and has received considerable attention both from the scientific community and from the mass media. The reasons for the drama inherent in the transition are, however, open to question, although they have been discussed at some length (i.e., Levinson (65); Gould (42). It might therefore be helpful to consider the meaning of the mid-life transition from the perspective of research and theory on transitions.

Central to the idea of transition is that each person develops, out of his or her unique set of experiences, what Parkes (93) calls an "assumptive world" and Levinson (65) calls a "life structure." The assumptive world guides our commerce with the environment and our perceptions of life. Its existence, however, is dependent on a relatively stable period of life, such as the "settling down" period (65) of the 30s. When we lose a cornerstone of the structure which underlies our assumptive world, the figurative walls come tumbling down, and Parkes (93) and others have described in detail the pain and agony which such a loss can generate—whether it be due to widowhood, slum clearance, migration, etc.

The pain and agony stem at least in part from the commitment people have to their assumptive worlds. Situations which continue for some time create an often intense involvement (7). Erikson (35) suggests that there may be an innate need for the regularity (or ritualization) of experience afforded by a worldview, and Parkes (93) notes that affectionate bonds develop to the way of life predicated by one's assumptive world. Loss, either real or threatened, of such a worldview can be disturbing, and may provoke a crisis (65, 76, 93, 106).

The actual scenario of the mid-life transition may vary widely from individual to individual. In the general case, the individual's assumptive world becomes increasingly disparate with new information, leading to a condition of *precarious homeostasis*. The challenge to the assumptive world is usually not from a single source, but several: children leaving the home, an illness, being passed over for promotion, the death of a friend, etc. Associated with this precarious homeostasis may be an increasing tension or anxiety as the soon-to-be middle-ager attempts to cope with the problem(s) in conventional ways that match with the increasingly mismatched assumptive world (for example, "I'm her father, so I can tell her to be home by midnight even if she is 21."). Next, there may be a precipitating event. Levinson (65) and others have called these "marker" events or signposts. In themselves, and occurring by themselves, these may have very little meaning. In the context of other major changes, they may initiate the quest for a more satisfying way of life. For example, the middle-aged worker whose career has peaked may begin to question his or her role in the world of work, and wonder if there is not something more rewarding in life. Whatever the new assumptive world may be, the quest may take place in the context of heightening tension, as old coping strategies continue to fail, but have not been supplanted by more effective strategies. This phase of the transitional experience can be very disruptive to those in middle age, since, unlike prior periods of transition, there are no clearly spelled out roles and activities awaiting them (20).

Finally, with the emergence of a more satisfying assumptive world, comes re-equilibration. Efforts are now directed at consolidating a life-style as implied by the new view: "I am a family person. I am here to enjoy life and not work so hard and risk another heart attack." The remainder of the new phase of life is then spent consolidating and refining the new assumptive world, until it too shows signs of increasing discrepancy.

The importance of nonnormative events

While the mid-life transition (or transitions—there can be more than one) may be dramatic, the more common and mundane stresses of everyday life may play an increasing role in the lives of the middle-aged.

The ordinary stresses of life have, in fact, been postulated to be one of the conditions for change that were mentioned briefly in the section on stability versus change. Baltes (6), for example, identifies three sources of change in the personality and behavior: normative age-graded sources such as maturation and socialization; normative history-graded sources such as the unique set of historical events experienced by members of a given cohort; and finally the nonnormative influences which do not occur to most people and do not follow an age-graded schedule of appearance. The normative age-graded influences appear to be most salient in childhood and adolescence; the influence of the history-graded sources may begin to wane in early adulthood; and the nonnormative may become increasingly salient in the middle and latter years (6) (see also Neugarten (82)).

These are, of course, normative events which still do occur in middle age, since people in mid-life can still expect certain events to occur: The empty nest, death of spouse, and retirement are examples. These latter events form part of what Neugarten (85) has called the "normal expectable life-cycle," and as such can be predicted and prepared for. The expectable events of later life are usually much less devastating than the unanticipated: death of a child, unemployment prior to retirement, divorce, loss of a wife (20, 22, 70, 82). Unexpected events have received far less attention, on the average, than the expected, and relatively little is known about them save for their disruptive qualities. If, therefore, we accept the perspective that in the later years we begin to lose our biological and social "programming," we should pay heed to the role of such stresses in everyday life. On the other hand, one should not ignore the lifetime of experience the middle-aged have had with themselves; perhaps by middle age we are more capable of writing our own programs!

Research perspectives on stress

During the past ten to 15 years, a number of studies have examined the stresses of later life. The usual measurement tool has been some form of a life events inventory (see, for example, Holmes and Rahe (50), wherein the occurrence of some 20 to 138 potentially stressful events is checked off by respondents. Although this research approach suffers from several methodological inadequacies (1, 13, 22), there are at least two conclusions about the stresses of middle and later life that can be drawn. First, at some point between young adulthood and middle age, there is a general decrease in the frequency of stressful life events (cf. 1, 23, 30, 71, 77, 81, 109). To what extent this decrease might be linked with theories of psychological and social disengagement (29, 49) is unclear, but the second conclusion is suggestive: Middle-aged and older respondents are less likely to rate equivalent stresses as disruptive (cf. 52, 56, 77). In other words, not only are life events less frequent, but in a sense the older person puts more psychological distance between the self and those events that do intrude. It may also be that older respondents, having experienced a greater variety of stresses than younger respondents over the course of their lives (71), are simply better prepared and more experienced.

Although on a strictly quantitative basis the middle-aged experience fewer of them, a variety of stresses make their presence felt during the second half of life. Children leave the home, health begins to decline, one's work career reaches a plateau, retirement draws near, friends have their first heart attacks, etc. In short, stress is obviously a social and personal reality of middle age.

A Longitudinal Study of Stress

In order to investigate the nature of stress experiences among the middle-aged as well as among younger adults, a longitudinal study was begun in 1969. The sample included high school seniors, newlyweds within one year of marriage, middle-aged parents whose youngest child was about to leave the home, the persons facing retirement.

The initial results confirmed that life in middle age is generally less eventful than during young adulthood. When a life events schedule was considered in tandem with other kinds of life experiences, such as distance from last or next important event, distance from last turning point, and retrospections about the eventfulness of past life, the results suggested that middle-aged respondents in the study had decreased in the overall level of life experiences, not simply those related to stress (73). Subsequent research suggested, however, that the nature of the stressful events experienced in middle age is quite different from those in earlier years. In one analysis life events reported at a five- and seven-year follow-up were compared. Stress was defined not only in terms of frequency, but in terms of whether the reported events were rated as good or bad, and whether respondents experienced intrusive thoughts about the events. At the five-year follow-up, the middle-aged respondents had reported fewer events and had been less preoccupied with them (23). When overall change scores were computed for positive and negative experiences, both the middle-aged groups reported greater change in the negative direction than did the two younger groups, and this difference was most obvious in the area of family functioning (22). In contrast, the middle-aged parental (now postparental) group showed the greatest increase in positive life experiences during the two-year period, while the (now) retired group reported the least. These differences were most apparent in the marital dimension. Taken in conjunction with the previously noted finding that the middle-aged postparental group had experienced considerable negative events in the family category, the results would seem to add to our knowledge concerning the issue of whether the empty nest is a crisis or a challenge: It would appear to have elements of both! In contrast, entry into the retirement phase of life would appear to be associated with more pain than pleasure.

CONCLUDING COMMENTS

Research on middle age is only beginning to emerge as a field. Most of the knowledge to be gleaned from the literature is not directly related to middle age, but represents life span studies which happened to include people in middle years of life. The situation is rapidly changing, but, somewhat ironically, the field of middle age is more like a newborn infant than the mature adult it studies.

There is a certain dualism in the characteristics of middle age reviewed in the preceding pages. On one level, middle age is the prime of life. Interviews with the middle-aged themselves suggest that they feel effective, competent, and at the peak of their powers. They assume responsibilities for others, as well as for themselves. Moreover, people of all ages, young and old, turn to those at mid-life for advice and aid. No longer driven to meet duties and responsibilities, they are truly the "dominant" generation.

For some, the major events associated with middle age assume a more ominous note. Disturbing body changes, loss of family members during the empty next phase, impending retirement, the death of parents and friends, a first heart attack, may underscore the approach of old age and emphasize the finitude of life. It is not entirely surprising, then, that with middle age, especially for men, comes an increase in the kinds of problems discussed in later chapters: alcoholism, suicide, first admissions to mental institutions, etc.

An individual's experience of middle age appears to depend on how the events associated with that period are interpreted. The problem—and the challenge—is to seek out the opportunities that are available, and to discard old ways of thinking and acting that are no longer appropriate to one's life stage. Since the decrements in cognitive and physical performance are relatively minor, at least in the beginnings of this life stage, most research indicates that these decrements can be compensated for quite readily. The overall conclusion one can draw from various studies of life in the middle years is that it is a time of contrasts, containing as it does the potential for both challenge and defeat. Behind every gain there may lie a defeat, and behind every defeat there may lie a gain. Perhaps, as Byron said, middle age is a time when "We hover between fool and sage."

BIBLIOGRAPHY

1. ANDER, S., LINDSTROM, B., and TIBBLIN, G. (1974). Life changes in random samples of middle-aged. In: Gunderson, E. K. E. and Rahe, R. H. (eds).). *Life Stress and Illness.* Springfield, Ill.: Charles C Thomas.
2. ANDERS, T. R. and FOZARD, J. L. (1973). Effects of age upon retrieval from primary and secondary memory. *Developmental Psychology, 9,* 411.
3. ARENBERG, D. and ROBERTSON-TCHABO, E. A. (1977). Learning and aging. In: Birren, J. E. and Schaie, K. W. (eds.). *Handbook of the Psychology of Aging.* New York: Van Nostrand Reinhold.
4. ATCHLEY, R. (1975). *The Sociology of Retirement.* Cambridge, Mass.: Schenkman.
5. BAER, D. M. (1970). An age-irrelevant concept of development. *Merrill Palmer Quarterly, 16,* 230.
6. BALTES, P. B. (1979). Life-span developmental psychology: Some converging observations on history and theory. In: Baltes. P. B. and Brim, O. G., Jr. (eds.). *Life-Span Development and Behavior, Vol. 2.* New York: Academic Press.
7. BECKER, H. S. (1968). Personal change in adult life. In: Neugarten, B. L. (ed.). *Middle Age and Aging: A Reader in Social Psychology.* Chicago, Ill.: University of Chicago Press.
8. BEESON, D. and LOWENTHAL, M. F. (1975). Perceived stress across life course. In: Lowenthal, M. F., Thurnher, M., Chiriboga, D. and Associates. *Four Stages of Life: A Comparative Study of Women and Men Facing Transitions.* San Francisco: Jossey-Bass.
9. BENGTSON, V. L., KASSCHAU, P. L., and RAGAN, P. K. (1977). The impact of social structure on aging individuals. In: Birren, J. E. and Schaie, K. W. (eds.). *Handbook of the Psychology of Aging.* New York: Van Nostrand Reinhold.

10. BLOCK, J. (1971). *Lives Through Time*. Berkeley, Ca.: Bancroft.
11. BOTWINICK, J. (1977). Intellectual abilities. In: Birren, J. E. and Schaie, K. W. (eds.). *Handbook of the Psychology of Aging*. New York: Van Nostrand Reinhold.
12. BOTWINICK, J. and STORANDT, M. (1974). *Memory, Related Functions and Age*. Springfield, Ill.: Charles C Thomas.
13. BROWN, G. W. and BIRLEY, J. L. T. (1968). Crises and life changes and the onset of schizophrenia. *J. of Health and Social Behavior, 9*, 203.
14. BÜHLER, C. (1935). The curve of life as studied in biographies. *J. of Applied Psychology, 19*, 405.
15. CAMERON, P. (1970). The generation gap: Which generation is believed powerful versus generational members' self-appraisal of power? *Developmental Psychology, 3*, 403.
16. CAMERON, P. (1973). Which generation is believed to be intellectually superior and which generation believes itself intellectually superior? *International Journal of Aging and Human Development, 4*, 157.
17. CAMERON, P. (1976). Masculinity/feminity of the generations: As self-reported as stereo-typically appraised. *Int. Journal of Aging Human Development, 7*, 143.
18. CATRON, L., CHIRIBOGA, D., and KRYSTAL, S. (1980). Divorce at mid-life: Psychic dangers of the liminal period, Part I. Empirical considerations. *Maturitas. 2*, 131-139.
19. CHIRIBOGA, D. A. (1979). Marital separation and stress: A life course perspective. *Alternative Lifestyles, 2*, (4): 461-470. Beverly Hills, Ca.: Sage.
20. CHIRIBOGA, D. A. (1979). Conceptualizing adult transitions: A new look at an old subject. (Guest Editor, Issue of life transitions), *Generations*, Western Gerontological Society, IV, 4.
21. CHIRIBOGA, D. (1966). Self actualization in middle aged roles: A preliminary examination. Unpublished research document. Committee on Human Development, University of Chicago, Chicago, Illinois.
22. CHIRIBOGA, D. A. and CUTLER, L. (1980). Stress and adaptation: Life span perspectives. In: Poon, L. (ed.). *Aging in the 1980's: Selected Contemporary Issues in the Psychology of Aging*. Washington, D.C.: American Psychological Association.
23. CHIRIBOGA, D. and DEAN, H. (1978). Dimensions of stress: Perspectives from a longitudinal study. *J. of Psychosomatic Research, 22*, 47.
24. CHIRIBOGA, D. A. and GIGY, L. (1975). Perspective on life course. In: Lowenthal, M. F., Thurnher, M., Chiriboga, D., and Associates. *Four Stages of Life: A Comparative Study of Women and Men Facing Transitions*. San Francisco: Jossey-Bass.
25. CHIRIBOGA, D. A. and THURNHER, M., (1975). Concept of self. In: Lowenthal, M. F., Thurnher, M., Chiriboga, D., and Associates. *Four Stages of Life: A Comparative Study of Women and Men Facing Transitions*. San Francisco: Jossey-Bass.
26. CLARK, M. M., and ANDERSON, B. G. (1967). *Culture and Aging*. Springfield, Ill.: Charles C Thomas.
27. COSTA, P. T. and McCRAE, R. R. (1978). Objective personality assessment. In: Storandt, M., Siegler, I. C., Elias, M. F., (eds.). *The Clinical Psychology of Aging*. New York: Plenum Press.
28. CRAIK, F. I. M. (1977). Age differences in human memory. In: Birren, J. E. and Schaie, K. W. (eds.). *Handbook of the Psychology of Aging*. New York: Van Nostrand Reinhold.
29. CUMMING, E. and HENRY, W. E. (1961). *Growing Old: The Process of Disengagement*. New York: Basic Books.
30. DEKKOR, D. J. and WEBB, J. T. (1974). Relationships of the social readjustment rating scale to psychiatric patient status, anxiety and social desirability. *J. of Psychosomatic Research, 18*, 125.
31. DENNY, N. W. (1979). Problem solving in later adulthood: Intervention research. In: Baltes, P. B. and Brim, O. G., Jr. (eds.). *Life-Span Development and Behavior, Vol. 2*. New York: Academic Press.
32. ELDER, G. H., Jr. (1979). Historical change in life patterns and personality. In: Baltes, P. B. and Brim, O. G., Jr. (eds.). *Life-Span Development and Behavior, Vol. 2*. New

York: Academic Press.
33. ELDER, G. H., Jr. (1974). *Children of the Great Depression: Social Change in Life Experience*. Chicago, Ill.: University of Chicago Press.
34. ERIKSON, E. H. (1977). *Toys and Reasons: Stages in the Ritualization of Experience*. New York: Norton.
35. ERIKSON, E. H. (1980). Themes of adulthood in the Freud-Jung correspondence. In: Smelser, N. and Erikson, E. (eds.). *Themes of Work and Love in Adulthood*. Cambridge, Mass.: Harvard University Press.
36. ERIKSON, E. H. (1950). *Childhood and Society*. New York: Norton.
37. FISKE, M. (1977). Toward a socio-psychological theory of change in adulthood and old age. In: Birren, J. E. and Schaie, K. W. (eds.). *Handbook of the Psychology of Aging*. New York: Van Nostrand Reinhold.
38. FISKE, M. (1980). Tasks and crises of the second half of life: The interrelationship of commitment, coping, and adaptation. In: Birren, J. E. and Sloane, R. B. (eds.). *Handbook of Mental Health and Aging*. Englewood Cliffs, N. J.: Prentice Hall.
39. FLAVELL, J. H. (1970). Cognitive changes in adulthood. In: Goulet, L. R. and Baltes, P. B. (eds.). *Life-Span Developmental Psychology: Research and Theory*. New York: Academic Press.
40. FOZARD, J. L. and THOMAS, J. C., Jr. (1975). Psychology of aging: Basic findings and some psychiatric applications. In: Howells, J. G. (ed.). *Modern Perspectives in the Psychiatry of Old Age*. New York: Brunner/Mazel.
41. FRENKEL-BRUNSWIK, E. (1968). Adjustments and reorientation in the course of the life span. In Neugarten, B. L. (ed.). *Middle Age and Aging: A Reader in Social Psychology*. Chicago: University of Chicago Press.
42. GOULD, R. (1978). *Transformations: Growth and Change in Adult Life*. New York: Simon and Schuster.
43. GROMBACH, H. H. (1976). Consistency and change of personality variables in late life. *Contributions to Human Development, 3*, 51.
44. GUTMANN, D. (1977). The cross-cultural perspective: Notes towards a comparative psychology of aging. In: Birren, J. E. and Schaie, K. W. (eds.). *Handbook of the Psychology of Aging*. New York: Van Nostrand Reinhold.
45. GUTMANN, D. (1975). Parenthood: Key to the comparative psychology of the life cycle? In: Datan, N. and Ginsberg, L. H. (eds.). *Life-Span Developmental Psychology: Normative Life Crises*. New York: Academic Press.
46. HAAN. N. and DAY, D. (1974). A longitudinal study of change and sameness in personality development, adolescence to later adulthood. *Int. Journal of Aging and Human Development, 5, 11*.
47. HAVIGHURST, R. J. (1957). The social competence of middle-aged people. *Genetic Psychology Monographs 56*, 297.
48. HAVIGHURST, R. J. (1948). *Developmental Tasks and Education*. New York: David McKay.
49. HOCHSCHILD, A. (1975). Disengagement theory: A critique and proposal. *American Sociological Review, 40*, 553.
50. HOLMES, T. H. and RAHE, R. H. (1967). The social readjustment rating scale. *Journal of Psychosomatic Research, 11*, 213.
51. HORN, J. L. and DONALDSON, G. (1976). On the myth of intellectual decline in adulthood. *American Psychologist, 31*, 701.
52. HOROWITZ, M. J. SCHAEFER, C., and COONEY, P. (1974). Life event scaling for recency of experience. In: Gunderson, E. K. E. and Rahe, R. H. (eds.). *Life Stress and Illness*. Springfield, Ill.: Charles C Thomas.
53. HULTSCH, D. F. (1974). Learning to learn in adulthood. *J. of Gerontology, 29*, 302.
54. HULTSCH, D. F. and PLEMONS, J. K. (1979). Life events and life-span development. In: Baltes, P. B. and Brim, O. G., Jr. (eds.). *Life-Span Development and Behavior, Vol. 2*. New York: Academic Press.

55. JAMES, W. (1950). *The Principles of Psychology, Vol. 1.* New York: Dover.
56. JEWELL, R. W. (1977). A quantitative study of emotion: The magnitude of emotion rating scale. Medical thesis, University of Washington, Seattle, Washington.
57. JUNG, C. G. (1969). *Collected Works, Vol. II, Psychology and Religion: West and East.* Princeton, N. J.: Princeton University Press.
58. JUNG, C. G. (1966). *Collected Works, Vol. 7, Two Essays on Analytic Psychology.* Princeton, N. J.: Princeton University Press.
59. JUNG, C. G. (1954). *Collected Works, Vol. 17, The Development of Personality.* New York: Pantheon Books.
60. JUNG, C. G. (1933). *Modern Man in Search of a Soul.* New York: Harcourt Brace.
61. KAGAN, J. and MOSS, H. A. (1962). *Birth to Maturity: A Study in Psychological Development.* New York: John Wiley and Sons.
62. KANGAS, J. and BRADWAY, K. (1971). Intelligence at middle age: A thirty-eight year follow-up. *Developmental Psychology, 5,* 333.
63. KELLY, E. L. (1955). Consistency of the adult personality. *American Psychologist, 10,* 659.
64. KRYSTAL, S. and CHIRIBOGA, D. (1979). The empty nest process in mid-life men and women. *Maturitas, 1,* 215.
65. LEVINSON, D. J. (1978). *The Seasons of a Man's Life.* New York: Alfred G. Knopf.
66. LIFTON, R. J. (1971). Protean man. *Archives of General Psychiatry, 24,* 298.
67. LIVSON, N. (1973). Developmental dimensions of personality: A life-span formulation. In: Baltes, P. B. and Schaie, K. W. (eds.). *Life-Span Developmental Psychology: Personality and Socialization.* New York: Academic Press.
68. LIVSON, N. and PESKIN, H. (1980). Psychological health at age 40: Prediction from adolescent personality. In: Eichorn, D., Mussen, P., Clausen, J., Haan, N., and Honzik, M. (eds.). *Present and Past in Middle Life.* New York: Academic Press.
69. LOWENTHAL, M. F. (1977). Toward a sociopsychological theory of change in adulthood and old age. In: Birren, J. E. and Schaie, K. W. (eds.). *Handbook of the Psychology of Aging.* New York: Van Nostrand Reinhold.
70. LOWENTHAL, M. F., BERKMAN, P., and ASSOCIATES. (1967). *Aging and Mental Disorder in San Francisco: A Social Psychiatric Study.* San Francisco: Jossey-Bass.
71. LOWENTHAL, M. F. and CHIRIBOGA, D. (1973). Social stress and adaptation: Toward a life course perspective. In: Eisdorfer, C. and Lawton, M. P. (eds.). *The Psychology of Adult Development and Aging.* Washington, D.C.: American Psychological Association.
72. LOWENTHAL, M. F. and CHIRIBOGA, D. A. (1972). Transition to the empty nest: Crisis, challenge or relief? *Archives of General Psychiatry, 26,* 8.
73. LOWENTHAL, M. F., THURNHER, M., CHIRIBOGA, D., and ASSOCIATES. (1975). *Four Stages of Life: A Comparative Study of Women and Men Facing Transitions.* San Francisco: Jossey-Bass.
74. MAAS, H. S. and KUYPERS, J. A. (1974). *From Thirty to Seventy: A Forty-Year Longitudinal Study of Adult Life-Styles and Personality.* San Francisco: Jossey-Bass.
75. MACFARLANE, J. (1964). Perspectives on personality consistency and change from the guidance study. *Vita Humana, 7,* 115.
76. MARRIS, P. (1974). *Loss and Change.* New York: Random House.
77. MASUDA, M., and HOLMES, T. H. (1978). Life events: Perceptions and frequencies. *Psychosomatic Medicine, 40,* 236.
78. MCKEE, J. P. and TURNER, W. S. (1961). The relation of drive ratings in adolescence to CPI and EPPS scores in adulthood. *Vita Humana, 4,* 1.
79. MODELL, J., FURSTENBERG, F. F., Jr., and STRONG, D. (1978). The timing of marriage in the transition to adulthood: Continuity and change, 1860-1975. In: Demos, J. and Boocock, S. S.(eds.), *Turning Points: Historical and Sociological Essays on the Family.* Chicago: University of Chicago Press.

80. MONGE, R. H. (1975). Structure of the self-concept from adolescence through old age. *Experimental Aging Research, 1, 281*.
81. NELSON, P., MENSH, I. N., HECHT, E., and SCHWARTZ, A. N. (1972). Variables in the reporting of recent life changes. *J. of Psychosomatic Research, 16,* 465.
82. NEUGARTEN, B. L. (1977). Personality and aging. In: Birren, J. E. and Schaie, K. W. (eds.). *Handbook of the Psychology of Aging.* New York: Van Nostrand Reinhold.
83. NEUGARTEN, B. L. (1974). Age groups in American society and the rise of the young-old. *Annals of the American Academy of Political and Social Science, 415,* 187.
84. NEUGARTEN, B. L. (1973a). Personality change in late life: A developmental perspective. In: Eisdorfer, C. and Lawton, M. P. (eds.). *The Psychology of Adult Development and Aging.* Washington, D. C.: American Psychological Association.
85. NEUGARTEN, B. L. (1973b). Continuities and discontinuities of psychological issues into adult life. In: Charles, D. C. and Looft, W. R. (eds.). *Readings in Psychological Development Through Life.* New York: Holt Rinehart and Winston.
86. NEUGARTEN, B. L. (1968). The awareness of middle age. In: Neugarten, B. L. (ed.). *Middle Age and Aging: A Reader in Social Psychology.* Chicago, Ill.: University of Chicago Press.
87. NEUGARTEN, B. L. and ASSOCIATES. (1964). *Personality in Middle and Late Life: Empirical Studies.* New York: Atherton Press.
88. NEUGARTEN, B. L. and GUTMANN, D. L. (1968). Age-sex roles and personality in middle age: A thematic apperception study. In: Neugarten, B. L. (ed.) *Middle Age and Aging: A Reader in Social Psychology.* Chicago, Ill.: University of Chicago Press.
89. NEUGARTEN, B. L. and PETERSON, W. A. (1957). A study of the American age-grade system. *Proceedings of the Fourth Congress of the International Association of Gerontology, 3,* 497.
90. NISBET, J. D. (1957). IV. Intelligence and age: Retesting with twenty-four years' interval. *Brit. J. Educ. Psych.,* 27, 190.
91. ODEN, M. H. (1968). The fulfillment of promise. Forty-year follow-up of the Terman gifted group. *Genetic Psychology Monographs, 7,* 3.
92. ORTEGA y GASSET, J. (1958). *Man and Crisis.* New York: Norton.
93. PARKES, C. M. (1972). *Bereavement: Studies of Grief in Adult Life.* New York: International Universities Press.
94. RABBITT, P. (1977). Changes in problem solving ability in old age. In: Birren, J. E. and Schaie, K. W. (eds.). *Handbook of the Psychology of Aging.* New York: Van Nostrand Reinhold.
95. ROSENBERG, S. D. and FARRELL, M. P. (1976). Identity and crisis in middle aged men. *Int. J. Aging and Human Development, 7,* 153.
96. RUBIN, K. H. and BROWN, I. D. R. (1975). A life-span look at person perception and its relationship to communicative interaction. *J. of Gerontology, 30,* 461.
97. ROSENBERG, S. D. and FARRELL, M. P. (1976). Identity and crisis in middle aged men. *Int. J of Aging and Human Development, 7,* 153.
98. SCHAIE, K. W. (1979). The primary mental abilities in adulthood: An exploration in the development of psychometric intelligence. In: Baltes, P. B. and Brim, O. G., Jr. (eds.). *Life-Span Development and Behavior, Vol. 2.* New York: Academic Press.
99. SCHAIE, K. W. (1977). Quasi-experimental research designs in the psychology of aging. In: Birren, J. E. and Schaie, K. W. (eds.). *Handbook of the Psychology of Aging.* New York: Van Nostrand Reinhold.
100. SCHAIE, K. W. and PARHAM, I. A. (1976). Stability of adult personality: Fact or fable? *J. of Personality and Social Psychology, 34,* 146.
101. SEARS, P. S. and BARBEE, A. H. (1978). Career and life satisfaction among Terman's gifted women. In: Stanley, J., George, W. and Solano, C. (eds.). *The Gifted and the Creative: A Fifty Year Perspective.* Baltimore, Md.: Johns Hopkins University Press.

102. SEARS, R. R. (1977). Sources of life satisfactions of the Terman gifted men. *American Psychologist*, *32*, 119.
103. SELYE, H. (1976). *Stress in Health and Disease*. Boston, Mass.: Butterworths.
104. TERMAN, L. M. and ODEN, M. H. (1959). *Genetic Studies of Genius: V. The Gifted Group at Mid-Life*. Stanford, Calif.: Stanford University Press.
105. THOMAE, H. (1976). Personality development in two cultures. A selected review on research aims and issues. Research memo. *Bonn Longitudinal Study of Aging*. Bonn, Germany.
106. THOMPSON, P. W. (1976). Individual adaptation in the middle years: Effects in middle age of 'forgetting' origins and roots. *Journal of Geriatric Psychiatry*, *9*, 5.
107. THURNHER, M. (1974). Goals, values, and life evaluations at the pre-retirement stage. *Journal of Gerontology*, *29*, 85.
108. TURNER, V. W. (1969). *The Ritual Process: Structure and Anti-Structure*. Chicago, Ill.: Aldine Publishing Co.
109. UHLENHUTH, E. H., LIPMAN, R. S., BALTER, M. B. and STERN, J. (1974). Symptom intensity and life stress in the city. *Arch. of General Psychiatry*, *31*, 759.
110. VAILLANT, G. E. (1977). *Adaptation to Life*. Boston, Mass.: Little, Brown and Co.
111. VAILLANT, G. E. and McARTHUR, C. C. (1971). A thirty-year follow-up of somatic symptoms under emotional stress. In: Roff, M., Robins, L. N., and Pollack M. (eds.). *Life History Research in Psychopathology, Vol. 2*. Minneapolis, Minn.: University of Minnesota Press.
112. VAN GENNEP, A. (1960). *The Rites of Passage*. London: Routledge & Kegan Paul.
113. WOHLWILL, J. F. (1970). The age variable in psychological research. *Psychological Review*, *77*, 49.
114. WOODRUFF, D. S. and BIRREN, J. E. (1972). Age changes and cohort differences in personality. *Develop. Psychol.*, *6*, 252.

2

PSYCHOLOGY OF THE WIDOW AND WIDOWER

MARCIA KRAFT GOIN, M.D., PH.D.

Clinical Professor of Psychiatry and the Behavioral Sciences,
University of Southern California School of Medicine.

and

RODNEY W. BURGOYNE, M.D., PH.D.

Professor of Clinical Psychiatry and the Behavioral Sciences,
University of Southern California School of Medicine.

INTRODUCTION

The death of a spouse is psychologically traumatic. The partner sharing the process of daily living is gone. Lost is a special person, whether loved or hated, with whom there are strong emotional ties. The spouse who lives on is no longer wife or husband, but instead has a new sociocultural role, that of widow or widower. An inescapable part of the adaptation to the death of a loved one is the confrontation with the inevitability of one's own death. Immersed as the bereaved is in the grieving process, he or she may be unaware of this deep-lying fear, but it is an inseparable part of the anxiety associated with death.

PHYSICAL AND PSYCHOLOGICAL MORBIDITY

Physical Morbidity

Greenblatt's article, "The Grieving Spouse" (12), contains an excellent review of the literature on the correlation of grieving and physical illness. Several investigators (1, 2, 17, 22) have documented the increase in morbidity which occurs in the year following bereavement, by measuring the

26

number of visits made by the bereaved person to a physician. Cox and Ford's (5) review of government actuary files showed that mortality in widows was higher than average in the second year after widowhood.

Investigations designed to determine if there is a variation in the intensity of these reactions, depending upon whether the spouse died following a brief or a prolonged illness, have produced conflicting answers. In a study of 132 widows, Maddison and Walker (18) found no significant difference in the morbidity whether the husbands had died suddenly or following a long illness. However, Gerber et al.'s (9) data on 81 widows and widowers showed that those bereaved after a chronic illness did not fare as well. They also reported that widowers had more medical problems than widows. Jacobs and Ostfeld's (13) epidemiological review also reported that widowers of all ages were at greater risk for medical illness than women. The peak risk time occurs about six months following the death of the spouse for men, and about two years following the husband's death for women. The reasons given to explain these reactions include: 1) that many of the visits to the medical doctor are actually stimulated by symptoms of depression (rarely did the bereaved see a psychiatrist); 2) the physiological stress caused by the crisis of loss; and 3) behaviors in response to the loss which result in the bereaved's failure to take adequate care of him/herself.

Psychological Morbidity

Lindemann (15) studied the psychological course of acute grief experienced by 101 people. Talks with the bereaved led to the identification of a group of symptoms which could be considered part of a "normal" acute grief reaction. These include sensations of physical distress, extreme hostility, guilt, and preoccupation with the image of the deceased. These were recognized as common reactions in the first few months following bereavement. But, what about the longer term effects?

Much less is known about the long-term psychological effects. We have found that there is a conspiracy of silence between the bereaved and those who have not experienced the death of a loved one regarding the long-range effects of the loss. Although theoretical hypotheses have been formulated, there has been little in-depth study. Marris (19), in his study of 72 widows, reported that many continued to have an active sense of their husbands' presence months after the death. But how long do the pain and the attachments continue? The bereaved somehow learn not to talk about their grief; others, not wanting to understand the intensity of the pain (which someday they themselves will have to face), are relieved to see a widow's or widower's cheerful smiling face. They are not inclined to probe beneath the surface. Some may avoid their bereaved friends altogether, thereby effectively preventing any awareness of what the loss is like.

In their work with patients, psychiatrists can learn much about the grieving process of those patients who suffer losses while in treatment. However, there is always the question whether the lengthy period of grieving is a "normal" reaction or instead a result of the patient's emotional instability.

Because of our interest in this subject, we have taken every opportunity to observe those who were bereaved (friends, colleagues, psychiatric patients and participants in psychological studies) and encouraged them to share their feelings about losses that had occurred years before. We found that the internal emotional attachment to a loved one, including subsequent recurrent episodes of painful grief, may remain for many years. One widow said that it was five years before she could enjoy any activity without feeling a sense of loss because she was neither actively sharing it with her husband nor able to anticipate retelling the experience to him when she returned home. Women, widowed for years, who had made apparent successful adaptations to their new lives, realizing they had an empathic listener, told us about the numbing pain they had for years hidden from others. They also confided that, following their own bereavement, friends, widowed for years, who had never before described their continuing struggle with feelings of loss, began to tell them about what might be called the "secrets of the bereaved." Within this group the secrets could be shared; outsiders would see it as "complaining." "No one," they said, "wants to know how difficult it is" (10).

The timeless, enduring attachment to a dead spouse is another aspect of bereavement. This forcibly came to our attention while conducting a prospective study of 50 female, face-lift patients (11). In the course of this study there was an opportunity to extensively interview several widows. Two, one widowed for five years and another for nine years, revealed that they still experienced a comforting sense of their dead husband's presence, especially during times of stress. Clinically, and in psychological tests (MMPI, FIRO-B, and Beck Depression Scale), these women showed no evidence of psychological disturbance. Their reactions appeared to be one means of achieving psychological adaptation to the loss of their loved ones.

Schaefer (24) writes about the "immortality" of object representations. He hypothesizes that since no living person has experienced death it cannot be conceived of in primary process ideation. "The . . . object of . . . (one's) unconscious or of (one's) psychic reality therefore cannot be 'lost' and is by implication immortal." Yamamoto (25), in his study of mourning in Japan, also addressed the subject of continued emotional attachment to a dead relative. He found that Shintoism and Buddhism permit and give institutional sanction for the mourner to maintain a relationship with the dead through ancestor worship. In Japan, where the mourner is encouraged to acknowledge and maintain ties with the dead loved one, 90% of the 20 Japanese widows in Yamamoto's study acknowledged that they had a sense of their husband's continued presence. In London, according to Marris (19), only 50% acknowledged this feeling. We can reasonably assume that this difference is a reflection of cultural acceptance and non-acceptance of the phenomena of a continued relationship.

THE EFFECT OF MID-LIFE

There has recently been considerable interest in the middle years of life, recognizing it as a period in life with its own particular problems and specific potential for emotional development. The successful mastery of mid-life difficulties, according to Erikson (6), results in "generativity": failure of mastery results in "stagnation." Kline reported Grotjahn as saying that "maturity is the mastery of reality—wisdom is the mastery of death" (14).

The middle-aged have a greater awareness of the finiteness of time and conceptualize their lives in terms of time remaining rather than time since birth (6). They realize that early hopes and dreams for unrealized goals must be accepted as just that—hopes and dreams. The menopause, failing physical strength and diminished vitality are the tangible evidences that time is passing. Fears of dependency reflected in concerns about the loss of health and income are paramount among the anxieties of the middle-aged.

It is a time when life patterns are changing. Children leave or have left home. Parents must deal with feelings of envy as they observe their children's vigor, their excitement about the first job, the availability of young, attractive partners and of marriage and procreation. Women may be going to work for the first time or returning to interrupted careers. In both cases, there are attendant anxieties. However, there is still a great deal of living to be done. Often the post-menopausal years carry with them a feeling of increased sexual freedom. This is not always adequately appreciated, for, as Gadpoille (8) writes, "our culture has been as negative and repressive toward sexuality in older people as toward that in children and in adolescents."

Another profound experience with which the middle-aged person frequently must deal concerns the relationship with parents. During these years there is often a reversal of the child-parent role. Parents may become ill or debilitated, and the responsibility for their care falls to their middle-aged children. One or both parents may die. These realities attack regressive desires and fantasies concerned with the wish to be a child again. Nemiroff and Colarusso (20) have written about the intrapsychic work linked with the death of one's parents. The loosening of the childhood introjects precipitates a great deal of anxiety, since these introjects had "as a central component the internalization of a sense of continuance and security, provided in childhood by the good-enough parent" (4). The adult must now identify that aspect of himself which is part of the true or authentic self, separate from dependence on parents—a developmental task the success of which is crucial to the achievement of emotional fulfillment. Intrapsychically there is a strong struggle waged against accepting this narcissistic injury imposed by the loss of parents. Nemiroff and Colarusso describe how some bereaved attempt to deny the loss of the intrapsychic ties by a regression and an attempt to achieve the type of complete gratification believed possible by infants. Recognition of the "limits imposed by the human condition" (4) can lead to a true sense of separation-individuation and opportunity for realistic achievements.

Socially, there are some special implications for those bereaved in midlife. Although the identified roles of men and women are changing, the core roles of the man as breadwinner and the woman as caretaker remain common. A woman who is widowed in her middle years may have to get her first job. She must do this while enduring the pain of her loss. Finding a job for the first time or returning to a previously abandoned career may prove to be a welcome distraction. In other instances, it may be extremely difficult in view of the limited energy remaining during the emotionally draining grieving experience.

Circumstances force the widow to return to the world of the single woman, but she is usually surrounded by the married couples that formed the basis of her previous social life. Friends often don't know what to do with her. Do they include her when the group gets together, or will it be too painful for her (or for them)? It is painful for her, riding alone in the back seat, but usually it is better than being excluded. Neugarten et al. (21) found that widows often suffer a decrease in their social status. They feel like members of a minority group, singled out for unequal treatment and social discrimination.

The widower may not experience this same social isolation. He often becomes the eligible extra man. There is usually a place for him at social events. In fact, he may feel overwhelmed by the sexual and emotional pressure of women if they cluster around to pursue, nurture and be nurtured by him.

On the negative side, he must cope with unfamiliar daily household tasks, each one of which reminds him of the loss of his wife. While men may appear to have greater resources and to be more socially desirable because of the relative scarcity of available older men, statistics show that they have a greater morbidity following bereavement than do women.

Character Structure and Bereavement

Both men and women who find themselves suddenly single during middle age will struggle with problems related to the process of meeting, getting to know and becoming involved with the opposite sex.

There are many different patterns which the course of bereavement may follow, depending upon the person's character structure. For example, a 58-year-old woman, widowed three years before her first psychiatric interview, had always been active, was engaged in a busy career, and had many interests different from those of her husband. She thought her husband boring and non-intellectual. She experienced his unexpected death from a heart attack as a relief. Now she could meet and spend time with other men. She seemed to have no lack of male companionship, and told the interviewer that she was enjoying many new sexual experiences. The only hint of a negative reaction to her loss was her determined statements that she had no intention of ever becoming emotionally involved again. The interviewer suspected that she was denying feelings of grief and loss and was not surprised when these emerged following a face-lift operation. Post-operatively she was delighted with her new appearance, but very depressed. She admitted that she felt exhausted "playing the dating game." When anyone commented on her youthful appearance, she was quick to reveal her age and the fact that she had had a face-lift. For the first time she began to talk about those aspects of her husband that she had valued, to grieve over his loss, and to wish for a replacement—all of which she had denied pre-operatively by her frantic and indiscriminate sexual encounters.

Another example is a 55-year-old attractive woman who was still actively grieving for her husband one and one-half years after his death. She and her husband had had a close relationship, sharing their lives at home, socially and in the business they ran together. Although she had known for months prior to his death that he had a fatal illness, the reality of his loss still came as a shock. At about the same time as her husband's death, her younger sister was divorced and the patient moved into the sister's home. For the first year she seemed unable to do much more than take care of the necessities of life. However, in the next six months she returned to work part-time and decided to have a face-lift. Before her husband's death, with his constant attention and the reassurance of his affection, she rearely looked at herself in the mirror. When she came in for the face-lift, she talked of worries about the physical restraints which the operation might impose. During her bereavement, she had found that unless she was active with housework, gardening, or other "busy work" she would be flooded with feelings of anxiety and grief. The post-operative surprise for her was the absence of this anxiety; intermittent sadness, painful thoughts, and tears about her husband's death continued, but the agitation was gone. She realized she was actually enjoying her gardening and not just driven to it as an escape. As she probed for a psychological understanding of this change, she became aware that the decision to have the operation represented, symbolically, the beginning of saying a "good-bye" to her dead husband and a decision to reenter the world of the living. It had taken her one and one-half years to reach that point. Six months later she had returned to full-time work. Although she had not yet dated, men were asking her out and she was trying to work up the courage to accept them. Her shyness and discomfort were especially intense because she and her husband had been childhood sweethearts and now, at 55, she was experiencing the anxiety about dating which she had avoided as an adolescent.

The second patient, in contrast to the first, had consciously experienced her loss and grief. Following a time of what Lindemann would call "grief work" she was becoming actively involved in many activities. Dating for the first widow had been a regressive escape—an attempt to deny her loss and her anxieties about her aging body and own mortality. The second patient was well aware of the pain of her loss and clearly expressed some of the special problems of middle age. Her recent concerns about her aging appearance had seemed not to exist when she had the reassurance provided by her devoted husband. Working full-time had previously been easy, but now facing the need to work and perform adequately was frightening in the face of coping with her lack of someone else to depend upon. And finally, loosening the emotional ties with her dead husband meant facing many of the problems which others ordinarily encounter during adolescence.

Sociocultural Effects of Mid-life Bereavement

Lopata (16) has called to our attention the differences in the grieving process that are related to socioeconomic class. These differences are especially clear in the widow's need to construct a new identity following the death of her husband. In contrast to those in the upper socioeconomic classes, women in the lower socioeconomic classes often lead a segregated existence, experiencing little in the way of companionship with their spouses. Their free time and relationships are frequently centered around women friends and there is less need to find a new way of life. An individual of any socioeconomic status will have reactions which are unique to the particular intensity and exclusiveness of the lost relationship. In some instances, class may have influenced the nature of the relationship. However, there do appear to be certain universals that cut across socioeconomic class, for in Maddison and Walker's study social class was not correlated with the incidence of physical illness following the death of a spouse (18).

The Clinician's Role

The problems for the bereaved are significant. The impact of the loss of a spouse lasts for a long time—longer in many respects than we may wish to believe. One of the greatest problems for the bereaved is the wish of well-meaning others to rush them along with their grief work, not recognizing that people must proceed at their own pace. The pressure from others for them to live in the present and look enthusiastically to the future can only lead to frustration and perhaps impede the grieving process. Raphael (23) found that those widows identified as being at high risk for post-bereavement morbidity, but who had the opportunity to share their ongoing feelings of rage, loss, guilt, etc., had decreased morbidity compared to a control group of high-risk widows who were not provided this same opportunity. These data reinforce the fact that the clinician's role is to encourage acceptance of the "normality" of these feelings. This relieves the bereaved of anxieties which may result when the feelings persist long beyond the time others think appropriate, sometimes causing them to believe they are "going crazy."

SUMMARY

We have described the mourning process in general, its longevity, the special problems of the middle-aged, and the difficulties imposed on the middle-aged widow or widower by the interrelationships of these factors.

The death of a loved one is traumatic for everyone. Careful studies of the immediate reactions to the loss have revealed a complex of symptoms during the stage of acute grief. Longer term morbid reactions are more difficult to document but have been indicated by the bereaved's increased number of visits to the physicians and the elevated death statistics in coroner's reports.

The reactions to the death of a spouse may last a long time, longer than many would wish to believe. The fact of the denial of the problem is, in and of itself, a problem for middle-aged widows or widowers. It pressures them to put aside their grief and place a smile on their faces in a hopeful and engaging manner.

The middle-aged are still involved in breadwinning, the nurturing of growing children and perhaps also the nurturing of ailing parents, or their loss.

Clinicians must be alert to the fact that concerns about the need to depend upon others, the awareness of the finiteness of living time remaining, and anxieties about failing health are primary worries of the middle-aged. It is necessary to appreciate this in order to avoid accepting the patient's cheerful attitude at face value. One must allow and encourage the bereaved to describe their deep-seated concerns which otherwise, for fear of rejection, would remain hidden. Do not become unreasonably concerned if their grief reactions continue longer than "expected." Listen, understand the depth of the problems, look for and analyze destructive attempts at denial and escape, but grant people in mid-life the reality that grieving a dead spouse is a long, painful process, fraught with special problems for the middle-aged. These special problems include children leaving home, unachieved life goals in work, responsibility for parents, fears about involvements with the opposite sex and a new awareness of the growing concern about the physical frailities imposed by aging.

REFERENCES

1. BORENSTEIN, P. E., CLAYTON, P. J., HALIKAS, J. A., et al. (1973). The depression of widowhood after thirteen months. *Br. J. Psychiat.*, 122: 561.
2. CLAYTON, P. J. (1974). Mortality and morbidity in the first year of widowhood. *Arch. Gen. Psychiat.*, 30(6): 747.
3. CLAYTON, P. J. (1978). Epidemiological review of the mortality of bereavement. *Psychosom. Med.*, 40(5): 435.
4. COLARUSSO, C. A., and NEMIROFF, R. A. The father at midlife: Crisis and the growth of paternal identity. Unpub. manuscript
5. COX, P. R., and FORD, J. (1964). The mortality of widows shortly after widowhood. *Lancet*, 1: 163.
6. ERIKSON, E. H. (1963. Eight stages of man. In: Erikson, E. H. *Childhood and Society*. New York: W. W. Norton (second edition).
7. FREEDMAN, A. M., KAPLAN, H. I., and SADOCK, B. S. The middle aged (chapter 47). In: Freedman, A. M. et al. (Eds.) *Modern Synopsis of Comprehensive Textbook in Psychiatry*. Baltimore: Williams and Wilkins.
8. GADPOILLE, W. (1975). *The cycles of sex*. New York: Scribners.
9. GERBER, I., RUSALEN, R., HANNON, N., BATTIN, D., and ARKIN, A. (1975). Anticipatory grief and aged widows and widowers. *J. Gerontol.*, 30(2): 225.
10. GOIN, M. K., BURGOYNE, R. W., and GOIN, J. J. (1979). Timeless attachment to a dead relative. *Amer. J. Psychiat.*, 136(7): 988.

11. GOIN, M. K., BURGOYNE, R. W., GOIN, J. M., and STAPLES, F. R. (April 1980). A prospective psychological study of 50 female face-lift patients. *Plast. & Reconstructive Surgery*.
12. GREENBLATT, M. (1978). The grieving spouse. *Amer. J. Psychiat., 43*: 7.
13. JACOBS, S., and OSTFELD, A. (1977). An epidemiological review of the mortality of bereavement. *Psychosom. Med., 39*(5): 344.
14. KLINE, F. Personal communication.
15. LINDEMANN, E. (1944). Symptomatology and management of acute grief. *Amer. J. Psychiat., 101*: 141.
16. LOPATA, H. Z. (1975). On widowhood grief work and identity reconstruction. *J. Geriatric Psychiat., 8*: 41.
17. MADDISON, D. (1968). The relevance of conjugal bereavement for preventive psychiatry. *Br. J. Med. Psychol., 41*: 223.
18. MADDISON, D., and WALKER, W. L. (1967). Factors affecting the outcome of conjugal bereavement. *Amer. J. Psychiat., 113*: 1057.
19. MARRIS, P. (1958). *Widows and their families*. London: Routledge and Kegan Paul.
20. NEMIROFF, R. A., and COLARUSSO, C. A. (1980). Authenticity and narcissism in the adult development of the self. *Annual of Psychoanalysis*. New York: International Universities Press.
21. NEUGARTEN, B., and DATAN, N. (1974). The middle years (chapter 29). In: Arieti, S. (Ed.) *American Handbook of Psychiatry*. New York: Basic Books (second edition).
22. PARKES, C. M. (1970). The first year of bereavement. *Psychiatry, 33*(4): 444.
23. RAPHAEL, B. (1977). Preventive intervention with the recently bereaved. *Arch. Gen. Psychiat., 34*: 1450.
24. SCHAEFER, R. (1968). *Aspects of Internalization*. New York: International Universities Press.
25. YAMAMOTO, J., OKONOGI, K., IWASAKI, T., and YOSHIMURA, I. (1969). Mourning in Japan. *Amer. J. Psychiat., 125*(12): 1660.

3

PARENTS AND THEIR PARENTS-IN-LAW

Eric Lager, M.D.

Clinical Assistant Professor
Department of Mental Health Sciences,
Hahnemann Medical College and Hospital, Philadelphia

INTRODUCTION

Current interest in the family seems hardly to have extended to the in-law relationships. These relationshps may, however, be of considerable clinical significance. They may, for instance, represent the other side of a defensive split in which the biologic parents are seen as all good or all bad. In some instances, the relationship between child and parent-in-law may have significantly contributed to the choice of spouse. Such marriages may be particularly vulnerable when disruptions occur in the in-law relationship. Commonly, the in-law child is not aware of the connection between problems in the marriage and what is occurring in the parent-in-law relationship. The recognition of this connection, at an appropriate time in treatment, may allow a spouse to reconsider his inclination toward divorce and so avert family breakup.

FREUD AND THE MOTHER-IN-LAW

A review of the literature indicates that only Freud (1) paid serious attention to the mother-in-law. *In Totem and Taboo,* he devoted several pages (pp. 12-16) to the subject. He showed that the totems and taboos of preliterate societies served to avoid the temptation to incest. "By far the most wide spread and strictest (and the most interesting from the point of view of civilized races) is that which restricts a man's intercourse with his mother-

36

in-law." In our own society the avoidances are internally reinforced. ". . . the fact that in civilized societies mothers-in-law are such a favorite subject for jokes seems to me to suggest that the emotional relation involved includes sharply contrasted components. I believe that this relation is in fact an ambivalent one, composed of conflicting affectionate and hostile impulses."

Freud quickly disposed of the hostile impulses, which are derived from the mutual feelings of possessiveness of husband and mother for the bride. His description of the development and fate of the affectionate impulses stands quoting at some length.

> A mother, as she grows older, saves herself from this (being left unsatisfied) by putting herself in her children's place, by identifying herself with them; and this she does by making their emotional experiences her own. Parents are said to stay young with their children, and that is indeed one of the most precious psychological gains that parents derive from their children. . . . . A mother's sympathetic identification with her daughter may go so far that she herself falls in love with the man her daughter loves . . . . . . and very often, the unkind sadistic components of her love are directed to the son-in-law, in order that the forbidden, affectionate ones may be the more severely suppressed.

In regard to the son-in-law's feelings, the connection between mother and mother-in-law seems obvious enough today. Freud explained, "The temptation in phantasy is set in motion through the agency of unconscious connecting links." We can add that these unconscious links may affect the relationship of the man and the woman toward either or both of their parents-in-law.

LINKS TO THE PAST

A person's wish to make up childhood deprivations, humiliations and defeats suffered at the hands of parents, or to undo aggressions real or imagined toward them, exerts a continuous if unconscious force on significant current relationships. It affects the relationship to the spouse directly, and also indirectly, through the relationship to the parents-in-law. In clinical practice we can find many instances where the parents-in-law represent a particularly strong link to the past. Frequently, the patient's initial complaint is directly connected to difficulties and distortions in that in-law relationship.

Choice of Spouse and Parents-in-law

The characteristics of the intended spouse's family may be a determinant in the choice of spouse. This includes not only the personal characteristics of family members, but also the configuration of the family and the relationships in the family. In some instances, the absence of the father-in-law may be a significant factor in making it possible for a woman to marry since it offers a condition for avoidance of temptation. In another instance, the father-in-law's relationship to potential rivals offers the opportunity to undo childhood trauma. The therapist can expect to find any of a variety of determinants which will contribute to his understanding of the case.

Avoidance of Guilt. In the following two cases, the patients were able to replace their mothers with their mothers-in-law. In their relationships to them they were able to avoid the guilt experienced toward their own mothers.

Mrs. A's mother had died when she was seven. She had experienced her mother's death as a desertion and unconsciously experienced guilt for the anger she felt toward her mother in that regard. Her feelings toward her father had been considerably sexualized. These had been acted out with a brother-in-law throughout adolescence. He had fondled her genitals while she feigned sleep. These experiences made her feel that an actual "Oedipal victory," that is, the elimination of mother and the sexual possession of father, was a real possibility. Her guilt toward mother, as well as toward her older sister, a mother figure, had thus been intensified. Her relationship to her mother-in-law offered an opportunity to atone for her guilt and to gain her mother-in-law's (mother's) love and forgiveness. *In the treatment, she recalled that she had actually thought that she could marry her husband-to-be because his mother was a widow. Therefore there would be no temptation or possibility for a sexual relationship with her father-in-law (father).*

Mrs. B found a somewhat different solution to a similar problem. She had engaged in sexual intercourse with her stepfather. Marriage had offered an escape from this traumatic situation. Guilt and fear of continued temptation forced her to sever her connection to her parents. She verbalized the feeling that her marriage had allowed her to replace her parents with her husband's parents. *Her mother-in-law's overprotectiveness and her father-in-law's distancing and religiosity were in clear contrast to her mother's permissiveness in regard to sex and her stepfather's seductiveness. This parental configuration protected her to a considerable degree from a repetition of the earlier experience.*

Aspects of her relationship to her mother-in-law made it possible for her to further avoid temptation and atone for guilt. She spent much time with her mother-in-law, specifically in the activity of eating. Her husband observed, with growing unease, her weight gain. She had come to resemble strikingly her obese mother-in-law. It seemed that out of a need for forgiveness by mother, she had identified with her mother-in-law (mother). She had shunted her sexual impulses to a regressive orality.

Bisexual Conflicts. Bisexual conflicts may enter importantly into the in-law relationship. In intensive therapy, such conflicts will become explicit if they appear and are verbalized in the transference. In less intensive situations, they will have to be inferred by the therapist.

Mr. C is an example of a male patient who was eventually able to verbalize his feeling of being feminine in a sexualized relationship to the therapist. This feminine attitude had represented an unconscious defensive maneuver toward his father whom he felt he had easily displaced in his mother's affection, but whose retaliation he feared. He recognized that he had sought the love of powerful male figures. This protected and reassured him from a repetition of retaliatory danger. He recalled how important his father-in-law-to-be was to him as such a figure. It seemed that this man was more significant to him in the marriage than his wife, for whom he was never able to feel much warmth. Even after he divorced her, he was struck by his continued relationship to his father-in-law. His wife's family also allowed for a safer victory. This was over her brother, whose life was a disappointment to the father-in-law in comparison to Mr. C's professional success. Such rewards made it possible for Mr. C to tolerate the humiliating feminine position. A series of frustrations in his father-in-law's love led to rebellious eruption which overturned the entire situation. We will elaborate on this in the section on marital disruptions.

Mrs. D's bisexual conflicts can be inferred. An unusually attractive young woman, she was preoccupied with what she considered defects in her anatomy. This implied masculine strivings which had been heightened by her mother's obvious preference for her brother, about which the patient complained bitterly. Her mother-in-law, in contrast, had been delighted by her feminine beauty. She had spoken to her about her son in ways that made her feel that she preferred her to him. For the first time, the patient felt loved and preferred as a female by a maternal figure. Unfortunately, it was not the patient's fate to be accepted as she was. Her mother-in-law's pleasure in her was motivated by a wish to make her into the kind of woman that she herself had wanted to be. The patient's masculine tastes, reflecting her masculine strivings, did not conform to that image. In addition, any compliance to authority was seen by Mrs. D as feminine submission and as vulnerability to rejection. The "honeymoon" between mother and daughter-in-law was short-lived.

The Biologic Child's Role. The therapist needs also to consider how the biologic child participates in setting up the relationship between the spouse and his/her parents. Mr. B, for instance, was pleased to be able to provide a daughter for his mother, though perhaps his complaint about the closeness of his mother and wife also reflected jealousy. This aspect was more striking with Mrs. D's husband who, though equally anxious to please his mother in this way, became quite sadistic toward the patient as toward a preferred younger sister.

When the use of the spouse to gain access to parent or parent-in-law is not considered in the marital turmoil, both therapist and patient may be confused about the marital difficulties. This was the case in the treatment of Mr. E. He was quite aware that he had been attracted to his wife's family and even converted to their religion to gain a sense of belonging. He was less aware of how much he looked to his wife as a mother. When she threatened divorce he was badly shaken and came to treatment. What was confusing was that while his wife was threatening divorce, she was also urging him to work for her father. This required their moving to another city. Mr. E would have to leave his job where he did highly technical work. Clearly she was contradicting her threat to dissolve the marriage. The patient took great pride in his work. Giving it up to do work for his father-in-law, for which he was overqualified, meant to him relinquishing the last vestiges of his sense of masculinity and ability to stand alone. He vacillated for some time, but when he finally made his decision not to give up his work, his wife asked him to leave her and the children.

In retrospect, the reason for his wife's conflicting messages could be reconstructed. She had been excluded from the family business in favor of a brother. Her husband's superior technical ability was a means of access. She both despised and needed his compliance. Phallic conflicts were apparent in that she both needed and hated her husband's masculinity. The case is reminiscent of a brutal hunting story by Hemingway (2) in which the wife taunts her husband, Macomber, for his lack of courage. Yet she needs him to be weak and to depend on her. When he finally finds his courage by standing his ground against a charging buffalo, she knows he will leave her.

She "accidentally" kills him. Her desire for his family's power as well as for his, represented here by money, is implied in the story.

Disruptions

Disruptions in the in-law relationship may significantly affect the individual and the marriage. Whether the in-law child becomes symptomatic or "acts out" to avoid symptoms depends for the most part on the character of the individual. The pattern will tend to follow that of the reaction to previous disappointments, in particular those with the parents. The disruption may result from a disappointment in love, or from a death.

Divorce. Lager (3) reported several cases which came to divorce following a disappointment with a parent-in-law. Characterologically, these patients reacted to narcissistic hurts with actions that warded off painful affects connected to fantasies of helplessness and castration.

Mr. C, who presented himself unconsciously in a feminine position toward his father-in-law, was able to tolerate this mortification as long as he was able to prove himself worthy of the special love and esteem of this father figure. A series of incidents, which involved him and other in-laws of this man, proved to him that the blood of biologic family was, to his father-in-law, thicker than the water of in-law relationships. At that point, he had to reclaim his masculinity by flaunting an extramarital affair. His rejection of his wife was also retaliatory for the rejection he suffered at the hands of his father-in-law. Both he and his therapist were unaware of these connections for some time. By that time it was already too late to hold together the family, which included three children. When he recognized the connections, he verbalized regret for his actions. His initial complaint had been only a vague sense that he was not in control of his actions.

Mrs. D, who complained initially about her mother-in-law's criticisms, was also a person who had to take action to avoid painful feelings. She also eventually left her spouse. There were a number of determinants for this, but clearly the loss of love of her mother-in-law was a most significant one. Subsequently, she avoided a repetition of disappointment by a woman. Instead she replaced her mother-in-law in an affair with an older man who provided a kind of maternal nurturance for her, and tolerated her narcissistically phallic pursuits in additional affairs with younger men.

Precipitation of Symptoms. The unconscious link of parent to parent-in-law may be particularly strong when a parent was lost through death in childhood. Depression and anxiety may break out after the death of a parent-in-law.

Such a reaction was dramatically demonstrated by a middle-aged grandmother. She became depressed not immediately following the death of her husband, but some months later. Her children, whose solicitousness had no apparent effect on her condition, connected the depression to their father's death. This was true, but only indirectly. The patient's mother had died when she was three years old, and it was her mother-in-law who had unconsciously replaced her. Her affection or rejection could make her well or ill. The patient and her husband had regularly visited the woman every week for 30 years. The patient thought the mother-in-law's expectation that they visit was as much motivated by a love for her as a daughter as it was out of love for the son. After her husband's death the mother-in-law told her that it was not necessary for her to visit so often. The patient experienced the loss as she had experienced the loss of her mother and became clinically depressed.

As is often the case with more severely depressed patients, it was difficult for her to acknowledge the stimulus for her depression. Only gradually was she able to relate the incident, and, even then, she tended to deny its impact.

Mrs. A, the patient who had felt she had to marry a fatherless man, had easier access to her feelings. She came to treatment following the death of her mother-in-law. She readily saw the connection between the loss of her mother-in-law and her symptoms. Predominant among these was anxiety generated in part by her search for a replacement. To that end her husband was now an obstacle, and his negative traits, which previously she had tolerated, now seemed intolerable. Her complaint about his lack of sexual interest in her lost its force as she recognized how she withdrew out of fear of his approaches, which, often coming after she had fallen asleep, replicated the forbidden sexual encounters with her brother-in-law. Her guilt had increased with the death of the mother-in-law, because the death was unconsciously equated with the fulfillment of death wishes toward her mother. As the various connections became clearer to her, the complaints decreased. As she was able to work through her guilt toward her actual mother, her anxiety decreased. She had wanted to keep her family, children and husband together and was able to do so.

Other Clinical Aspects

Many parent/child-in-law relationships are mutually rewarding and stabilizing. Here we are concerned with problems, common in clinical practice. These grow out of intense unconscious conflicts and lead to distortions of current relationships. Such common pathological defenses as splitting and parentification play a part here. Sociocultural differences must also be considered in regard to what significance the in-law relationship may have in a family and what defenses allow for such significance.

Splitting. In a number of the previous examples the defense of splitting relationships into good and bad helped patients maintain a relationship with their parents-in-law. Frequently, in such cases, family members and even parents had been sexually abusive toward the patient during childhood or adolescence. Commonly, patients also split relationships so that the parents-in-law become the objects of their rage in order to protect the parents from it, so to maintain the relationship. The patient's psychological growth may reflect itself in the change that such perceptions undergo. A middle-aged patient may in the initial history report that he/she has come to accept the limitations of a parent-in-law which early in the marriage had been reacted to with hurt and resentment.

Distancing. Few other relationships make it possible for participants to invest so much transference expectation in what appears to be so casual a situation, even to them. This was true for Mrs. F and her father-in-law who lived with her and her family. Mrs. F broke off with her own father after he refused her a small amount of money which would have allowed her to complete her education. Her father-in-law, on the other hand, had been generous from the outset toward her and had given the couple money for the downpayment for the house. In the most overtly intimate moments of their otherwise laconic relationship over the years, the father-in-law would come into the kitchen before dinner and approvingly sniff her cooking. Nevertheless, after he died she left her husband and almost grown children for a man almost her father-in-law's age. Important to her was that he too was generous toward her. Her husband easily fit the part of the miserly father. Despite the importance of the father-in-law, she said that she had not been close to him, but then she added, correctly, that she had after all not been close to anyone. This was true also in the therapy, where it seemed that the therapist was not particularly important to her. Significantly, she soon ran up a balance of unpaid fees equal to the amount her father had not given her.

Sociocultural factors affect the possibility for such relationships. In the American blue-collar family, for instance, three-generational homes are not uncommon, and seem to be made possible by the patriarchal structure of such families. This protects against the possibility of the more regressive and dangerous mother (mother-in-law)-son incest. The difficulty in maintaining the patriarchy and the seesawing balance thus established were the basis of much of the humor in the successful television comedy series "All in the Family."

In contrast, in many black ghetto matrifocal families, distance may have to be maintained actually as well as psychologically. Meers (4) has described how the danger of mother-son incest has propelled sons into the street, with its drug and alcohol addictions. A similar effect may be exerted on the mother/son-in-law relationship. One patient from a ghetto community told how he broke off with his girlfriend because she would only marry him if he moved in with her mother and her children from a prior marriage. He feared the mother-in-law's domination but also verbalized his concern about being drawn into other sexual relationships in the household. Thus, the possibility of a strong maternal figure, who is also available sexually, offers a dangerously regressive temptation. Its avoidance contributes to a perpetuation of the fragmentation of the family. This seems true for the many single-parent families appearing recently in all strata of society.

Parentification. A parent may force a child to take care of him/her through intimidation. Such a tactic will not work with an in-law child or grandchild because the hold cannot be complete. The parent-in-law (grandparent) may resort to a kind of nonsexual seductiveness toward them. In this the parent-in-law (grandparent) abandons the injunctions imposed on his/her child. If that child had identified with those injunctions, even imposed them on her own children, the family may now see him/her as demanding, and the parent-in-law (grandparent) as kind, further isolating and burdening the now confused parentified member. The therapist may, however, be able to demonstrate to that person that the inconsistencies reflect parental self-interest, rather than a set of inherent values. It should be added that such parental tactics are often also out of the awareness of the perpetrator.

In a different kind of parentification, the biologic child may, after his/her marriage, suddenly become the object of favors, in contrast to the in-law child who is ignored or rejected. The in-law child is seen as the intruder who deprives the parents of their child's care. The birth of grandchildren may, in the healthier of such families, reduce this animosity. The in-law child becomes accepted as the provider of grandchildren. When the grandparents are sicker, the birth of grandchildren may be perceived as such a threat to their dependency that they withdraw from their child or become ill.

CONCLUSION

The importance of parents-in-law, both in stabilizing and destabilizing marriages, may be underestimated. Routine investigation of that relationship is indicated when marital problems predominate in the initial complaint. Whenever connections between those difficulties and disturbances in the in-law relationship are found, it will be helpful to bring them to the attention of the patient. The regressive aspects, the links to the past, cannot be interpreted until a manageable transference has been established. In fact, such interpretations, prematurely made, may further destabilize the situation as the patient acts out outside the marriage in an attempt to substitute for the parent-in-law, whom he can no longer invest with regressive needs.

Parent and child-in-law offer to each other opportunity to rework unconscious conflicts—a second chance family. A side effect of the ever increasing divorce rate is loss of such an opportunity. It is not clear what institutions, if any, are taking the place of this relationship.

REFERENCES

1. FREUD, S. (1913), *Totem and Taboo* Standard Edition, Vol. 13, London, Hogarth Press, 1968,p. 1-17.
2. HEMINGWAY, E. (1938) The Short Happy Life of Francis Macomber. In: *The Fifth Column and the First Forty-nine Stories,* New York: Charles Scribner's Sons.
3. LAGER, E. (1977) Parents-in-law: Failure and divorce in a second chance family, *Journal of Marriage and Family Counselling,* 3, 4, 19-23.
4. MEERS, D. R. (1972) Crucible of ambivalence: Sexual identity in the ghetto. In: Muensterberger, W. (Ed.) *The Psychoanalytic Study of Society,* Vol. V, New York: International Universities Press.

4

FEMINISM: A RETURN TO PARITY

Virginia Abernethy, Ph.D.

*Professor of Psychiatry (Anthropology) and Director,
Division of Human Behavior, Department of Psychiatry,
Vanderbilt University School of Medicine
Nashville*

INTRODUCTION

The Women's Movement has compelled attention within the mental health field not only because some patients come predisposed to challenge any perceived sex-role stereotyping, but also because the salience of feminism in the culture has made gender role a symbol as well as the context for conceptualizing and expressing numerous identity and interpersonal conflicts. As a corollary, it is increasingly difficult for young women to disregard feminist ideology in their self-definition; its values are confronted almost of necessity, whether all, part or none are subsequently assimilated.

This paper addresses selected issues associated with feminism, including gender role as a state of mind, biologically determined behaviors that distinguish between male and female, the distribution of sociopolitical power as a function of sex, male/female relationships in contemporary society, views of women within the mental health profession, and the female backlash against feminism. An overview suggests that socialization alone can produce stereotypic sex-role behavior, but that experiential and biological factors are probably mutually reinforcing in most cases. It is further proposed that urbanization and industrialization in a mobile, modern society have had far from benign effects on women, and that the Women's Movement can be seen as a corrective force within this milieu.

GENDER AS STATE OF MIND

There is more than one avenue for discovering inner meanings. Both naturalistic language and research findings have been used to plumb the concept of femininity in traditional western culture.

Sex-Role Stereotypes

Many authors agree that women have been viewed, and often think of themselves, as passive, gentle, sometimes irrational, and ineffective (except in providing for the needs of others). It also has been noted that other attributes are systematically denied through conventional usage of terms to denote the human female. To be persuaded that linguistic patterning is real, the reader should test "woman," "lady" and "girl" as alternate completions to the following sentences (from Lerner (37)):

1. She feared that after her hysterectomy she might no longer feel like a real —————.
2. Jane is sweet, soft-spoken, and modest. She is truly a —————.
3. When Sue began to menstruate, she knew she was on the road to becoming a —————.
4. Why are you always fighting and screaming? Can't you behave like a —————?
5. She felt very passionate with him—he made her feel very much like a —————.

To the native English speaker, the term "woman" is obligatory where there is attribution of aggressivity or sexuality, but it comes as a jolt where the traditional image of femininity is invoked. By contrast, "girl" and "lady" imply childishness, docility, and asexuality. Lerner, a psychologist, suggests that there is resistance to relinquishing the latter terms because the habit and need to think of women as innocent and malleable are deeply entrenched, even among mental health professionals (36, 37). Feminists, on the contrary, insist upon the wholeness of their persons and ask to be known as "women."

Awareness of how women and interactions with women are constrained by the culture is further focused by research on sex-role stereotypes. It appears that in Western culture these stereotypes are pervasive, exert a major influence on self-concept and behavior, and may be an obstacle to growth and mental health in both men and women, although they are particularly damaging to women (3, 17).

A number of research teams working in the United States have reported congruent findings relative to ideas of what is archetypically male and female (6, 7, 29, 31, 39). Especially impressive is the work of Broverman and her associates, who developed a Sex-Role Questionnaire consisting of 41 empirically derived items that distinguish at highly significant levels (p < .001) between popular conceptions of the "average man" and the "average woman." Testing nearly 1,000 subjects in samples that cover a broad spectrum of religious, socioeconomic, sex and age categories, the Broverman team was consistently able to replicate findings. Stereotypically masculine traits identified in this way cluster around the concept of competency; stereotypically female traits cluster around the dimensions of warmth and expressiveness (3, 17).

Social Desirability

The isolation of sex-role stereotypes is in itself not so striking as Broverman's discovery that the masculine cluster of attributes is more socially desirable than the female cluster: In 29 of the 41 stereotypic traits, the masculine pole of the scale was not only judged to be more desirable, but also more desdriptive of a "healthy adult." By comparison, the female pole was judged as more desirable and part of the healthy adult profile for just 12 of the 41 items (3, 17).

A sampling of the socially desirable items that cluster at the masculine pole are: aggressive, independent, not emotional, hides emotions, objective, not easily influenced, dominant, active, competitive, logical, worldly, etc. The complete list of the socially desirable items describing the feminine pole are: doesn't use harsh language, talkative, tactful, gentle, aware of feelings of others, religious, interested in own appearance, neat, quiet, needs security, enjoys art and literature, and easily expresses tender feelings (3, 17).

Self-concept

The Broverman data further suggest that the skewed social desirability of the stereotypes impinges in a negative way on women's self-concept. Not only are there fewer positively valued feminine traits, but women, unlike men, appear to incorporate the devalued characteristics attributed to their sex along with the positive items. It appears that women see themselves not only as sensitive, gentle, expressive, etc., but also as *not* independent, subjective, easily influenced, passive, *ir*rational, etc. On the contrary, men describe themselves as possessing the positively valued competency attributes that are stereotypic for the "average man," and *also* those traits of the warmth-expressiveness cluster that are positively valued in the "average woman's" personality (3, 17).

Androgyny

As exemplified by the Broverman group, the traditional culture has predisposed many, including social scientists, to conceptualize masculinity and femininity at opposite ends of a single gender-role continuum. More recently, however, a research team has developed the concept of androgyny. This term describes the condition of being high on *both* masculinity and femininity, as measured on two independent scales (12, 13). Androgynous women (the evidence for androgynous as opposed to masculine men is mixed) appear to be more flexible than sex-typed individuals in terms of performing stereotypically opposite-sex tasks (14, 33). Moreover, androgynous males and females and masculine males appear to have greater self-esteem than those who score low on the masculinity scale (49). Not surprisingly, androgyny has become the ideal for many feminists who wish to be assertive, active and rational without renouncing positive feminine attributes, as well as for men who value in themselves not only traditional masculinity but also traits such as sensitivity and the capacity for nurturance and empathy.

Achievement as a Function of the Traditional Female Stereotype

It is not known to what extent poor self-concept may be crippling. Nonetheless, it seems a reasonable hypothesis that a woman's internalization of the traditional negative evaluation of female capabilities promotes her withdrawal from competition, so that this would be a factor in the well-known tendency for girls' school performance to deteriorate beginning around high school age, and in the associated downgrading of achievement goals during adolescence (3, 7, 31).

This hypothesis suggests that performance follows from expectations. In addition, however, Horner (31) has proposed that achievement carries a negative valence for women because it is associated in the culture with social rejection: Whereas a successful man is more sought after, a bright and successful woman may eliminate most if not all her potential suitors, so that she is likely to be unpopular and ultimately alone. On the basis of research carried out in the mid-sixties, Horner cites threat of rejection as the underlying dynamic in the "fear of success" motive among college women. Her findings subsequently received independent support, particularly from research protocols that simulated competition in traditionally opposite-sex occupations (16). The hypothesis is also congruent with O'Leary's (43) analysis of internal, or psychological, barriers to female advancement in industrial and business settings. Nonetheless, recent attempts to test the "fear of success" hypothesis have had equivocal or negative results (50, 58).

It is possible that the impact of feminism on the culture has, in fact, changed the reality for many young women today. It is equally true, however, that the results of Horner's study resound with intuitive validity to women whose adolescence spanned the fifties or sixties: This was the era of the "dumb blond" stereotype, the folk wisdom that "Gentlemen Prefer Blondes," and the "Nobody loves a smart ass" aphorism.

Selective Incompetence

Other scholars have suggested that women's intellectual and occupational limitations stem from inhibitions in acquiring specifically quantitative and mechanical skills. For example, Tobias has shown that "math anxiety" afflicts both sexes but women in particular, and that this derives from cultural expectations about boys being good in mathematics while girls are not. This assumption is epitomized by one of the great put-downs in any mathematics class, "You think like a girl" (56, p. 88). Interestingly, the sexes perform approximately equally in mathematics at age nine, but by 13 girls begin to fall behind, a trend that eventually extends to all academic subjects except writing ability and music (55).

Until very recently in the United States, differential skills in quantitative and mechanical skill have been reinforced not only through culturally transmitted expectations but also by school curricula and tracking. Talented girls have typically not been encouraged to take the fourth year of high school mathematics whereas boys are; similarly, there has been differential assignment by sex to workshop or home economics, and encouragement for boys but not girls to use recreational time in sports that teach practical physics through experience with motion, force and trajectory (56).

This socialization process is said to endow males with greater self-esteem and trust in their own competence and rationality so that they are predisposed to achieve in the higher paying occupations that require mechanical and quantitative skills. On the contrary, traditionally reared females tend to have lower self-esteem, appear less flexible than individuals with "masculine" traits in performing opposite-sex activities, fail to acquire quantitative skills, withdraw from competition, and may even be conflicted about the worthwhileness of success in intellectual and occupational spheres.

BIOLOGY AND SEX-ROLE STEREOTYPES

Justification for rigid sex roles hinges usually on the protest, "This is the natural order so nothing can be done." Thus, it is necessary to confront a different order of question: whether in fact the stereotypes are an accurate reflection of male and female potentials independent of socialization pressure. Are these differences between men and women innate or learned? And if innate, do they exist in small degree, or in the magnitude suggested by the stereotypes (3)?

Some assert that innate differences on any of the stereotypic traits must be negligible because observable variations within a sex are of greater magnitude than the difference between the average of each sex, i.e., there is enormous overlap of male and female distributions. Clearly, the evidence that will resolve this hard question is not in, and may never be (3).

It is a "problem" for those who believe that differences in competence are innate to find that girls perform academically at least as well as boys up to the age when career choices begin to be made, so that only after adolescence do discrepancies in male-female achievements favor the male (31, 55). Similarly, statistics on the prevalence of various mental disorders in childhood show that boys greatly outnumber girls in every category, be it learning difficulties, behavior disorders, or childhood psychoses. However, among adults the prevalence of almost all categories of mental illness is reversed: Women are sicker than men (3, 39).

What causes this shift? Are adult, but not developing, females weaker than men? Is labeling applied differentially to men and women? Or is the environment perhaps more pathogenic for women than for men? It is at least a plausible explanation of these related phenomena that the dawning realization of culturally-determined expectations for women, and choices closed to them, *causes* young women to constrict their horizons, thus increasing their susceptibility to psychological disorders (3).

Anthropological Case Studies

The issue of innate differences is addressed both by Mead in *Sex and Temperament in Three Primitive Societies* (40), and by Tiger and Shepher in *Women in the Kibbutz* (54). They reach opposite conclusions.

Tiger and Shepher found that kibbutz women had reverted to maternal and familistic roles despite kibbutz ideology that male and female participation in the economy should be equal (54). This writer, however, suspects that their unqualified conclusion in support of biologically determined sex roles rests upon misinterpretation of their own data: They ignore the impact of differential assignment of women to kitchen and maintenance functions, over the women's protests, during the critical formative period of the 1930s. Once women were cast into de facto domestic roles that already limited their productive activities in the larger economy, it seems unsurprising that they would revive an emphasis on maternal functions and familistic values.

The "biology is destiny" position is challenged by Mead's description of a New Guinea society. Here, women assumed responsibility for the management as well as productive functions of the economy and exhibited, to a greater degree than men, characteristics associated with the competency cluster. Men, on the contrary, were passive, narcissistic and, to the extent that they dwelled on jealous intriguing for the women's attentions, could be seen as masochistic. These findings suggest that male-female differences along the specific dimensions of our cultural stereotype are not so great as to be immutable and, indeed, that role reversal is possible (3, 40).

An intermediate position in the nature/nurture controversy emerges from Draper's (21) controlled comparison of two !Kung (African Bushmen) bands. The first band was studied while continuing its nomadic, foraging existence; the second had become sedentary and semi-agricultural about ten years before Draper's observations were made. Her conclusion is that small differences between boys' and girls' spontaneous behavior are "picked up" and exaggerated into sex-role stereotypes in settings where it is economically advantageous to have specialists in domestic versus other activities.

The nomadic !Kung band was characterized by minimal subsistence needs so that adults worked just a few days a week and essentially no chores were assigned to children. Plant foods gathered by women formed the dietary staples; meat was more valued but less dependably provided through men's hunting. Children were discouraged from accompanying adults on either gathering or hunting expeditions and were casually supervised by any adult remaining in camp. Under these undemanding conditions, it was observed that girls remained somewhat closer to camp and were more often in the company of adults (either sex) than were boys. Boys ranged farther and showed a somewhat greater affinity for peer groups. Draper suggests that these differences occurred spontaneously, without adult suggestion or role models for female domesticity, because women without male protection traveled up to ten or 15 miles from camp on gathering expeditions. Moreover, there was no rigid sex differentiation in play groups because the smallness of !Kung bands (about 30 individuals total) precluded such exclusivity(21).

The sedentary !Kung presented a different aspect. Male and female specialization in animal and plant products, respectively, had been extended so that women took responsibility for cereal cultivation, storage and preparation. This involved them in a major domestic commitment, whereas men assumed the less demanding work of livestock herding and retained free time to interact with adjacent groups. The labor associated with agriculturalism had greatly increased the effort required for subsistence, and children were put to work. Apparently in efforts to escape adult notice, both boys and girls spent more time out of camp than was true of nomadic children, although the sex differential (girls in camp more) persisted. Comparisons within the group of sedentary children also showed girls, more often than boys, becoming the target of commands that required interrupting their activities in order to assist an adult. Boys, when they could be found, were put to work on the longer-term chore of herding livestock (21).

Draper suggests that sex-role stereotyping had been absent among these newly sedentary !Kung (as with their nomadic brethren), but that the different innate proclivities of boys and girls with respect to attachment to adult company and likelihood that they would be within call lead to girls' being differentially socialized to accept commands, tolerate frequent interruptions, easily shift concentration, and restrict activities to the domestic sphere. Ergo, a sex-role stereotype; very small, naturally occurring differences between sexes had been exaggerated when this became economically advantageous (21).

Medical and Experimental Evidence

Also germane for separating biological from experiential factors are controlled, albeit small sample size, studies of individuals with hormonal anomalies. This research suggests that normal females are somewhat more nurturant and have more fantasies related to parenting than either females androgenized in utero or normal males. Testosterone influences are thought to underlie this variability because nurturant behaviors are exaggerated beyond normal female tendencies both among genetic males with testicular feminizing syndrome (end-tissue insensitivity to testosterone) and among X0 females in whom absence of ovaries results in minimal circulating androgens (41).

More easily observed behavioral differences between sexes are tangential to the stereotypic sex-role attributes, although easily incorporated within it. These differences include the male primate's higher activity level (28, 41), and from the embryonic stage onward, the female's greater tolerance for stress (35, 53). In addition, the cyclicity of female hormonal production probably exaggerates and inhibits certain traits in a rhythmic way, there being some evidence for increased sexual drive, sense of competence and well-being around time of ovulation (3, 11, 41, 57).

Finally, there is evidence of a structural basis for males' higher average performance on spatial tasks. Spatial ability appears to be a function of greater lateralization of the brain, and this, in turn, has been shown in one study to correlate with delayed maturation. That is, late maturers of either sex evince greater lateralization and greater spatial ability. When boys and girls are matched on age of puberty, there appears to be no difference in their spatial ability. In the population at large, however, boys tend to mature later, a biological, developmental factor that may account in part for observed differential performance by sex (58).

Hormones and neural structures aside, it appears likely that many, if not all, individuals are sufficiently malleable before about 18 months of age to make a successful adjustment in a gender role opposite to their genetic sex. This is suggested clinically both by transsexuals who are chromosomally and physiologically normal but have been reared in an identifiably pathogenic family setting (51), and by the rare instance where loss of the penis during infancy (e.g. at Johns Hopkins, secondary to circumcision) necessitated rearing a male infant as a female (41).

Learning appears to be a potent influence not only during infancy but also at later stages in the life-cycle. For example, in connection with spatial abilities, it has been reported that, whereas males generally are more "field indpendent" than females, Kikuyu girls without brothers have field independence scores equivalent to those of males in the society. Because these girls have the responsibility of herding the family livestock, they acquire experience in orienting themselves in large open spaces and also are not subject to the constant supervision and interruption that would occur in the home. The inference is that field independence, one measure of spatial abilities, is learned in the context of socialization practices usually associated with males (59).

Thus, although the data are characterized by small sample sizes and either soft or contaminated measurements, it appears that most of sex-role stereotyping is under cortical control, mediated either through idiosyncratic or culturally-transmitted experiential factors. Nonetheless, there is evidence for genetically-based behavioral variability between the sexes. It appears that these relatively small biologically determined differences can be elaborated and magnified under particular environmental conditions.

THE DISTRIBUTION OF POWER BY SEX

Part of the impetus for the Women's Movement derives from a sense that women are unfairly and unnaturally deprived of power in contemporary society. The present attempt to unravel this issue 1) distinguishes between public power (better identified as authority) and de facto power; 2) adduces evidence about the natural predispositions of primate females with respect to power; and 3) examines environmental (socioeconomic) factors that differentially favor male or female power.

Non-human Primates

If reproductive success accrues differentially and positively to more dominant animals, natural selection for assertiveness would be expected. The argument that female as well as male non-human primates are benefitted by assertiveness and power is compelling: Dominant animals in many species, including primates, regularly have preferential access to valued resources, resulting in better rates of offspring survival (2); numerous independent studies of non-human primates show both that stable female hierarchies exist and that dominant females are more likely to consort and mate with the most dominant males (15, 32, 44); logically, too, it is self-evident that no species that selects strongly against females can long survive (15). Therefore, it seems highly probable that selection for assertiveness and striving is independent of sex.

It is true, however, that female non-human primate hierarchies have low visibility compared to male hierarchies and were uniformly overlooked in early field studies (20). Few professionals or nonprofessionals expressed surprise at the "finding" that primate female hierarchies were non-existent: On the contrary, the writer (4) and others viewed it as congruent with women's apparently minimal preoccupation with personal status: "The hierarchical principle doesn't correspond with women's reality . . ." (23, p. 54). Nonetheless, it has recently become clear that powerful matriarchal groups are often extremely stable and consequential in non-human primate species (32, 44). This contrasts with the male pattern of brilliant individual, albeit short, careers.

Human Social Relations

The ease with which female hierarchies were overlooked in non-human primate studies was paralleled by the widespread consensus in anthropology that, cross-culturally, women rarely wield power. More recently, the distinction is being made between authority (public power) and real influence over decision-making and outcomes. It appears that women have been active in the latter aspect of human social relations in many socioeconomic environments, although almost always without concerning themselves about their personal status and, on the contrary, while fostering the view of male authority (47).

Rogers' (47) ethnography of a traditional French peasant farming community illustrates 1) female control over all decisions where villagers can influence outcomes (election to local public office; children's marriages; disposition of the family income), 2) the incumbency of males in all positions of authority (public office and head of household), and 3) the collusion of both sexes in perpetuating the myth of male power.

The lack of correspondence between authority and real power in Rogers' study community is brought home by concrete examples such as the household head's (father) being unable to exercise sanctions over whom a daughter married whereas in another family the mother was; and purchase of equipment desired only by the wife after (wink), "Pierre changed his mind" (47, p. 741). As with the household heads, the village council exercised no power except to elect the equally functionless mayor (47).

The bases for female power in this society, according to Rogers, are that 1) women's economic contribution was at least equal to men's (the traditional family's cash income derived from the wife's dairy work), 2) women controlled the flow of vital information in the society, and 3) women maintained active kinship networks.* Women control information in part because of the geography of French farming communities: Arrayed like a pinwheel, residential areas are the hub; fields, where men spend their days, radiate outward. Not only do kitchens face the street, but women gather regularly at the community water wells, and during the evenings at the barns where women without cows come for milk. Moreover, when men are present, women serve them and listen, but if a man comes upon a group of women, conversation ceases or turns to trivia. Thus, women know most of men's concerns, but the reverse is not true. Much of the information and opinions that men have has been selectively passed on to them by their wives (47).

The balance of power described by Rogers is subject to transformation by a number of social structural and economic factors. She suggests that when women are associated primarily with the domestic sphere, they retain power only so long as the society is domestically oriented, including productive as well as consumer functions, so long as most important interactions concern the community, and where face-to-face communication predominates. When this is balanced by preferential male access to positions of jural authority, an approximation to equality between the sexes appears to exist (47).

It is immediately obvious that these conditions do not obtain in a highly mobile, urban society: Women are still primarily associated with the domestic sphere, but households are isolated from the locus of major economic

---

*One woman without female relatives in the community seemed relatively unable to influence her husband.

and political decision-making as well as from the sources of earned income. Information contained in the women's network is thus relatively trivial and gives them limited influence. Moreover, female kinship networks tend to be fragmented and marginally functional, further undermining women's traditional source of power. In modern society, so long as women remain at home, male power is no myth. It is reality.

It is not surprising that the present distribution of power is a source of discontent for women and fosters social instability. Female primates do not appear to be genetically predisposed to accept powerlessness. On the contrary, female matriarchies, although unobtrusive, appear to be the most stable and cohesive element of non-human primate societies and to exist as a viable form in at least one type of human agricultural economy. In modern urban society, power inheres in the public, nondomestic sphere. In order to acquire power, individuals must participate and compete in this sector, as women are doing in increasing numbers.

Contingency Factors

Women's competitiveness in the public sphere continues to be limited both by expectations as to their work commitment and by the actual constraint of child-bearing. Thus, culturally-transmitted biases and reality factors are often confounded, but jointly create barriers to the advancement of women in many circumstances. For example, a national sample survey of managers and executives showed that job discrimination against women correlates with: "1. less managerial confidence in the ability of women to balance home and career responsibilities; and 2. less expectation that career women's husbands should sacrifice for the sake of their (wives') careers" (48, p. 565).

The respect husbands and wives accord each other's careers is possibly the most modifiable element in this situation. The traditional view that the husband's occupation is automatically of overwhelmingly greater importance is altering, particularly among young professional couples, where it is agreed either that one will locate only where the other can find a suitable job, or that professions must be followed even at the cost of temporary separation in distant cities. Taking the first option, there still remains the decision of what is a minimally "suitable" job, and whether it is the husband or wife who will be underemployed. Decisions are sometimes reached by comparing the *best* offer that each has received and supporting that career; alternatively, the best *combination* may be chosen; or the more traditional choice of favoring the husband's career is often made.

Research is confirming that husbands' attitudes are a major element influencing women's career orientation. It appears that a wife's elective employment is facilitated, and marital satisfaction for both partners is enhanced, when a husband is supportive of his wife's career commitment and also ranks family above career in his personal ordering of priorities. Since women almost always rank family above career, this results in congruence in spouses' value systems. Paradoxically, husbands' average marital satisfaction appears greater when a wife follows a life-style different from that of his own mother—that is, if his mother was career-oriented, happier with a wife who remains at home, and vice versa (10).

Husbands' attitudes toward wives' elective employment appears particularly important when consideration is given to the decision process followed by most potentially career-oriented women. Whereas men are reared with the expectation that they will work during the majority of their lifetime and have only to select a vocation, most women decide *whether* to prepare themselves for a serious work commitment; only then do they consider what to do. Moreover, the consideration of "what" is often limited by stereotypes about gender-appropriate fields, and by anticipation that after marriage one might have little control over geographic location or mobility. Therefore, instead of selecting a career for its intrinsic interest and maximum opportunity, a woman might "realistically" choose a field where relocation is easy. These conflicting criteria force a nonrational decision in terms of career advancement. Finally, if a husband's income is adequate, married women with children or of child-bearing age cannot escape awareness that they have a continuing alternative to career. Their becoming a full-time mother will be applauded by many, including, not infrequently or insignificantly, a husband. When a career is in a difficult or unrewarding phase, the temptation is great. Thus, in the present cultural milieu women's career motivation is assaulted by the tenuous nature of the original commitment, its frequent incompatibility with other valued goals, and its reversibility during a long and crucial stage of the life-cycle (9). Dissatisfaction with the role of housewife, either experienced firsthand or perceived through one's mother, needs to be indelible to persevere against such opposite pressures.

Given that motivation, training, and husband's attitude are all positive, child-rearing remains as a major deterrent to women's occupational achievement. Without abundant energy as well as good options for substitute child care, a mother of young children is severely pressed to maintain a full-time work commitment. The long period of infant dependency among higher-order primates forces a surprisingly similar and restricted life-style upon mothers in dissimilar environments. For example, cross-cultural data show that women with children participate significantly more in home-centered and sex-segregated activities compared either to men or to women without children (18). Similarly, chimpanzee females with infants cluster in relatively stationary groups, whereas males and unemcumbered females roam in mixed-sex bands over much larger territories (25). Moreover, it appears that labor force participation by women with young children in the United States is highly contingent upon the "convenience factors" of particular occupations: These factors all conduce to home-centeredness of life-style, including availability of work at home, close proximity of home to work, and short or flexible working hours (19). Even among modern professional couples who have a long established, dual career life-style and where both careers are successful, in-depth studies (45) and informal observation suggest that it is the wife who typically interrupts her workday when children and household emergencies arise; the husband's work is tacitly accorded greater importance so that he is less likely to become housebound by competing responsibilities.

Given the negative impact of children on women's occupational achievement, the advent of effective female contraception can be seen as a necessary (albeit not sufficient) condition for coalescence of a Women's Movement. It also is unsurprising that feminists strongly support the right of women to terminate unwanted pregnancies. A woman who cannot choose whether to become a mother or not, or at least time a birth to her least detriment, is effectively barred from the vineyards of a modern, urban, mobile society.

CHANGING SOCIAL RELATIONSHIPS

Women's relationships with other women and with men both appear to change as a result of feminist influences. These shifts appear healthy and vital in the long run, although, as will be discussed, for some women the prerequisite for integration of relationships at a more creative level is destruction of existing intimate ties.

In the urban or suburban, mobile environment experienced by many, significant and trusting relationships among women have been rare, contrasting with the good fellowship and loyalty supposedly characterizing men's informal social groups. Subjective reports and research findings suggest that a major obstacle to formation of satisfying relationships among women is low self-esteem. Correlations have been shown between a woman's low self-esteem and 1) a sense of alienation from other women and 2) a low assessment of relationships with women (1). The underlying dynamic appears to be that seeing the self as worthless leads, by identification, to perceiving other women as of no value and consequently feeling that friendships with them are meaningless.

This hypothesis predicts that raising a woman's self-esteem will increase her receptivity to other women's companionship and support. Such an outcome has indeed been reported from countless women's consciousness-raising groups. Initial participation in women's groups is often tentative, somewhat ashamed, and skeptical; as the group moves to the discovery that each member's unsatisfying life situation is not totally her own fault or the result of her incompetence (i.e., blame is externalized onto the culture, the parents, the husband, etc.), women begin to look upon themselves *and* other women as worthwhile individuals who have coped adequately, or perhaps heroically, under adversity. The accuracy of this reinterpretation is not at issue here, but only the process by which some women have discovered self-worth and then become able to attribute positive qualities to other women and ultimately to relate to them as valued friends.

The evolution of women's heterosexual relationships follows a different course. Assuming a like beginning, with men acknowledged as the primary arbiters of value and sought after as offering the only avenue for self-definition available to women, the feminist movement ushered in a reaction that initially generated immense anger toward the culture and society, most often personified in husbands who were identified as major actors in the subjugation of wives. Attainment of the greater psychological and physical comfort attributed to men became a feminist goal, and severance of relationships in which women were dependent, and therefore exploited, an end in itself. Considerably later it began to be discovered, and was eventually reflected in the Women's Movement, that integration of an identity requires more than cutting loose from prior commitments; it requires effort, self-discipline, acquisition of skills, and integrity through adherence to a personal value system or set of principles.

Much of this process has been portrayed in the late Victorian through contemporary literature. The dilemma in which women are traditionally and often realistically portrayed stems from their having no " 'world outside of loving' " (George Eliot, *The Mill on the Floss*) to give them personality and quality, and from the characteristic of loving that is expressed in self-effacement and concern for others (30). Thus, the traditional woman is limited to identity and self-realization founded on selflessness—a contradiction in terms, or at least a dangerously passive stance, dependent for meaning on husband's and children's voluntary response. Thus, the problem for a married woman was (is) self-integration, because her role too often foreclosed fulfillment of any intellectual, physical or emotional needs outside of marriage, and a wife and mother was not supposed to intrude *her* needs into marriage.

The early feminist heroines asserted themselves by leaving a stifling marriage (e.g., Henrik Ibsen's Nora, and Thomas Hardy's Sue Bridehead), an oversimplification repeated (with the variant of adultery) in numerous contemporary novels. The more difficult issue of personal growth is addressed by a limited number of contemporary authors, including Doris Lessing and Margaret Drabble. It is recognized that, in today's society, blaming men and marriage for women's failures is little more than a subtler manifestation of dependency. Thus, persons, male and female, are portrayed as responsible for defining their own occupational, social, and domestic identities(30). The theme that men and women may undertake these goals creatively, together, is apparently not moot for literature, but is nonetheless an optimistic note sounded within the feminist movement and, with increasing frequency, in the culture generally.

The traditional view is that a marriage necessarily suffers if a woman does not put her own needs last. On the contrary, a more negotiated ranking of priorities may have psychologically healthier outcomes for a woman and therefore for the family. Positive effects should be increasingly evident as equality is accepted, so that women are less often pushed into positions of reactive militancy. The basis for healthier male-female relationships is that women who acquire social power for themselves in a career or professional setting are able to empathize in a new way with their mates. Not only are there new areas of common experience, but also a woman who carries a sense of independence and competence within herself is not threatened by, and is actually more open to, another's occasional needs to be passive, emotional, and cared for (3).

In the traditional culture, permission to express passivity and vulnerability is denied to men. This is inevitable so long as husbands bear sole responsibility for the security of dependent, stereotypically feminine wives. The artificial and rigid rules for masculine behavior are beginning to relax, however. A reprieve for woman is a reprieve for man because, as the culture comes to allow women greater scope for exercise of competence, men will benefit from a complementary permission to be more expressive and less determinedly, exhaustingly invulnerable (3).

PSYCHOTHERAPY AND FEMINISM

Although still difficult and alien to many, the social pattern embodied in renewed agitation for women's rights can be seen as an effort to innovate and grow that is fundamentally creative and in harmony with the underlying tenets of the mental health professions. Moreover, the history and ideology of the Women's Movement are germane because, just as psychoanalysis has the goal of exposing and thereby freeing one from determination by developmental history, so, too, an awareness of cultural forces can also enlarge the individual's range of free choice. In the Women's Movement, the process of becoming aware is being called "consciousness raising" (3).

The evidence is mixed as to whether the average mental health professional provides constructive and appropriate support to a female patient. Haan and Livson's (29) findings suggest that female therapists are more critical of close adherence to sexual stereotypes by either male or female patients, while male therapists are more concerned by deviance from sexual stereotypes. However, other data suggest that both male and female therapists evaluate patients against an idealization of the stereotypes (3, 8, 26, 34).

The Broverman team (see above) found not only that male and female mental health professionals reflect the cultural sex-role stereotypes and therefore agree with each other on descriptions of characteristic differences between men and women, but also that comparison of clinicians' profiles of the "average man" and the "average woman" reveal a negative evaluation of the female character: "The clinicians' ratings of a healthy adult and a healthy man did not differ from each other. However, a significant difference did exist between the ratings of the healthy adult and the healthy woman. Our hypothesis that a double standard of health exists for men and women was thus confirmed: the general standard of health (adult, sex-unspecified) is actually applied to men only, while healthy women are perceived as significantly *less* healthy by adult standards" (17, p. 71).

From these data it appears that some clinicians share the general cultural sex-role stereotypes. The further inference is that the stereotypes color perception of patients, clinical judgments about prognosis, and most vitally, interactions with female patients so that the net effect is probably to promote a choice for the traditional female role and self-concept. The *less healthy* aspects of the feminine personality may be reinforced because so much of what is healthy is considered to be specifically masculine, and therefore, inappropriate for a woman. It is difficult to allay the suspicion that, in therapy just as in the culture generally, a woman is rewarded for unaggressiveness, irrationality, dependence, passivity, and emotionality, whereas she may be attacked for exhibiting the opposite traits—those very traits which are judged by clinicians to be healthy in the "socially competent, adult person" (3).

There are limits to inferences which can be drawn from therapists' responses to questionnaires or to hypothetical patient profiles, and clinical evidence that treatment varies systematically with the sex of therapist and patient is usually anecdotal. However, those who wish to be sensitized to this area of doctor-patient interaction will find a mass of documentation in the American Psychological Association's casebook compiled by the Task

Force on Sex Bias and Sex-Role Stereotyping in Psychotherapeutic Practice (3, 8).

Overall, patients' complaints focus on the male therapist's tendency to view women's problems in terms of unfeminine assertiveness, lack of compliance, inattentiveness to a husband's emotional requirements, and failure to put the needs of the marriage above personal satisfactions. The patient's career or aspirations may be depreciated, while therapeutic goals are set by the therapist in terms of acceptance and adjustment to the roles of wife and mother. In addition, a woman's assertiveness is not infrequently interpreted as penis envy, while her attitudes toward child-bearing or rearing may be used as indices of emotional maturity (3).

The Relevance of Psychotherapy

Such value judgments carry a therapist a vast distance from the currents of the new subculture which is gradually legitimizing a broad range of roles for women. Many women no longer docilely accept that their psychological difficulties lie within themselves, and that they must therefore strive to adapt to difficult environmental situations; instead of trying to change themselves, women's newly legitimized objective is to change or reject that difficult social environment (3, 24).

Specifically, it is beginning seriously to conflict with the culture to view "feminine assertiveness as a neurotic phenomenon . . . aimed at overcompensation for and denial of the lack of penis" (34, p. 90). On the contrary, it is accepted by large numbers of women, i.e., it is part of their subculture, that women envy men for their *social power;* it is the cultural permission to be competitive, rational, competent, and sometimes just plain ornery that is important and worth having (3).

In order to be relevant to women today, therapists are asked to be creative, open, and nondirective. If, as an individual, a therapist is a product of the traditional culture, this does not prevent him or her from recognizing, as a professional, that attitudes toward women have been culturally-determined and do not necessarily represent truth. In the service of promoting mental health, a therapist can support women's endeavors to think and feel better about themselves, so that they will not become (in a self-fulfilling prophecy) dependent, passive and ineffective *non*-adults (3).

Feminism and Mental Health

Feminism may already have had and has still considerable potential for promoting mental health (46). This is both observable and modifiable by the clinician.

For example, it appears that sexuality is no longer the problem for women that it was in the 1950s. Comparing a series of 25 outpatients in each of two periods (recent and 25 years ago), Moulton (42) found that 18 patients in the early series reported frigidity or great reluctance with respect to sex even though nearly half of these women were married. She continued, "One woman (from the 1950s series) denied her husband sexual access for over a year and refused to see it as a problem." In contrast, few of the recent series reported sexual problems and, "Sex as an important part of the marital battle has also sharply declined." On the other hand, although sexually active, ten women of the recent series chose not to marry at all, seeing marriage as "a trap that makes women 'sick' rather than safe" (42, pp. 2, 3).

These clinical observations are congruent with research findings suggesting that feminists, compared to more traditional women of like marital status, tend to take greater sexual initiative. They also appear to be more satisfied with ongoing heterosexual relationships, a finding possibly explained by the likelihood that feminists will be self-supporting and therefore relatively free to avoid, and do avoid and withdraw from, emotionally damaging commitments (5).

Self-assertion was a second major problem area for women of the 1950s, many appearing "literally phobic" about assorted mundane activities that required them to express themselves or take control. This symptom, too, has diminished. However, as women feel pressure to achieve occupationally, anxiety associated with assertiveness is being discovered at a new level—for example, in relation to public speaking, recognition of their achievements and intra-office politics or aggression (42).

Describing similar trends in a clinical practice, Kronsky (34) suggests that envy of the male role often vanishes as women begin to take control of their own lives. In particular, emphasis in the therapeutic context on acceptance of their own sexuality and possibilities for self-assertion is seen as useful for increasing women's pleasure in being female. (34)

At the same time, it is recognized that women are distributed along a continuum, some finding that the best adjustment for them lies within the dependent, stereotypic role model. Lerner warns that flexible sex roles may not be for everyone. Her clinical experience suggests that *rigid* sex-role stereotyping is *adaptive* for individuals of either sex who have not ". . . consolidated a stable and clear sense of gender identity" (38, p. 48). These limited individuals are helped by the rigid structuring of a sex role that affirms for them their maleness or femaleness.

However, it may be noted that many patients are as unaware as any traditional therapist that their treatment goals are susceptible to being culturally prescribed and sex-specific. Because of gender stereotyping, which until recently virtually all women accepted for themselves, both patient and therapist may misinterpret the presenting complaints, and thus treatment may fall short of its potential to stimulate growth. Increasing numbers of women are questioning, distressed, or raging at the confines in which their life-style places them. The constructive therapist can provide support or insight for change compatible with each patient's strengths and wishes.

BACKLASH AGAINST FEMINISM

One of the more interesting phenomena associated with feminism is the backlash, energized primarily by women, that it has inspired. In historical perspective, this reaction is not surprising because women in many societies have long been known to ". . . participate as vigorously in their own depreciation as do men"; however, as Lerner notes, ". . . the reasons behind the complicity of both sexes are less than clear" (36, pp. 539-40). Demographic and then psychodynamic hypotheses are advanced as explanations. As with most complex phenomena, multiple causes should probably be sought.

The Demographic Hypothesis

The geographic distribution of supporters and detractors of feminism may shed light. In the United States, the 15 states* that have failed to pass the Equal Rights Amendment (ERA) have without exception a strong rural base and little more than one major metropolitan center. Moreover, four states** that passed but now wish to rescind the amendment approximate these criteria. The anti-abortion movement has also found its greatest support in predominantly rural states. Conversely, supporters of the Women's Movement appear much more likely to have grown up in large cities (52). Thus, demographically, it appears that feminism is spawned in an urban environment and resisted in the hinterland.

These findings recall the description (above) of a French peasant community where women exercised real power but nonetheless promoted their husbands' public display of authority and the myth of male dominance. Reviewing that analysis, conditions conducive to female power were said to

---

*Alabama, Arizona, Arkansas, Florida, Georgia, Illinois, Louisiana, Mississippi, Missouri, Nevada, North Carolina, Oklahoma, South Carolina, Utah, and Virginia.

**Idaho, Kentucky, Nebraska, and Tennessee.

be 1) a domestic-centered society with production as well as consumption activities performed by the family unit, and 2) primacy of face-to-face interactions (47). In large measure, these conditions prevail in rural and small town America, particularly in stable communities where family farms are numerous, much business activity transpires among family enterprises, and religion is a vital force and facilitates regular communication among women. Even where it is no longer the reality, American tradition grows out of this pattern: Not until 1930 were more than half of native-born white Americans living in an urban setting (22). Thus, it might be argued that American women have spearheaded resistance to the ERA and feminism in precisely those settings where they retain real power, and where, for reasons of balance, harmony and family prestige, promotion of the myth of male dominance is compatible with their interests. Thus, they might be expected to resist feminism both 1) because of failure to appreciate that women have been exploited and are powerless in many settings, and 2) because overt challenge to male authority destabilizes their system.

The Psychodynamic Hypothesis

A psychodynamic explanation of resistance to feminism by women complements and amplifies other material covered in this chapter. For example, it could resolve what is a mystery for this writer, viz. why, in societies where women have real power, do they go to lengths to preserve male authority and the myth of male dominance? Men have shown little of such niceties where the environment and social structure have favored them.

Lerner suggests that, for both men and women, ". . . the devaluation of women as well as the very definitions of 'masculine' and 'feminine' behavior stem in large part from a defensive handling of the powerful and persistent affects of the early infant-mother relationship" (36, p. 540). Lerner reasons that the child's helpless dependency on an all-powerful maternal figure arouses negative affects, including envy, fear, rage and shame.

Envy is perhaps the earliest and central affect because the infant perceives the mother as controlling all valued resources within herself. The mother gives all gratification, but is therefore also the source of frustration. " (Melanie) Klein has suggested that spoiling and devaluing are inherent aspects of envy and that the earliest and most important objects of envy and devaluation are the mother and her breast" (36, p. 542). This affect and defensive maneuver appear to be exaggerated in less well-functioning individuals. Otto Kernberg has found that a conspicuous characteristic of borderline and narcissistic patients is "intense envy and hatred" of women, and that this is dealt with defensively by their depreciation and devaluation (36).

Lerner further suggests that the impulse to devalue women is not only pervasive because of the ubiquity of the mother-child relationship, but also sufficiently strong to be reflected in the values and institutions of societies worldwide. In order to neutralize affects engendered by the all-powerful mother, cultures represent women as passive, childish, helpless and dependent. The resulting definition of the traditional husband-wife relationship allows men to experience ". . . a defensive reversal of an early matriarchy" (36, p. 543). Christian David and Karen Horney see this reversal as a manifestation of revenge, the need for which is felt no less by females than by males. Theoretically, these responses should be the more powerful where the child is most targeted for the mother's attention—for instance, when she has sole responsibility for child-rearing and limited alternate outlets for energy and exercise of power (36).

It is clear that, for women, devaluation of the female sex is tantamount to self-devaluation. Yet, this neurotic impulse is sufficiently dynamic so that it is expressed repeatedly in individuals and in whole cultures. In this light, it is proposed that the Women's Movement, through contemplation of the still greater wrongs perpetrated against adult women in modern urban society, represents an effort to replace neurotic defenses with reality-based goals. It may also be noted that, to the extent that the wish for revenge fuels the original impulse, anger may be a necessary stage in every woman's transition to a positive self-image. Moreover, to the extent that women expend their energies and satisfy needs for competence and control on targets other than children, the experiences of childhood should be more benign. Thus, a self-perpetuating cycle in which men and women collude in the devaluation of women could, theoretically, step down to a lower level of intensity.

CONCLUSION

Diverse bodies of data have been applied to explication of the Women's Movement. Biology, anthropology, social psychology, political demography and psychoanalysis have been brought in as seemed appropriate. Only limited conclusions can be drawn, however. It does seem clear that there are innate predispositions to learn particular behaviors which, when socially useful, can be picked up and developed into sex-role stereotypes. It appears untenable, however, to assert that the sex-role stereotypes accurately reflect innate characteristics that distinguish between male and female, either as to the degree of the differences, or in the majority of cases, as to the designated traits. For example, the burden of proof would be on those who see women as weak, when biology unambiguously and repeatedly illustrates the female's capacity to withstand stress.

Feminism specifically challenges negative assumptions about women, viewing this correction as a prerequisite for women's obtaining equal access to education, jobs, and other rights. A more recent goal of feminism has been to show that men, as well as women, are unfairly constrained by the stereotypes and thereby prevented from maximizing both individual potential and the quality of interpersonal relationships.

The basis of some women's resistance to feminism has also been explored. In this context, it seems relevant that women are not everywhere so powerless as they appear in a contemporary, mobile, urban society, but that even in social contexts where women have decisive influence, a myth of male dominance persists. Psychodynamics underlying male and female devaluation of women have been proposed, from which the inference is drawn that movement of women into full-time occupations outside the home could bring unanticipated benefits by mitigating the negative effects of early mother-infant interactions.

In summary, the Women's Movement appears from many perspectives to be a force toward mental health. It can only partially, however, free individuals from the constraints of birth, infant dependency, and parental investment in the young with the consequences that this entails for male-female relationships.

REFERENCES

1. ABERNETHY, V. (1973). The abortion constellation. *Arch. of Gen. Psychiat., 29,* 346.
2. ABERNETHY, V. (1978). *Population Pressure and Cultural Adjustment.* New York: Human Sciences Press.
3. ABERNETHY, V. (1976). Cultural perspectives on the impact of women's changing roles on psychiatry. *Am. J. Psychiat., 133*(6), 657.
4. ABERNETHY, V. (1978). Female hierarchies: An evolutionary perspective. In: Tiger, L. (ed.), *Female Hierarchies.* Chicago: Aldine Press.
5. ABERNETHY, V. (1978). Feminists' heterosexual relationships; More on dominance and mating. *Arch. Gen. Psychiat., 35:* 435-438.
6. ABRAMOWITZ, S. I.; ABRAMOWITZ, C. V.; JACKSON, C., and GOMES, B. (1973). The politics of clinical judgment: What nonliberal examiners infer about women who do not stifle themselves. *J. Consult. Clin. Psychol., 41*(3), 385.
7. ALPER, T. G. Achievement motivation in college women. Manuscript. Wellesley College, Wellesley, Massachusetts.
8. ASHER, J. (1975). Sex bias found in therapy. *Am. Psychol. Assoc. Monitor, 6:* 1,4.
9. BAILYN, L. (1964) Notes on the role of choice in the psychology of professional women. *Daedalus, 93,* 700.
10. BAILYN, L. (1970). Career and family orientations of husbands and wives in relation to marital happiness. *Human Relations, 23*(2), 97.

11. BARDWICK, J. (1970). Psychological conflict and the reproductive system. In: Walker, E.L
. (ed.), *Feminine Personality and Conflict*. Belmont, CA: Brooks-Cole Publishing Company.

12. BEM, S. L. (1974). The measurement of psychological androgyny. *J. Consult. Clin. Psychol.*, 42(2), 155.

13. BEM, S. L. (1975). On sex role adaptability: One consequence of psychological androgyny. *J. of Personality and Social Psychol.*, 31(4), 634.

14. BEM, S. L. and LENNEY, E. (1976). Sex typing and the avoidance of cross-sex behavior. *J. of Personality and Social Psychol.*, 33(1), 48.

15. BERNSTEIN, I. S. (1978). Sex differences in the behavior of nonhuman primates. *Social Science and Medicine, 12B,* 151.

16. BREEDLOVE, C. J. and CICIRELLI, V. G. (1974). Women's fear of success in relation to personal characteristics and type of occupation. *J. Consult. Clin. Psychol.*, 44(3), 444.

17. BROVERMAN, I. K., et al. (1972). Sex-role stereotypes: A current appraisal. *J. of Social Issues, 28(2),* 59.

18. BROWN, J. K. (1970). A note on the division of labor by sex. *American Anthropologist, 72,* 1073.

19. DARIEN, J. C. (1975). Convenience of work and the job constraint of children. *Demography, 12(2),* 245.

20. DEVORE, I. (1965). *Primate Behavior*. New York: Holt, Rinehart and Winston, Inc.

21. DRAPER, P. (1975). Cultural pressure on sex differences. *American Ethnologist, 2(4),* 602.

22. EASTERLIN, R. (1971). Does human fertility adjust to the environment? *American Economic Review, 61(2),* 399.

23. Editorial. (1975). Feminism. *Human Behavior,* 54. (April).

24. ELIAS, M. (1975). Sisterhood therapy. *Human Behavior,* 56. (April).

25. GOODALL, J. (1965). Chimpanzees of the Gombe Stream Reserve. In: DeVore, I. (ed.), *Primate Behavior*. New York: Holt, Rinehart and Winston.

26. GOODALL, K. et al. (1973). Garden-variety sexism: Rampant among psychologists. *Psychology Today,* 9. (February).

27. GOVE, W. R. (1978). Sex differences in mental illness among adult men and women: An evaluation of four questions raised regarding the evidence on the higher rates of women. *Social Sciences and Medicine 12B,* 187.

28. GOY, R. W. (1970). Experimental control of psychosexuality. In: Harris, G. W. and Edwards, R. G. (eds.), *A Discussion of the Determination of Sex*. London: Philosophical Transactions of the Royal Society, series B, vol 259, 149.

29. HAAN, N. and LIVSON, N. (1973). Sex differences in the eyes of expert personality assessors: Blind spots? *J. of Personality Assessment,* 37(5), 486.

30. HASSAN, E. L. (1978). Marriage and divorce in contemporary literature. In: Asbury, B. (ed.), *Marriage-Divorce*. Nashville, Tennessee: Committee for the Humanities.

31. HORNER, M. S. (1970). Femininity and successful achievement: A basic inconsistency. In: Walker, E. L. (ed.), *Feminine Personality and Conflict*. Belmont, California: Brooks-Cole Publishing Co.

32. IMANISHI, I. (1965). The origin of the human family—A primatological approach. In: Altman, S. A. (ed.), *Japanese Monkeys*. Atlanta: Yerkes Regional Primate Center, Emory University.

33. JONES, W. H.; CHERMOVITZ, M. E. O'C., and HANSSON, R. O. (1978). The enigma of androgyny: Differential implications for males and females? *J. Consult. Clin. Psychol.*, 46(2): 298.

34. KRONSKY, B. J. (1971) Feminism and psychotherapy. *J. Contemp. Psychother.*, 3(2), 89.

35. LANE, E. A. (1968). The sex ratio of children born to schizophrenics and a theory of stress. *Psychology Rec.*, 19, 579.

36. LERNER, H. E. (1974). Early origins of envy and devaluation of women: Implications for sex role stereotypes. *Bull. Menninger Clinic,* 38(6), 538.

37. LERNER, H. E. (1976). Girls, ladies, or women? The unconscious dynamics of language choice. *Comprehens. Psychiat.*, *17*(2), 295.
38. LERNER, H. E. (1978). Adaptive and pathogenic aspects of sex-role stereotypes: Implications for parenting and psychotherapy. *Am. J. Psychiat.*, *135*(1), 8.
39. LEVINE, S. V.; KAMIN, L. E., and LEVINE, E. L (1974). Sexism and psychiatry. *Am. J. Orthopsychiat.*, *44*(3), 327.
40. MEAD, M. (1963). *Sex and Temperament in Three Primitive Societies*. New York: William Morrow.
41. MONEY, J. and EHRHARDT, A. A. (1972). *Man and Woman, Boy and Girl*. Baltimore: Johns Hopkins University Press.
42. MOULTON, R. (1976). Some effects of the new feminism—On men and women. Paper presented at the Joint Meeting of the American Academy of Psychoanalysis and the American Psychiatric Association. May 11, 1976. New York: Department of Psychiatry, Columbia University Medical School.
43. O'LEARY, V. E. (1974). Some attitudinal barriers to occupational aspirations in women. *Psychol. Bull.*, *81*(11), 809.
44. RANEY, D. and ABERNETHY, V. (197). Female dominance among non-human primates. Vanderbilt Medical School. In preparation.
45. RAPOPORT, R. and RAPOPORT, R. N. (1969). The dual career family. *Human Relations, 22*(1), 3.
46. RICE, J. K. and RICE, D. G. (1973). Implications of the women's liberation movement. *Am. J. Psychiat.*, 130(2), 191.
47. ROGERS, S. C. (1975). Female forms of power and the myth of male dominance: A model of female/male interaction in peasant society. *American Ethnologist, 2*(4), 727.
48. ROSEN, B.; JERDEE, T. H. and PRESTWICH, T. L. (1975). Dual-career marital adjustment: Potential effects of discriminatory managerial attitudes. *J. of Marriage and the Family*, 565. (Aug)
49. SPENCE, J. T. and HELMREICH, R. L. (1978). *Masculinity and Femininity: Their Psychological Dimensions, Correlates and Antecedents*. Austin: University of Texas Press.
50. STAKE, J. E. (1976). Effect of probability of forthcoming success on sex differences in goal setting: A test of the fear of success hypothesis. *J. Consult. Clin. Psychol.*, *44*(3), 444.
51. STOLLER, R. J. (1971). Transsexualism. *Psychiatric Annals, 1*(4), 61.
52. STOLOFF, C. (1973). Who joins women's liberation? *Psychiatry, 36*(3), 325.
53. TEITELBAUM, M. S. and MANTEL, N. (1971). Socioeconomic factors and the sex ratio at birth. *J. Biosocial Science, 3*(1), 23.
54. TIGER, L. and SHEPHER, J. (1975). *Women in the Kibbutz*. New York: Harcourt Brace Jovanovich.
55. *Time Magazine*, October 27. (1975). Testing the creed. p. 60.
56. TOBIAS, S. (1978). *Overcoming Math Anxiety*. New York: W. W. Norton.
57. UDRY, J. R. and MORRIS, N. H. (1968). Distribution of coitus in the menstrual cycle. *Nature* 220, 593.
58. WABER, D. (1976). Sex differences in cognition: A function of maturation rate? *Science, 192:* 572-574.
59. WHITING, B. (1969). Personal communication. Harvard University, Cambridge, Massachusetts.
60. ZUCKERMAN, M. and WHEELER, L. (1975). To dispel fantasies about the fantasy-based measure of fear of success. *Psychol. Bull.*, *82*(6), 932.

5

WORKING WOMEN
TODAY AND TOMORROW

JOYCE SULLIVAN, PH.D.

Manager, West Coast Branch,
Batten, Batten, Hudson & Swab, Inc.,
Irvine, California

and

KAREN G. ARMS, PH.D.

Assistant Dean, College of Fine and Professional Arts
and Assistant Professor, School of Home Economics,
Kent State University, Kent, Ohio

INTRODUCTION

Outdated before it can be written is the profile of the contemporary working woman. The transition from the dead-end clerical job in which she was frustrated, underpaid, and underutilized to the female executive has only begun. The present picture and relevant statistical information with the accompanying trends will be addressed in this chapter. However, this limited view is too restrictive to portray an accurate perception of the undercurrents. Massive waves resulting from the Women's Movement are projecting women into the full spectrum of the working world roles, including top positions in corporate management.

To assist helping professionals in understanding the transitional pressures experienced by career women, their families and their employers, the content of this chapter will incorporate information and insights not ordinarily packaged together. Gainful employment in a consistent pattern is an element of the adult world; therefore, adult development and life phases as they reflect on work and family decisions will be examined.

71

An emphasis will then be focused on a select group of women emerging as the trendsetters of tomorrow, rather than on the majority of working women. Without precedent, the mid-life, highly committed, married career woman is sculpting a life-style which will undoubtedly influence the direction and acceptance of sex-role changes for generations to come. These changes will have profound impact on societal, governmental and corporate policies. The mid-life married career woman, in addition, represents a model which will exemplify possibilities which were impossibilities a mere decade ago.

STATISTICAL TRENDS

The volume of women of all ages embarking into the labor force is unprecedented. From 1950 to 1977, the number of women working doubled to 40 million (49), and in the year 1978 increased by another million (3). Women now comprise 40% of the total work force in the United States, with over three-fourths of them married. At the turn of the century, a woman's life expectancy was 47 years, 18 of which, on the average, were devoted to giving birth and caring for children. In 1977, these averages converted to 77 years of life expectancy with an average of 10 years devoted to child-rearing (49). This temporal differential is almost 40 years, a startling revolution which has occurred during the period of one lifetime.

The number of mid-life women is significant. It is estimated that American women between ages 45 and 64 will peak numerically at about 36 million around the year 2000 as the post-World War II baby boom reaches this stage of life (10). Over half this number of women, 18.6 million, are anticipated to be dependent upon federal aid programs for their subsistence at that same point in time (5).

In 1920, the typical working woman was 30 years old, from the working class, and single. Currently, the majority of working women are married; half are 40 years of age or older (46), and 30% are age 45 and over (3). Between 1950 and 1974, participation in the labor force by married women living with their husbands increased 80% (46).

Some women must work to survive economically. In 1977, 14% of all families were headed by a female with no husband present (1). As of 1976, 62% of these single female heads of household had children under 18 years of age, and 56% of these women participated in the labor force (1).

Other women work for a multitude of reasons. The psychosocial change of the meaning of success and self-fulfillment affects people in all walks of life and from every economic and social stratum. Included are the symbols of success, such as money, possessions and stable family life, and an emphasis on self-fulfillment (49). Further, there is an increase in decisive commitment to lifetime careers by many highly qualified women (17, 22).

In 1955, families with both spouses in the labor force constituted 26% of all two-parent families; by 1975, this percentage increased to 41% of husband/wife intact families. This figure was equal, for the first time in history, to the percentage for male-wage-earner-only families (1).

Families with the wife in the paid work force with an annual family income of $25,000 and over (in constant 1974 dollars) increased from 19 to 51% in the 20-year span from 1954 to 1974 (1). If the husband earned more than $30,000, the wife's participation in the labor force from 1967 to 1974 jumped 38% (25). Families with a combined income of $22,000 represent the top 20% of all families in earning power; of these income elites in American families, 44% of the wives worked in 1965, and 54% worked in 1978 (25). The Population Reference Bureau reported that one of every five gainfully employed wives brings home a paycheck as large as or larger than that of her husband (43).

ADULT DEVELOPMENT AND THE WORKING WOMAN

Age can be arbitrarily defined as specific periods in one's life; for instance, middle age has been identified as the years of life between 40 and 65. Chronological age per se, however, is not the most meaningful measure (36). Age may be better identified by the events which shape periods of the life course. For the highly motivated, married career woman, middle age is better described as one of the most demanding, most productive and free periods of life. It is the time when she has launched her children and has the potential to reach the peak in her chosen profession. For others, it is the time for identity crisis (6), a time for psychiatric disaster, a prolonged interval of deadening routine (27), and a time to assume responsibility for the young and the old.

The contemporary middle-aged woman may look both backward and forward. In retrospect, she has reached the point when many choices made while a young adult are finite for the remainder of her life. She may have chosen to bear no children and relinquished the option of wonderment at this epitome of creation, a heritage of herself. Or, having chosen the singular struggle of rearing children and excluding gainful employment, she may now question if it has been worth the social strain and hardship of increased demands on the available family resources. If she concomitantly chose marriage, family, and career, she may question the past toll on her energy and time, balancing this against improved family economic status and/or career advancement. The middle-aged married woman is caught between theories that claim middle age as "potentially the most exciting period of life" (9, p. 323) and theories which identify this stage of the life-cycle with feelings of despair, disenchantment, and decline.

Many theorists have compared the ages of adolescence and middle age as times of instability and searching for the meaning of life. "Crisis" has been used to define this transitional phase in the life span. However, the mid-life crisis may be more myth than fact. Specific tests (12, 32) and a review of crisis theory research (13) have not found evidence to support mid-life crisis as a developmental stage through which all adults must proceed.

Predictors (10, 37) concur that mid-life experiences for women will change drastically and progressively with each successive group of women entering mid-life. Increasing education, more refined skills, and the snowballing precedent of changing combinations of family and work roles are influential factors. The claim has been made that three in five American working wives would work even if they had enough money to live comfortably without working (41), reflecting their reinforcing experiences in the working world and the resulting shifts in the statistics of working women. While most women will have jobs rather than careers, an increasing number will be involved in careers (24). Well-educated women are more likely to have worked before marriage and before child-bearing and for a longer period of time (46). Reasons given are that family consumption patterns become adjusted to two incomes, family management patterns within the family stabilize, and there are more opportunities for women to climb career ladders.

Emerging Models

In terms of defining oneself and one's role in society and the family, the middle-aged woman has faced a paucity of women models who have successfully combined family life and a career. However, this coalition of roles is a logical evolution considering the stability of high marriage rates (96% in the United States) and the increasing involvement of women in the work force. Although modeling has been accepted as an important behavioral learning phenomena, models for the mid-life woman have for the most part been isolated heroines. For example, Margaret Mead, a modern-day idol, might be questioned as a viable model considering the elitism of her contributions (38). Presently, there is a segment of more typical women surfacing in this modeling role capacity who are likely to be the predictors of lifestyles of tomorrow.

An exploration will be made of the pressures on and potential of a specific group of women—the mid-life, highly committed, married professional women—as they experience new avenues made possible through the human liberation movement. An emphasis will be placed upon the professional woman, often the wife of the corporate executive, with an assumption that these women, in general, possess personal resources and have access to influential factors that are basic ingredients for success. They have the rearing and the skills necessary to respond socially to situations, the intelligence to be perceptive and to learn quickly, and the capability and self-confidence to adapt to and progress rapidly within an environment geared for success.

Additionally, these women have the relationships and social contacts to be influential, including a marital partner who is a successful businessman in his own right. His receptiveness to his wife's concerns can and do affect his business decisions, as well as his informal conversations with peers who also make policy decisions. Her husband's business contacts aside, the professional wife of the executive has a well-developed network of contacts of her own.

FUTURISTIC IMPLICATIONS FOR FAMILY AND CORPORATE STRUCTURAL CHANGES

The multiple changes resulting from societal attempts to eliminate sex-role biases in the world of work have occurred so rapidly that there has been little time to assess the ramifications of these changes on traditional structures of family practice and corporate policies. The ideology of equality for women has begun to have an impact upon the concept of conjugal equality, the concept of masculinity, and traditional career development paths. There is growing evidence to suggest that work patterns, family life-styles and corporate policy will simultaneously expand horizons to formulate variegated models designed for more optimal integration of the demands and rewards of work and family for both females and males. According to noted writers in this field, the dual-career couple represents a "corporate time bomb" which will exert its greatest impact five years from now as these employees advance to more responsible, critical positions of management (21, p. 76).

Frustrations are mounting as more and more dual-career couples attempt to combine the multifaceted demands of career and family. Resistance to various corporate practices, ranging from policies pertaining to nepotism to traditional corporate expectations for relocation of family as a result of upward mobility, is mounting. New vocabulary emerges to define alternative approaches to traditional eight-to-five patterns, such as flexitime, permanent part-time, temporary mobility and job-sharing. Dual professional couples are more willing to experiment with a wider variety of life-styles at various stages of life to permit higher levels of mutuality in the sharing of careers and family. Alternative career development models and long-distance marriages are being attempted by some vanguard dual-career couples as wives and husbands search for deeper meaning in life and greater self-realization.

This movement is headed, in large part, by those who can best afford to lose the battle if necessary—the mid-life, dually employed, economically stable professional couple. Although it is frequently the younger generation which is first to point out fallacies in value systems and practices, it is often the middle-aged generation which is in the most appropriate position to facilitate change. More and more representatives of this group are thinking in terms of self-actualization and mid-life career changes rather than "making it in the corporation." The gains sought through the Women's Movement have offered the greatest advantages and, perhaps at the same time, the greatest dilemmas for the highly qualified, highly committed, dually employed professional couple.

Bailyn claims that ". . . women and men from dual-career families are at a disadvantage today. . . . They are faced with choices that men in top positions have previously not had to make" (4, p. 20). More and more two-career couples are declining promotions and transfers if it means moving, more work, longer hours and additional responsibilities (21, 30). Increased salary differentials offered as incentive for job transfers frequently do not compensate for the loss of a spouse's salary. Professional couples have formulated a new set of criteria upon which to select and/or maintain careers. Marital/career conflicts and alternatives which have resulted from these changes are considered in the following discussion.

The Corporate Picture

One of the earliest reflections of shifting priorities of dual-career couples has been a reevaluation of the "executive transfer." The changes which have widened occupational horizons for women have also contributed to the "acceptability of employment" of upper-middle-class women. Executive wives are no exception. It has been estimated that one-third of the wives of corporate executives are currently employed full-time and another one-third are employed on a part-time basis. Many of these women are involved in the development of their own businesses or in management of large corporations. It is becoming increasingly apparent to more and more corporations that a wife with a career can drastically reduce the male executive's geographical mobility or vice versa. In the past few years, numerous executives have chosen to limit options for geographical mobility because of the careers of their wives. Several major corporations are exercising caution about transferring employees with employed spouses, although they continue to recognize that the two-career family can "create a problem in upward mobility." One representative of an international executive recruiting firm claims, "Our clients are learning that to attract many of today's brightest young executives, they've got to find career opportunities for the spouse as well" (8, p. 94).

Other illustrations of changing corporate practices are beginning to surface. One oil company is currently utilizing six-month offshore assignments rather than permanent transfers in an effort to reduce the necessity of family relocation. This particular company flies the scientist back to the family every couple of weeks. Another company offers couples child-care or live-in expenses incurred in managerial out-of-town business trips. Several companies have launched the practice of job-hunting or paid placement search services for the spouses of transferred executives (21).

Rosebeth Moss Kanter, in her critical review of work and family in the United States, claimed that corporations in the future will change social aspects of their functions to a more businesslike approach. For example, she predicts that out-of-town business meetings will be shorter and will not include the executive wives. In addition, says Kanter, wives will no longer be asked to plant rumors or seek corporate information at cocktail parties (26).

Perhaps the most devastating corporate practice exerted on executive families is that of a family relocation as a result of the "move-up-or-move-over syndrome." This practice is no doubt ingrained in the assumption that the corporate wife is an extension of her husband's identity, a social hostess for the corporation and a community witness to her husband's success and prestige. Her role is often indirectly assigned in a set of unwritten expectations ranging from social secretary and party hostess to travel companion. If the corporation deems it advisable to transfer the executive, the family is expected to move without question. The expectation has been so widely accepted as a necessary fact of life for executives and their families that, ironically, the phenomenon received very little research attention until the 1970s. In an attempt to better understand this phenomenon, a brief historical overview will follow, accompanied by research findings pertaining to the impact of male occupational mobility on family life.

Executive Gypsies: Impact of Upward Mobility on Families

Traditional career mobility has, for men, implied the possibility of residential mobility for the family (23, 46). As early as 1949, Parsons predicted that marriage between dually employed professionals would not be an appropriate way to emancipate American married women from domesticity and claimed that this would result only in high stress levels for the woman and would place her in a destructive competitive role with her husband (42). Numerous legal and social sanctions have arisen to reinforce this expectation. Corporations consider the image created by their executives and their families of utmost importance. Cuber and Harroff described the typical white middle-class American professional male in the corporate structure:

> To many career men the home is almost an adjunct to the job. It is not simply that he needs a place to entertain—although this can be important. It is a status symbol, at once evidence of his past successes and a recommendation to support his bid for more . . . Many corporations and some independent professions say that he is practically required to maintain a "certain kind" of home. He often has to trade on his home and family as he does his personality. It is all part of a package which you present to your public (14, p. 115).

Several researchers (34, 40) have traced male occupational mobility and have noted that the wives have had virtually little or no impact on the decisions to move. Duncan and Perrucci (15) concluded from a review of research that a husband's occupational mobility places an overall deleterious effect on career-minded wives, but the employment concerns of the wife were not influential in a male's geographical mobility decision.

The incidence of actual geographic reassignment for males is difficult to ascertain and varies widely from corporation to corporation. Pahl and Pahl (40) found in a sample of managers that 22% had moved their workplace once every two or three years, and 33% of these men changed residential locations once every four to five years. Marshall and Cooper (34) reported studies by others in which 2,000 British Institute of Management members changed employers 2.7 times per career and changed jobs within a company 2.9 times. Approximately one-fourth had changed jobs and locations five or more times in their careers. In another study (34), 66% of the managerial sample anticipated moving every three years.

From an interview study of 50 British mobile managers, Marshall and Cooper (34) described the typical occupationally mobile family, which they termed "executive gypsies." These families were middle-aged couples with two or three children. They had lived in three or more areas of the country and had never allowed themselves to become too attached to any one place. The husband was heavily absorbed in his job, and it was the primary source of his satisfaction. He devoted much of his spare time to his profession. The wife placed a high priority on providing the husband with a good home. She most likely had some professional training, usually as a nurse or a teacher. The younger the wife, the more likelihood she would be contemplating returning to her profession after the children were launched.

Slightly over 20% of these women had been employed prior to their last moves on either a full-time or part-time basis. The relocation meant a break from work and occasional difficulties in reentry due to the unavailability of new employment or changes in regional employment requirements. For women who were in training programs prior to relocation, the disruption meant either delay or possible cessation of training. None of the women in this British study felt resistant enough to prevent their husbands from accepting the transfers.

While the majority of wives in the Marshall and Cooper study accepted the occupational necessity for geographical relocation as a mere fact of their husband's employment, a significant number of them expressed a feeling of resentment about restrictions placed upon their own career development. Younger wives were more resentful than older wives, many of whom did not apparently conscientiously evalute the impact of the husband's job relocation upon their own lives.

Dual-professional Couples: Whose Career Determines Place of Residency?

The preceding discussions highlight the growing resistance and resentment toward corporate upward mobility requiring geographical relocation and the traditional corporate assumptions imposed on executive families. While approximately one-third of the corporate executive wives hold the view that one must accept this traditional concept if one has become a corporate wife, a growing majority of these wives are refusing to play the role. Some who attempt to carry the former role expectations along with their own career demands have, according to Eugene Jennings, Professor of Management at Michigan State University, become "executive workhorses" (8). Many of the new breed of dual-career executives are searching for new life-styles which will enable them to have the best of both marriage and career.

Relocation is no longer a factor for males only. The highly qualified, mature woman, as a result of affirmative action programs, is in top demand in the United States. In fact, it is now the woman who may have the greatest potential for career advancement if she is mobile. The president of a large Dallas bank recently stated, "So great is the demand for bright career women that there's hazard in losing them after you have trained them. There's a greater tendency for a woman to get outside alternative opportunities than for a man" (30).

Since many highly qualified, career-oriented men select for marriage highly educated and highly motivated women (17), it is becoming increasingly apparent that the waves of the liberation movement will continue to create a backlash on marital and career decisions for the upwardly mobile. It would indeed be unfortunate if the liberation movement resulted in gains in the marketplace for women at the expense of their marriages. For some, this has already become a reality. Others are attempting to analyze their priorities and commitments to their marriages and careers and are seeking alternatives to allow them to maintain both.

Long-distance Marriages—A Viable Approach for Some

In response to marital/career conflicts and pressures for career mobility, some contemporary couples have elected to enter into a relatively new life-style termed commuter marriage, weekend marriage, two-location marriage, married-singles, dual-career variant, or long-distance marriage. Whatever the term employed, this life-style connotes a relationship in which marital spouses voluntarily live apart, maintaining separate residences in distant cities, for the purpose of pursuing individual careers while at the same time maintaining their marital relationship and family obligations.

The incidence of long-distance marriages has not been assessed, primarily because this life-style has not been considered widespread. In fact, Kirschner and Walum (28) pointed out that accepted social definitions imply either intrinsically or extrinsically that a family, to be a family, must live together. According to definitions, a married single is assumed not to exist. Although long-distance marriage might have been used to describe life-styles necessitated by immigration, economic necessity, imprisonment, war or traveling sales jobs, it has more recently been used to describe the family life-style of dual-career couples who voluntarily live in separate locations. Because of career commitment and economic needs, spouses pursue their careers while maintaining a communicative network and a "home base" with periodic visitations. There is growing evidence to suggest that this way of life may eventually become an acceptable alternative to prolonged postponement of marriage, singlehood, or constant marital/career conflict. Tightened job markets, increased inflation and employment patterns may increase the probablity of two-location marriages, especially among highly trained specialists.

Data from recent studies on long-distance marriages (16, 18, 19, 28, 39) suggest that these marriages are viable for spouses who have developed a strength in the marital bond and who are strongly committed to their professions. Since it is a relatively expensive life-style, it is most popular among professionals involved in law, medicine, public relations, business and journalism. Commuter marriage is also becoming common in academia among both faculty and graduate students.

The majority of couples involved in long-distance marriages rate their marriages as relatively satisfactory or quite satisfactory at the onset of the long-distance arrangement and are even more enthusiastic about their marital relationship following the two-location life-style. Contrary to popular belief, these marriages were not on the verge of splitting up prior to involvement in long-distance relationships. Many of these couples stressed the fact that their marriages were on solid ground and that there was an inner trust which enabled them to cope with the loneliness of separate living arrangements. They claimed that the idea for a long-distance marriage "just evolved" as they attempted to work through alternatives which would offer the greatest career opportunities for both.

The respondents in these studies did not perceive their long-distance marriages as basic factors in either a decision to divorce or involvement in extramarital sex. The rate of divorce for couples in long-distance marriages was no higher than it was for couples in traditional marriages. When divorce did occur for long-distance marrieds, the majority of couples blamed factors other than the living arrangement for the divorce. Likewise, the rate of extramarital involvement was no higher for the long-distance marrieds than for traditional groups. In fact, one respondent claimed that although he was involved in extramarital sex prior to the long-distance marriage, he discontinued the practice as a result of the new life-style. The majority of couples studied said that neither their attitudes nor behaviors toward extramarital sex changed as a result of the long-distance marriage.

One of the major supports for the viability of long-distance marriages was the perceived benefits which respondents attributed to their decision to live apart for the majority of time. The respondents believed that they had been able to optimize career opportunities and gain an increased sense of independency, freedom, autonomy and self-confidence as a result of being a married single.

Many of the long-distance married respondents reported a decrease in the trivial conflicts in marriage and an increased sense of appreciation and romantic feeling for their spouses. Several attributed the life-style as responsible for a chance to rediscover each other. Others claimed it was the best of both worlds. Women in general were more enthusiastic about the life-style than were men, claiming that it gave them a greater sense of independency and privacy than provided in traditional marriage. Men had a tendency to complain about the necessity of doing household routines as a result of the living-apart arrangement.

Forty-eight percent of the participants in one study (39) had children ranging from infancy to young adults. In the majority of cases, children still living at home remained at the primary residence, most often with the mother. The most frequently mentioned complaint of the result of the long-distance marriage in regard to children was that the separated parent missed the children. Weekends often did not provide ample time to develop close relationships with both spouse and children.

In general, the vast majority of long-distance marrieds had favorable opinions about the life-style. Several couples had been involved in previous long-distance arrangements and found them satisfactory enough to enter into the life-style for a second or third time. Although the majority of these couples would overwhelmingly favor living together again if the chance arose, the self-gains and the career advantages evidently offset the disadvantages of the two-location marital life-style (39).

Ten years ago, Holmstrom (23) suggested that as long as geographical mobility is a critical issue of employment, it would be to each spouse's advantage to choose a geographic residence independently of the other's interest. "Career opportunities may beckon the husband and wife in opposite directions. And yet presumably they wish to remain together as a family" (23, p. 517). Thus emerges a life-style for some career-committed couples, which, although not necessarily completely desirable, may be more viable than existing alternatives.

Alternative Career Development Models

Corporations have, during the past few years, become more aware of the impact of occupational mobility on contemporary family life-styles and have decreased the incidence of transfers among executives. However, changes in occupational mobility patterns alone will not be a sufficient remedy to cure the problematic symptoms which modern marrieds face. Greater flexibility and wider alternatives will be demanded within the corporate structure to allow both women and men to combine personal and family priorities with occupational responsibilities. One of these alternatives might be a drastic change in the traditional career path.

The work ethic avenue to career success has typically been college degree entrance into a position and onto the proving grounds. This necessitated working through many phases of the organizational structure while under constant and stringent evaluation. The harder one worked, the more optimum the performance, the more dedication to the job, then the more likely one would be recognized and rewarded with advancements and promotions. These advancements, in turn, demanded more responsibility, more time and energy devoted to the job and greater job pressure. The climb to the top leaves little time for family togetherness or consideration of the development of the spouse's career. Bailyn (4) defined this scenario as the career success model and suggested other models which might be considered viable for career development and perhaps more appropriate for family development.

The apprenticeship model outlined by Bailyn (4) involves a fairly long period of continued learning and training during the early phase of career development and operates at a slower pace than the traditional career success model. Commitment to the job and involvement in the corporation would increase with time and age of the employee as child-rearing responsibilities lessened or other personal goals had been realized.

A culture which measures male success through the size of the paycheck leaves little room for occupational experimentation. The launching of women into higher paying positions will ultimately reduce this pressure on the male and will allow for more flexible models leading to career success and fulfillment for women and men. It will provide possibilities of rotational models which permit one person in the coupleship to further career training and development while the other places concern on earning the family income. It will virtually double the opportunities for couples to elect to accept promotions, transfers, career shifts, job changes, sabbaticals, and so forth. Corporations have already begun to change some of the traditional criteria for career success. What was once a sign of personal instability and referred to as job-hopping may now be evaluated by some business concerns as an indication of personal drive and breadth of experience (4).

Changes in Work Schedules, Work Space and Place

Changes in the place of work and in work shifts are bound to occur. As the cost of transportation increases, it may be more advantageous to work out of the home or at locations other than the traditional "office." Home offices would save time and energy without decrease in productivity for certain types of positions, at least on a limited basis.

A fuel-tight future may demand and produce many changes in work scheduling. Analysts predict a heavy increase in utilization of the home telephone as fuel shortages and increased fuel costs impact on business and industry. The necessity of many business trips could be drastically reduced as new technology enables us to make face-to-face visitations with clients in distant cities without leaving the home. According to experts of AT&T, new technology will soon enable us to connect home telephone lines with home computers and television screens (48). The opportunity for one or both marital partners to work out of the home will without doubt offer additional opportunities but at the same time be a potential source for new career/marital/family conflicts.

Work shifts are already becoming more flexible and may eventually emulate some of the European models. Part-time shifts have become very popular for women in many countries. In Melbourne, for example, women have choices of ten different shifts, seven of which call for 20 to 30 hours per week(11). Other plans operate on a four-day work week. Some United States companies are experimenting with a four-day week rather than resorting to layoffs. Thousands of business concerns and governmental agencies have adopted the concept of flexitime, which allows individuals to elect work times most appropriate to the demands of the family. Flexitime may be defined in two ways: either the starting and quitting hours may be altered, or the 40-hour week may be condensed into four days or perhaps expanded into six days per week (44).

Permanent part-time employment has been instituted in some companies. This concept permits employees to work fewer than 40 hours per week, without a set minimum number of hours. Permanent part-time is becoming more attractive to two-income families as well as to single heads of household. These positions offer benefit packages that were previously unavailable for part-timers in the past. This nation's campuses have experienced a rapid growth in this type of employment. In the past four years, full-time faculty positions increased by 9% while the number of part-time positions has grown to 38% of the total college and university faculties (2).

Job-sharing is another flexible concept which offers individuals the rewards of job commitment and yet reduces the demands on their time. Employers are unreceptive to the idea in most cases because it doubles the work for the personnel and payroll departments. According to Carol Parker of Job Sharers, Inc., a non-profit organization in Arlington, Virginia, job sharers are committed and enthusiastic people (35).

The Right Not to Work

An estimated six million unemployed Americans are not necessarily looking for work. These are not free floating hippies. For the most part, they are middle-class professionals who have become disillusioned with work as a way of life. They have lost belief in what they were doing and voluntarily chosen to stop in the midst of the cradle-to-the-grave work path while they take time to rethink their values and goals in life (31).

Some women choose not to be gainfully employed in deference to the traditional role of wife and mother. Women in this once-honored position need not feel inadequate or defensive. Their contributions can be extensive, and with care and attention they can prepare for self and family security if that should become solely their responsibility. Similarly, role reversals in which the wife is the breadwinner with a support system of a househusband may be the better alternative for some.

THE FAMILY THERAPIST'S ROLE

The reasons why women work are not precisely clear. Although many may work because they feel a financial necessity to do so, many also readily indicate that they would work even if the financial need did not exist. Other women claim that they work only to achieve a specific family goal, such as educating the children, but continue to remain in the labor force long after this goal has been realized. The reasons given for men's work in our society have a clearer, however assumed, focus.

It should be noted that research pertaining to why men and women work and the kind of work they perform has been accomplished under the auspices of a very limited spectrum of sex roles. Women who foresee occupational mobility, equal salary, and chances for career advancement may realize a different set of motivations for entering and remaining in the work force than did women who perceived only limited employment opportunities at two-thirds the salary of their male counterparts. By contrast, men who have traditionally perceived economics as the primary motivation for employment may reflect other criteria as incentives for employment if their wives enjoy the capability of commanding top positions and top salaries.

The misconceptions which have been so neatly and tightly woven into the fabric of sexual asymmetry will be difficult indeed to disentangle. The entrance of women into every level of corporate operation is beginning to weaken the fundamental assumptions which provided the framework for a society based upon predetermined sex roles. We have been reared in a culture which relegated work to men as a primary motivating force in life and the family to women as their salient domain. We have been conditioned to accept the fact that unemployment for men was a social problem and employment for women resulted in social problems for their children. We have lived to witness married men and single women rising to the top. And now we must pause to realize that values taught and put into practice before the dawn of human equality may have to be laid to rest.

Caution must now be exerted as we begin to reinterpret human behavior in the light of a more open environment. What are the processes by which men and women make occupational decisions? To what extent will we allow work to impact on families and, by the same token, families to impact on work? Will married men begin to choose to work or not to work in the same luxury that has been provided for married women? Will men seek more meaningful family bonds and reap greater personal rewards from the family in a future where they are not solely responsible for family income? What changes will occur in the very nature of marriage as women and men seek higher levels of satisfaction from marriage and career? What will be the stumbling blocks for those couples who search for uniqueness in family life-styles, individual self-discovery and, at the same time, a mutual sharing of love and understanding of each other's career?

The mid-life professional woman will without doubt be instrumental in the initiation of these changes. Most apparent may be the immediate increased commitment which she devotes to her career as she finds open doors replacing dead-end positions. Will she become over-committed to her career at the expense of other aspects of her life as she tries to make up for lost time? What will be the toll on her personal strengths and on her husband as he begins to search for a new identity in mid-life which becomes necessary as a result of shifting sex roles?

The period between the asking of these questions and the finding of answers will be strenuous and will require guidance and assistance. The psychic costs for husbands and wives will be high. Not incidentally, it will be the mid-life, middle- and upper-middle-class professional woman who will seek guidance in these dilemmas from the family therapist. These clients will be first to recognize imbalance in their lives and most willing and able to seek professional services.

There has been a documented need for raised consciousness concerning sex bias on the part of therapists (29). The biases of therapists are alleged to be rigid sex roles imposed upon women clients and an allegiance by the therapist to sex-biased social institutional policies which hinder career progress of women. These attitudes are reflected in counselor perceptions of the characterisitcs of the healthy male as disparate from those of the healthy female and prevail in large measure in the therapeutic treatment of individual and family relationships (7).

If family therapy is to make a real difference in the lives of individuals and families, it must do so with a deemphasis on the authoritative power of the therapist and with increased emphasis on the feeling of control and decision-making power on the part of the female client. The models for the new breed of women may not exist; individualized roles are being designed through the knowledge of old constraints and visions of new freedoms in the minds of the women who are no longer complacent with "the way it is." The family therapist who is freed from the narrow concepts of yesterday will be instrumental in helping working women and their husbands journey from traditional "wedlock" to a marriage which allows a commitment to each other as well as a commitment "to each other's need and right to pursue a career" (22).

REFERENCES

1. American Council of Life Insurance. (1978). *Data Track 4: Households and Families*. Washington, D.C.: Social Research Services, 1850 K Street, N.W. 20006.
2. *Association of American Colleges*. (1978). Part-time employment is on the increase. No. *20*, 1.
3. ATCHLEY, Robert C. (1978). Retirement preparation for women. In: *Women in Midlife—Security and Fulfillment (Part I)*, a compendium of papers submitted to the Select Committee on Aging and the Subcommittee on Retirement Income and Employment, U. S. House of Representatives, Comm. Pub. No. 95-170. Washington, D.C.: U. S. Government Printing Office.
4. BAILYN, Lotte. (1979). How much acceleration for career success? *Management Review, 68*, 18.
5. BLAU, Zena Smith, ROGERS, Pamela P., OSER, George T. and STEPHENS, Richard C. (1978). School bells and work whistles: Sounds that echo a better life for women in later years. In: *Women in Midlife—Security and Fulfillment (Part I)*, a compendium of papers submitted to the Select Committee on Aging and the Subcommittee on Retirement Income and Employment, U. S. House of Representatives, Comm. Pub. No. 95-170. Washington, D.C.: U. S. Government Printing Office.
6. BRAYSHAW, A. J. (1962). Middle-aged marriage: Idealism, realism and the search for meaning. *Marriage and Family Living, 24*, 358.
7. BROVERMAN, I., BROVERMAN, D., CLARKSON, F., ROSENKRANTZ, P. and VEGEL, S. (1970). Sex-role stereotypes and clinical judgments of mental health. *Journal of Consulting and Clinical Psychology, 34*, 1.
8. *Business Week*. (1979). The new corporate wife goes to work. April 9, 88.
9. BUTLER, Robert N. (1978). Prospects for middle-aged women. In: *Women in Midlife—Security and Fulfillment (Part I)*, a compendium of papers submitted to the Select Committee on Aging and the Subcommittee on Retirement Income and Employment, U. S. House of Representatives, Comm. Pub. No. 95-170. Washington, D.C.: U. S. Government Printing Office.
10. CAHN, Ann Foote (ed.). (1978). Highlights of eighteen papers on problems of midlife women. In: *Women in Midlife—Security and Fulfillment (Part I)*. a compendium of papers submitted to the Select Committee on Aging and the Subcommittee on Retirement Income and Employment, U. S. House of Represenatives, Comm. Pub. No. 95-170. Washington, D. C.: U. S. Government Printing Office.

11. COOKE, Alice. (1975). *The Working Mother. A Survey of Programs in Nine Countries*. Ithaca, New York: New York State School of Industrial and Labor Relations, Cornell University.
12. COOPER, M. W. (1977). An empirical investigation of the male midlife period: A descriptive cohort study. Unpublished honors thesis. Boston: University of Massachusetts.
13. COSTA, P. T. and McCRAE, R. R. (1978). Objective personality assessment. In: Storandt, M., Siegler, I. C. and Elias, M. F. (eds.). *The Clinical Psychology of Aging*. New York: Plenum Publishing Corporation.
14. CUBER, John and HARROFF, Peggy. (1965). *Sex and the Significant Americans*. New York: Appleton-Century.
15. DUNCAN, R. Paul and PERRUCCI, Carolyn. (1976). Dual occupation families and migration. *American Sociological Review, 41*, 252.
16. FARRIS, Agnes. (1978). Commuting. In: Rapoport, R. and Rapoport R. (eds.). *Working Couples*. New York: Harper and Row.
17. FOGARTY, M., RAPOPORT, R. and RAPOPORT, R. (1971). *Sex, Career and Family*, Beverly Hills, California: Sage.
18. GERSTEL, Naomi. (1977). The feasibility of commuter marriage. In: Stein, Peter J., Richman, Judith, and Hannon, Natalie (ed.). *The Family: Functions, Conflicts and Symbols*. Reading, Massachusetts: Addison-Wesley.
19. GROSS, Harriet E. (1978). Couples who live apart: The dual-career variant. Mimeo paper presented at the American Sociological Association Annual Meeting, San Francisco, California, September 4.
20. HALL, Francine S. and HALL, Douglas T. (1978). Dual careers—How do couples and companies cope with the problems? *Org. Dyn.*, Spring, 57.
21. HALL, Francine S. and HALL, Douglas T. (1979). *The Two Career Couple*. Reading, Massachusetts: Addison-Wesley.
22. HOFFMAN, Lois W. and NYE, F. Ivan. (1974). *Working Mothers*. San Francisco: Jossey-Bass Publishers.
23. HOLMSTROM, Linda L. (1970). Career patterns of married couples. In: Theodore, Athena (ed.). *The Professional Woman*. Cambridge: Schenkman.
24. HOPKINS, J. and WHITE, P. (1978). The dual-career couple: Constraints and supports. *The Family Coordinator, 27*, 3.
25. IGNATUS, David. (1978). Women at work, the rich get richer as well-to-do wives enter the labor force. *Wall St. J.*, September 8, 1.
26. KANTER, R. M. (1977). *Men and Women of the Corporation*. New York: Basic Books.
27. KASTENBAUM, Robert. (1979). *Humans Developing: A Lifespan Perspective*. Boston: Allyn and Bacon, Inc.
28. KIRSCHNER, Betty and WALUM, Laurel. (1978). Two location families: Married singles. *Alternate Lifestyles, 1*, 513.
29. KNAPP, Jacquelyn J. (1975). The problem of gender-role bias in mental health practitioners: A position paper. Paper presented at the First International Workshop of Groves Conferences on Marriage and the Family and co-sponsoring organizations. Dubrovnik, Yugoslavia, June.
30. KRONHOLZ, June. (1978). Women at work, management practices change to reflect role of women employees. *Wall St. J.*, September 13, 1.
31. LEFKOWTIZ, Bernard. (1979). *Breaktime: Living Without Work in a Nine-to-Five World*. New York: Hawthorn.
32. LOWENTHAL, M. F. and CHIRIBOGA, D. (1972). Transition to the empty nest. *Archives of General Psychiatry, 26*, 8.
33. MADAN, Homai and COOPER, Cary. (1977). The impact of dual career family development on organizational life. *Mgt. Decision, 15*, 487.
34. MARSHALL, Judi and COOPER, Cary. (1976). The mobile manager and his wife. *Mgt. Decision, 14*, 180.

35. MERKIN, Ann. (1978). Job sharing. *Women's Work, 1,* 19
36. NEUGARTEN, Bernice L. (1973). Personality change in late life: A developmental perspective. In: Eisdorfer, C. and Lawton, M. P. (eds.). *The Psychology of Adult Development and Aging.* Washington, D.C.: American Psychological Association.
37. NEUGARTEN, Bernice L. and BROWN-REZANKA, Lorill. (1978). Midlife Women in the 1980's. In: Women in Midlife—*Security and Fulfillment (Part I),* a compendium of papers submitted to the Select Committee on Aging and the Subcommittee on Retirement Income and Employment, U. S. House of Representatives, Comm. Pub. No. 95-170. Washington, D. C.: U. S. Government Printing Office.
38. O'BRIEN, Patricia. (1979). Is Margaret Mead a good role model? Knight-Ridder News Service Columnist, *Akron Beacon Journal.* Akron, Ohio, April.
39. ORTON, John and SULLIVAN, Joyce. (1979). Long distance marriage: Is it a viable lifestyle for couples? Research completed, Florida State University, publication pending.
40. PAHL, J. M. and PAHL, R. E. (1971). *Managers and Their Wives.* London: Allen Lane.
41. PARENS, H. S., SHEA, J. R., SPITZ, R. S., ZELLER, F. A. and Associates. (1970). *Dual Careers.* Manpower Research Monograph 21. Washington, D. C.: U. S. Department of Labor.
42. PARSONS, T. (1949). *Essays in Sociological theory: Pure and Applied.* Glencoe, Illinois: The Free Press.
43. SMITH, Lowell. (1979). Are you an average American? Newspaper column, *Akron Beacon Journal.* Akron, Ohio, January 27, B23.
44. STEIN, Barry, COHEN, Allan and GADON, Herman. (1976). Flextime: Work when you want to. *Psychol. Today, 10,* 40.
45. TROLL, Lillian E. and TURNER, Joanne. (1978). Overcoming age-sex discrimination. In: *Women in Midlife—Security and Fulfillment (Part I),* a compendium of papers submitted to the Select Committee on Aging and the Subcommittee on Retirement Income and Employment, U. S. House of Representatives, Comm. Pub. No. 95-170. Washington, D. C.: U. S. Government Printing Office.
46. VAN DUSEN, Roxann A. and SHELDON, Eleanor B. (1977). The changing status of American women: A life cycle perspective. In: Skolnick, Arlene and Skolnick, Jerome. *Family in Transition.* Boston: Little, Brown and Company.
47. VELIE, L. (1973). Where have all the fathers gone? *Reader's Digest, Vol. 102,* 155.
48. *Wall St. J.* (1979). Analysts see Americans staying at home more. July 3, *1,* 1.
49. YANKELOVICH, Daniel. (1978). Jobs and work. Presentation for preliminary meeting of the Aspen Institute for Humanistic Studies on the subject, "Financing the future," Aspen, Colorado, October.

6

MIDDLE-AGED MEN AND THE PRESSURES OF WORK

Cary L. Cooper, Ph.D.

Professor of Organisational Psychology,
Department of Management Sciences,
University of Manchester Institute of Science and Technology
Manchester, England

INTRODUCTION

Stress-related illnesses such as coronary heart disease have shown a steady upward trend over the past couple of decades in the U.K. and other developed countries, particularly for the middle-aged. In England and Wales, for example, the death rate for men between 35 and 44 nearly doubled between 1950 and 1973, and has increased much more rapidly than that of older age ranges (e.g., 45-54). By 1973, 41% of all deaths in the age group 25-44 were due to cardiovascular disease, with nearly 30% due to cardiac heart disease. In fact, in 1976 the American Heart Association estimated the cost of cardiovascular disease in the U.S. at $26.7 billion a year.

In addition to the more extreme forms of stress-related illnesses, there has been an increase in other possible stress manifestations, such as alcoholism (hospital admissions in the U.K. increased from roughly under 6,000 in 1966 to over 8,000 in 1974), industrial accidents, and short-term illnesses (through certified and uncertified sick leaves), with an estimated 300 million working days lost at a cost of £55 million in national insurance and supplementary benefits payments alone. The total cost to industry of all forms of stress-related illness and other manifestations, a large slice of which can be attributed directly or indirectly to the working environment of the middle-aged, must be enormous, beyond the scope of most cost accountants to begin to calculate. Some Americans estimate that it may represent in the order of 1% to 3% of GNP in the United States (19).

Many of these stress-related illnesses obviously affect the middle-aged more than the young, regardless of occupational grouping (as Table 1 indicates and other morbidity and mortality data would support). The purpose of this chapter will be to highlight the *sources* of stress acting on the middle-aged in a work context.

A survey of literature reveals a formidable list of over 40 interacting factors which might be sources of stress among middle-aged workers. Those to be dealt with here were drawn mainly from a wider body of theory and research in a variety of fields—medicine, psychology, management sciences, etc. Additional material has been drawn from exploratory studies carried out by Cooper and Marshall (5). Five major categories of work stressors can be identified (see Figure 1).

WORK LOAD AND THE MIDDLE-AGED

One of the most important sources of job stress for middle-aged individuals is their tendency to work long hours and to take on too much work. Research into work overload has been given substantial empirical attention. French and Caplan (7) have differentiated overload in terms of *quantitative* and *qualitative* overload. Quantitative refers to having "too much to do," while

TABLE 1

Acute Sickness and Consultations with General Medical Practitioners, 1974-75, in Great Britain

	Average number of restricted activity days per person per year (males)			Average number of consultations per person per year (males)		
	15-44	45-64	All ages	15-44	45-64	All ages
Professional	9	16	12	2.1	2.7	2.7
Employers and managers	11	13	14	1.8	2.4	2.7
Intermediate and junior non-manual	10	21	15	2.0	4.3	3.1
Skilled manual and own account non-professional	15	24	17	2.8	4.0	3.2
Semi-skilled manual and personal service	16	23	18	2.7	4.5	3.7
Unskilled manual	21	28	20	3.5	4.8	3.6
All persons	13	21	16	2.4	3.8	3.1

Source: General Household Survey, 1974 and 1975

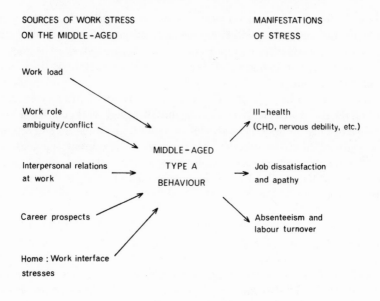

Figure 1

qualitative relates to work that is "too difficult." In one of their early studies, French and Caplan (6) found that objective quantitative overload was strongly linked to cigarette smoking (an important risk factor or symptom of CHD). Persons with more phone calls, office visits, and meetings per given unit of work time were found to smoke significantly more cigarettes than persons with fewer such engagements. In a study of 100 middle-aged coronary patients, Russek and Zohman (28) found that 25% had been working at two jobs and an additional 45% had worked at jobs which required (due to work overload) 60 or more hours per week. They add that prolonged emotional strain preceded the attack in 91% of the cases, while similar stress was observed in only 20% of a control group. Breslow and Buell (1) have also reported findings which support a relationship between hours of work and death from coronary disease. In an investigation of mortality rates of men in California, they observed that workers in light industry under the age of 45, who are on the job more than 48 hours a week, have twice the risk of death from CHD as similar workers working 40 or under hours a week. Another substantial investigation on quantitative work load was carried out by Margolis et al. (20) on a representative national U.S. sample of 1496 employed persons. They found that overload was significantly related to a number of symptoms or indicators of stress: escapist drinking, absenteeism from work, low motivation to work, lowered self-esteem, and an absence of suggestions to employers.

There is also some evidence that "qualitative" overload can be a source of work stress for the middle-aged. French et al. (8) looked at qualitative work overload in a large university. They used questionnaires, interviews, and medical examinations to obtain data on risk factors associated with CHD for 122 university administrators and professors. They found that one symptom of stress, low self-esteem, was related to work overload but that this was different for the two occupational groupings. Qualitative overload was not significantly linked to low self-esteem among the administrators but was significantly correlated for the professors. The greater the "quality" of work expected of the professor, the lower the self-esteem. Other studies have reported an association of qualitative work overload with cholesterol level (9). French and Caplan (7) summarise this research by suggesting that both qualitative and quantitative overload produce at least nine different symptoms of psychological and physical strain: job dissatisfaction, job tension, lower self-esteem, threat, embarrassment, high cholesterol levels, increased heart rate, skin resistance, and more smoking.

It is also interesting to note that overload is not always externally imposed. Many middle-aged professionals react to overload by working longer hours. For example, in an American study (33) it was found that 45% of the executives investigated worked all day, in the evenings, and during weekends, and that a further 37% kept weekends free but worked extra hours in the evenings. In many companies this type of behavior has become a norm to which executives feel they must adhere.

WORK ROLE AMBIGUITY/CONFLICT

Another major source of work stress among middle-aged individuals is associated with a person's role at work. Role ambiguity exists when an individual has inadequate information about his work role, that is, when there is *"lack of clarity* about the work objectives associated with the role, about work colleagues' expectation of the work role and about the scope and responsibility of the job" (17). Kahn et al. (17) found in their study that men who suffered from role ambiguity experienced lower job satisfaction, higher job-related tension, greater futility, and lower self-confidence. French and Caplan (6) found, at one of NASA's bases, in a sample of 205 middle-aged engineers, scientists, and administrators, that role ambiguity was significantly related to low job satisfaction and to feelings of job-related threat to one's mental and physical well-being. This also related to indicators of physiological strain, such as increased blood pressure and pulse rate. Margolis et al. (20) also found a number of significant relationships between symptoms or indicators of physical and mental ill health, on the one hand, and role ambiguity, on the other, in their national U.S. sample. The stress indicators related to role ambiguity were depressed mood, lowered self-esteem, life dissatisfaction, job dissatisfaction, low motivation to work, and intention to leave job.

Role conflict exists when an "individual in a particular work role is torn by conflicting job demands or doing things he really does not want to do or does not think are part of the job specification" (17). The most frequent manifestation of this is when an individual is caught between two groups of people who demand different kinds of behaviour or expect that the job should entail different functions. Kahn et al. (17) found that men who suffered more role conflict had lower job satisfaction and higher job-related tension. It is interesting to note that they also found that the greater the power or authority of the people "sending" the conflicting role messages, the more job dissatisfaction produced by the role conflict. This was related to physiological strain as well, as the NASA study (6) illustrates. The NASA group telemetered and recorded the heart rate of 22 men for a two-hour period while they were at work in their offices. They found that the mean heart rate for an individual was strongly related to his report of role conflict. A larger and medically more sophisticated study by Shirom et al. (30) found similar results. Their research is of particular interest, since they tried to look simultaneously at a wide variety of potential work stresses. They collected data on 762 male kibbutz members aged 30 and above, drawn from 13 kibbutzim throughout Israel. They examined the relationships between CHD, abnormal electrocardiographic readings, CHD risk factors (systolic blood pressure, pulse rate, serum cholesterol levels, etc.), and potential sources of job stress (work overload, role ambiguity, role conflict, lack of physical activity). Their data were broken down by occupational groups: agricultural workers, factory employees, craftsmen, and managers. It was found that there was a significant relationship between role conflict and CHD (specifically abnormal electrocardiographic readings), particularly for the middle-aged managers.

Another important potential source of middle-aged stress associated with work role is responsibility for people, as differentiated from responsibility for things (equipment, budgets, etc.). Wardwell et al. (34) found that responsibility for people was significantly more likely to lead to CHD than responsibility for things. Increased responsibility for people frequently means that one has to spend more time interacting with others, attending meetings, working alone and, in consequence, as in the NASA study (6), more time in trying to meet deadline pressures and schedules. Pincherle (26) also found this in his U.K. study of 2000 executives attending a medical centre for a medical checkup. Among the 1200 managers sent by their companies for annual examinations, there was evidence of physical stress being linked to age and level of responsibility; the older and more responsible the executive, the greater the probability of the presence of CHD risk factors or symptoms. French and Caplan (6) support this in their NASA study of managerial and professional workers—they found that responsibility for people was significantly related to heavy smoking, raised diastolic blood pressure, and increased serum cholesterol levels; however, the more the individual had responsibility for things as opposed to people, the lower were each of these CHD risk factors.

Having too little responsibility, lack of participation in decision-making, lack of managerial support, having to keep up with increasing standards of performance and coping with rapid technological change are other potential middle-aged role stressors found at work.

INTERPERSONAL RELATIONS AT WORK

Another major potential source of stress for the middle-aged worker has to do with the nature of the relationships with other people in the work environment. Behavioural scientists have long suggested that good relationships among members of a work group are a central factor in individual and organisational health (4).

Buck (2) focused on the attitude and relationship of middle-aged workers and managers to their immediate boss, using Fleishman's leadership questionnaire on consideration and initiating structure. The consideration factor was associated with behaviour indicative of friendship, mutual trust, respect and a certain warmth between boss and subordinate. He found that those managers who felt that their boss was low on consideration reported feeling more job pressure. Managers who were under pressure reported that their boss did not give them criticism in a helpful way, played favourites with subordinates, "pulled rank" and took advantage of them whenever he got a chance. Buck concludes that the "considerate behaviour of superiors appears to have contributed significantly inversely to feelings of job pressure."

Morris (22) encompasses this whole area of work relationships in one model, which he terms the "cross of relationships." While he acknowledges the differences between relationships on two continua—one axis extends from colleagues to users and the other intersecting axis from senior to junior staff—he feels that the focal middle-aged manager must bring all four into dynamic balance in order to be able to deal with the stress of his position. Morris's suggestion seems only sensible when we see how much of his work time the middle-aged manager spends with other people. In a research programme to find out exactly what managers do, Minzberg (21) showed just how much of their time is spent in interaction. In an intensive study of a small sample of chief executives, he found that in a large organisation a mere 22% of time was spent in desk work sessions, the rest being taken up by telephone calls (6%), scheduled meetings (59%), unscheduled meetings (10%), and other activities (3%). In small organisations, basic desk work played a larger part (52%), but nearly 40% was still devoted to face-to-face contacts of one kind or another.

CAREER PROSPECTS

Two major clusters of potential work stressors can be identified in this area: 1. lack of job security, fear of redundancy, obsolescence or early retirement, etc.; and 2. status incongruity, under- or over-promotion, frustration at having reached one's career ceiling, etc. For many middle-aged workers, career progression is of overriding importance—by promotion they earn not only money but also status and the new job challenges for which they strive. However, career progression is, perhaps, a problem by its very nature. For example, Sofer (32) found that many of his sample believed that "luck" and "being in the right place at the right time" play a major role in career advancement.

Typically, in the early years at work, ambition and the ability to come to terms quickly with a rapidly changing environment are fostered and suitably rewarded by the company. At middle age, and usually middle management levels, carrer advancement becomes more problematic and most workers find their progress slowed, if not actually stopped. Job opportunities become fewer, those jobs that are available take longer to master, past (mistaken?) decisions cannot be revoked, old knowledge and methods become obsolete, energies may be flagging or demanded by the family, and there is the press of fresh young recruits to face in competition. Both Levinson (18) and Constandse (3)—the latter refers to this phase as "the male menopause"—depict the manager as suffering these fears and disappointments in "silent isolation" from his family and work colleagues.

The fear of demotion or obsolescence can be strong for those who know they have reached their "career ceiling"—and most will inevitably suffer some erosion of status before they finally retire. Goffman (10), extrapolating from a technique employed in the con-game "cooling the mark out," suggests that the company should bear some of the responsibility for taking the sting out of this (felt) failure experience.

From the company perspective, on the other hand, McMurray (19) presents the case for not promoting a manager to a higher position if there is doubt that he or she can fill it. In a syndrome he labels "the executive neurosis," he describes the over-promoted manager as grossly overworking to keep down a top job and at the same time hiding his insecurity, and points to the consequences of this for the manager's work performance and the company. Age is no longer revered as it was; it is becoming a "young man's world." The rapidity with which society is developing (technologically, economically, and socially) is likely to mean that individuals will now need to change career during their working life (as companies and products are having to do). Such trends breed uncertainty, while research suggests that older workers look for stability (31). Unless the middle-aged adapt their expectations to suit new circumstances, career development stress, especially in later life, is likely to become an increasingly common experience.

HOME/WORK INTERFACE STRESSES

This section covers those interfaces between life outside and life inside the organisation that might put pressure on the middle-aged worker: family problems, life crises, financial difficulties, conflict of personal beliefs with those of the company, and the conflict of company with family demands.

The area which has received most research interest here is that of the middle-aged worker/manager's relationship with his wife and family. This individual has two main problems vis-à-vis his family: The first is that of time-management and commitment-management. Not only does his busy life leave him few resources with which to cope with other people's needs, but in order to do his job well the middle-aged man usually also needs support from others to cope with the details of house management, etc., to relieve stress when possible, and to maintain contact with the outside world. The second, often a result of the first, is the spillover of crises or stresses from one system which affect the other.

Marriage Patterns

The arrangement the middle-aged man reaches with his wife will be of vital importance to both problem areas. Pahl and Pahl (24) found that the majority of wives in their middle-class sample saw their role in relation to their husband's job as a supportive, domestic one; all said that they derived their sense of security from their husbands. Gowler and Legge(11) have dubbed this bond "the hidden contract," in which the wife agrees to act as a "support team" so that her husband can fill the demanding job to which he aspires. Handy (13) supports the idea that this is "typical" and that it is the path to career success for the middle-aged male manager. Based on individual psychometric data, he describes a number of possible marriage-role combinations. In his sample of top British executives (in mid-career) and their wives, he found that the most frequent pattern (about half the 22 couples interviewed) was the "thrusting male/caring female." This he depicts as a highly role-segregated combination, with the emphasis on separation, silence and complementary activities. Historically, both the company and the manager have reaped benefits from maintaining the segregation of work and home implicit in this pattern. The company thus legitimates its demand for a constant work performance from its employee, no matter what his home situation, and the manager is free to pursue his career but keeps a safe haven to which he can return to relax and recuperate. The second and most frequent combination was "involved/involved"—a dual career pattern, with the emphasis on sharing of responsibility. This, while potentially extremely fulfilling for both parties, requires energy inputs which might well prove so excessive that none of the roles involved is fulfilled successfully.

Mobility

Home conflicts become particularly critical in relation to work relocation and mobility among the middle-aged. Much of the literature on this topic comes from the United States, where mobility is much more a part of the national character for the middle-aged managers and other workers than in the U.K. (25), but there is reason to believe that in the U.K., too, it is an increasingly common phenomenon.

At an individual level, the effects of mobility on the manager's wife and family have been studied (5). Researchers agree that whether she is willing to move or not, the wife bears the brunt of relocations, and they conclude that most husbands do not appreciate what this involves. American writers point to signs that wives are suffering and becoming less cooperative. Immundo (15) hypothesizes that increasing divorce rates are seen as the upwardly aspiring manager races ahead of his socially unskilled stay-at-home wife. Seidenberg (29) comments on the rise in the ratio of female to male alcoholics in the United States from 1:5 in 1962 to 1:2 in 1973 and asks, provocatively, "Do corporate wives have souls?" Descriptive accounts of the frustrations and loneliness of being a corporate wife in the U.S. and U.K. proliferate. Increasing teenage delinquency and violence are also laid at the door of the mobile, middle-aged manager and the society which he has created.

Constant moving can have profound effects on the life-style of the people concerned—particularly on their relationships with others. Staying only two years or so in one place, mobile families do not have time to develop close ties with the local community. Immundo (15) talks of the "mobility syndrome," a way of behaving geared to developing only temporary relationships. Packard (23) describes ways in which individuals react to the type of fragmenting society this creates, e.g., treating everything as if it were temporary, being indifferent to local community amenities and organizations, living for the present and becoming adept at instant gregariousness. He goes on to point out the likely consequences for local communities, the nation, and the rootless people involved.

Pahl and Pahl (24) suggest that the British reaction is, characteristically, more reserved and that many middle-aged mobiles retreat into their nuclear family. Managers, particularly, do not become involved in local affairs due both to lack of time and to an appreciation that they are only short-stay inhabitants. Their wives find participation easier (especially in a mobile rather than a static area) and a recent survey suggested that, for some, involvement is a necessity to compensate for their husband's career involvement and frequent absences. From the company's point of view, the way in which a wife adjusts to her new environment can affect her husband's work performance. Guest and Williams (12) illustrate this by an example of a major international company who, on surveying 1800 of their executives in 70 countries, concluded that the two most important influences on overall satisfaction with the overseas assignment were the job itself and, more importantly, the wife's adjustment to the foreign environment.

THE MIDDLE-AGED TYPE A

Sources of pressure at work evoke different reactions from different people. Some are better able to cope with these stressors than others; they adapt their behaviour in a way that meets the environmental challenge. On the other hand, some middle-aged workers are psychologically predisposed to stress; that is, they are unable to cope or adapt to the stress-provoking situations. Many factors may contribute to these differences—personality, motivation, being able or ill-equipped to deal with problems in a particular area of expertise, fluctuations in abilities (particularly with age), insight into one's own motivations and weaknesses, etc. It would be useful to examine, therefore, those characteristics of the individual that research evidence indicates are predisposers to stress. Most of the research in this area has focused on personality and behavioural differences between high and low stressed individuals.

The major research approach to individual stress differences began with the work of Friedman and Rosenman (9, 27) in the early 1960s and later showed a relationship between behavioural patterns and the prevalence of CHD. They found that individuals manifesting certain behavioural traits showed a significantly greater risk of CHD. These individuals were later referred to as the 'coronary-prone behaviour pattern Type A' as distinct from Type B (low risk of CHD). Type A was found to be the overt behavioural syndrome or style of living characterised by "extremes of competitiveness striving for achievement, aggressiveness, haste, impatience, restlessness, hyperalertness, explosiveness of speech, tenseness of facial musculature and feelings of being under pressure of time and under the challenge of responsibility" (27). It was suggested that "people having this particular behavioural pattern were often so deeply involved and committed to their work that other aspects of their lives were relatively neglected" (16).

In the early studies, persons were designated as Type A or Type B on the basis of clinical judgments of doctors and psychologists or peer ratings. These studies found higher incidence of CHD among Type A than Type B. Many of the inherent methodological weaknesses of this approach were overcome by the classic Western Collaborative Group Study (27). A prospective study (as opposed to the earlier retrospective studies) of a national sample of over 3400 men free of CHD was undertaken. All these men were rated Type A or B by psychiatrists after intensive interviews, without knowledge of any biological data about them and without the individuals being seen by a heart specialist. Diagnosis was made by an electrocardiographer and an independent medical practitioner, who were not informed about the subjects' behavioural patterns. They found the following result: After two and a half years from the start of the study, Type A men between the ages 39-49 and 50-59 had 6.5 and 1.9 times, respectively the incidence of CHD than Type B men. They also had a large number of stress risk factors (e.g., high serum cholesterol levels, elevated beta-lipoproteins, etc.). After four and a half years of the follow-up observation in the study, the *same* relationship of behavioural pattern and incidence of CHD was found. In terms of the clinical manifestations of CHD, individuals exhibiting Type A behavioural patterns had a significantly higher incidence of acute myocardial infarction and angina pectoris.

From the perspective of middle-aged managers, the most significant work was carried out by Howard et al. (14). In this study, 236 middle-aged managers from 12 different companies were examined for Type A behaviour and for a number of the known risk factors in CHD (blood pressure, cholesterol, triglycerides, uric acid, smoking and fitness). Those managers exhibiting extreme Type A behaviour showed significantly higher blood pressure (systolic and diastolic) and higher cholesterol and triglyceride levels. A higher percentage of these managers were cigarette smokers and, in each age group studied, Type A managers were less interested in exercise (although differences in cardio-respiratory fitness were found only in the oldest age group). The authors conclude that Type A managers were found to be higher, on a number of risk factors known to be associated with CHD.

CONCLUSION

In summary, the sources of stress among middle-aged workers are many and varied, but an awareness of these is critical if we are to minimise their adverse effects, both for the individual and the organisation. As Wright (35) so aptly suggests, "the responsibility for maintaining health should be a reflection of the basic relationship between the individual and the organisation for which he works; it is in the best interests of both parties that reasonable steps are taken to live and work sensibly and not too demandingly."

REFERENCES

1. BRESLOW, L. and BUELL, P. (1960). Mortality from coronary heart disease and physical activity of work in California. *J. Chron. Dis.*, *11*, 615.
2. BUCK, V. (1972). *Working Under Pressure*. London: Staples Press.
3. CONSTANDSE, W. J. (1972). A neglected personnel problem. *Personnel J.*, *51*, 129.
4. COOPER, C. L. (1979). *The Executive Gypsy: The Quality of Managerial Life*. London: Macmillan. New Jersey: Petrocelli Books.
5. COOPER C. L. and MARSHALL, J. (1978). *Understanding Executive Stress*. London: Macmillan.
6. FRENCH, J. R. P. and CAPLAN, R. D. (1970). Psychosocial factors in coronary heart disease. *Indus. Med.*, *39*, 383.
7. FRENCH, J. R. P. and CAPLAN, R. D. (1973). Organizational stress and individual strain. In: Marrow, A. J. (ed.), *The Failure of Success*. New York: AMACOM.
8. FRENCH, J. R. P., TUPPER, C. J. and MUELLER, E. I. (1965). *Workload of University Professors*. Unpublished Research Report. Ann Arbor, Michigan: The University of Michigan.
9. FRIEDMAN, M., ROSENMAN, R. H. and CARROLL, V. (1958). Changes in serum cholesterol and blood clotting time in men subjected to cyclic variations of occupational stress. *Circulation*, *17*, 852.
10. GOFFMAN, E. (1952). On cooling the mark out. *Psychiat.*, *15*, *451*.

11. GOWLER, D. and LEGGE, K. (1975). Stress and external relationships—the 'hidden contract'. In: Gowler, D. and Legge, K. (eds.), *Managerial Stress*. Epping: Gower Press.
12. GUEST, D. and WILLIAMS, R. (1973). How home affects work. *New Society*, January.
13. HANDY, C. (1978). The family: help or hindrance. In: Cooper, C. L. and Payne, R. (eds.), *Stress at Work*. London: John Wiley & Sons.
14. HOWARD, J. H., CUNNINGHAM, D. A. and RECHNITZER, P. A. (1976). Health patterns associated with Type B behaviour: a managerial population. *J. Hum. Stress*, March, 24.
15. IMMUNDO, L. V. (1974). Problems associated with managerial mobility. *Personnel J.*, 53, 910.
16. JENKINS, C. D. (1971). Psychologic and social precursors of coronary disease. *N.E.J.M.*, 284, 307.
17. KAHN, R. L., WOLFE, D. M., QUINN, R. P., SNOEK, J. D. and ROSENTHAL, R. A. (1964). *Organizational Stress*. New York: John Wiley & Sons.
18. LEVINSON, H. (1973). Problems that worry our executives. In: Marrow, A. J. (ed.), *The Failure of Success*. New York: AMACOM.
19. MCMURRAY, R. N. (1973). The executive neurosis. In: Noland, R. L. (ed.), *Industrial Mental Health and Employee Counselling*. New York: Behavioral Publications.
20. MARGOLIS, B. L., KROES, W. H. and QUINN, R. P. (1974). Job stress: an unlisted occupational hazard. *J. Occup. Med.*, 16, 654.
21. MINZBERG, H. (1973). *The Nature of Managerial Work*. New York: Harper & Row.
22. MORRIS, J. (1975). Managerial stress and 'the cross of relationships'. In: Gowler, D. and Legge, K. (eds.), *Managerial Stress*. Epping: Gower Press.
23. PACKARD, V. (1975). A Nation of Strangers. New York: McKay.
24. PAHL, J. M. and PAHL, R. E. (1971). *Managers and Their Wives*. London: Allen Lane.
25. PIERSON, G. W. (1972). *The Moving Americans*. New York: Knopf.
26. PINCHERLE, G. (1972). Fitness for work. *Proc. Roy. Soc. Med.*, 65, 321.
27. ROSENMAN, R. H., FRIEDMAN, M. and JENKINS, C. D. (1967). Clinically unrecognised myocardial infarction in the Western Collaborative Group Study. *Am J. Cardiol.*, 19, 776.
28. RUSSEK, H. I. and ZOHMAN, B. L. (1969). Relative significance of hereditary, diet and occupational stress in CHD of young adults. *Am. J. Med. Sci.*, 235, 266.
29. SEIDENBERG, R. (1973). *Corporate Wives—Corporate Casualties*. New York: American Management Association.
30. SHIROM, A., EDEN, D., SILBERWASSER, S. and KELLERMAN, J. J. (1973). Job stress and risk factors in coronary heart disease among occupational categories in kibbutzim. *Soc. Sci. Med.*, 7, 875.
31. SLEEPER, R. D. (1975). Labour mobility over the life cycle. *Brit. J. Indus. Rel.*, 13.
32. SOFER, C. (1070). *Men in Mid-Career*. Cambridge: Cambridge University Press.
33. URIS, A. (1972). How managers ease job pressures. *Int. Mgt.*, June, 45.
34. WARDWELL, W. I., HYMAN, M. and BAHNSON, C. B. (1964). Stress and coronary disease in three field studies. *J. Chron. Dis.*, 17, 73.
35. WRIGHT, H. B. (1975). *Executive Ease and Dis-ease*. Epping: Gower Press.

7

THE DIVORCED IN MIDDLE AGE

Henry J. Friedman, M.D.

Associate Professor in Psychiatry,
Tufts University School of Medicine;
Director, Outpatient Psychiatry,
New England Medical Center Hospital, Boston

INTRODUCTION

To write about either divorce or mid-life should, as a prerequisite, require that one have something to offer from a specific point of view. Both subjects have been prominent in the popular and professional literature; the concepts that adult life has phases and that mid-life with its crises of adjustment is a particularly important phase have influenced most minds exposed to books, movies and television (1-4, 6). A psychiatric perspective, however, while open to these ideas, is often somewhat pressed as to how the generalized concepts actually apply to individuals treated in analytically-oriented psychotherapy. There has been some tendency to equate well presented descriptions of existentially relevant phases of life with the etiologically significant factors in neurosis (5, 7, 10, 12). For instance, Gail Sheehy concludes her excellent descriptions of depression, sadness and anxiety in her interview subjects by ascribing these symptoms to the phase of the life-cycle (11). This is an understandable and perhaps acceptable conclusion for a journalist to make; it is an ineffectual and therapeutically nihilistic conclusion for a psychiatrist. The difficulty of integrating the presence of neurotic conflict into any scheme of adult development is frequently overlooked—sometimes to the detriment of both sets of data.

On the subject of divorce even more formidable problems exist in the process of adding material from a psychiatric point of view. Mid-life, while a subject of general interest, lacks the controversial quality of divorce (8, 9). It has been difficult, even for professionals working in psychiatry, to view

103

divorce as a fact of life to be accepted as an experience which is there and can be quite advantageous. Mounting statistics of divorce are seldom viewed as the result of a beneficial change in societal values which has increased the options available to married people (13).

The purpose of this paper, then, is not to link the so-called stresses of mid-life with the growing incidence of divorce in mid-life. Certainly, for those who wish such a correlation, Sheehy's account of the mid-life couple covers the possibilities for this hypothesis from several angles, e.g., the sexual differences between men and women ("the sexual diamond"), and the so-called "switch forties." Her approach utilizes much of the work on adult life-cycle and includes the traditional belief that the preservation of the intact couple and family is the most desirable of outcomes. To this end, she is willing to accept Jung's mythology of sexual reversal within the individual as an explanation of the problems with continued intimacy which many mid-life couples are reported to experience. The opposite sex loses its magical powers over us after we discover that we have that opposite within ourselves. "To be sure," says Jung, quoted by Sheehy, "it takes half a lifetime to arrive at this stage."

THE CLINICAL PERSPECTIVE

People who get divorced in mid-life may questionably represent a special group of individuals. Their adult stage may be considered important by them or others. There is no question that publicly very few people are able to accept this particular change in life-style without feeling and expressing opinions, usually negative. Many basically stylistic decisions, like early retirement, moving to Florida or traveling extensively, fail to elicit so much emotional opposition and comment. If we utilize a chronological definition of mid-life, then we are likely to be dealing with individuals who range in age from about 35 to 50. It is clear immediately that the 15-year span is such that middle-aged individuals may be in entirely different life situations. What they do have in common, however, as far as marriage and divorce are concerned, is a mature identity and usually a marital history lengthy enough to have established a definite pattern of life and a shared set of experiences. Undoubtedly, natural forces favor the continuation of any marriage that persists beyond five years. Again, the problem of gathering meaningful data on the quality of a marriage, on the positive aspects both individuals derive from the partnership, is formidable. Since I do not know of any other discipline which allows for the measurement of such complex variables with any accuracy, I feel that data of individual and couples psychotherapy deserve to be reviewed and included in an essay on the topic of divorce in middle age.

It is safe to say that no one ever seems to want or approve of divorce, particularly not for marriages with some tenure and in individuals who are not considered young. The generalized moralistic disapproval of divorce has been modified; young people are allowed their mistake (very much in the singular). For the middle-aged the picture changes considerably; this is far from remarkable, since divorcing couples do indeed represent a threat to the societal status quo. Even more significant are the profound emotional dislocations that are activated in both parties to a divorce when they have shared their lives over many years, no matter how disillusioned and angry they have been. Weiss (13) has amply, perhaps even excessively, stressed the inevitability of this feeling state. However, he fails to see that some of the discomfort described by his group of respondents had to do with neurotic attachments to the separating spouse, unconscious guilt about being free from binding, burdensome attachments, and unresolved infantile fears and dependency. He also neglects to locate those individuals who, while not free from emotional responses, do not require the intervention of "Parents Without Partners" or some equivalent support group. Men are usually seen as responsible for the failure of long-term marriages. The societal anger at an older man who either leaves his wife and remarries a younger woman or remains free of a romantic commitment seems to be particularly great.

Psychiatric consultation provides a different point of view on marital relationships. It would appear that marriage favors the status quo, even if one or both partners have been involved in extramarital relationships for a varying period of time. From the viewpoint of psychoanalytic theory of the unconscious, it should be apparent that a marital choice is always indebted to the oedipal attachment in either one or the other of its polarities. Whatever the incidence of divorce in mid-life, there is reason, from a clinical point of view, to believe that far more non-adaptive marriages that survive into mid-life continue into old age than are dissolved during the period of mid-life crisis. A good deal of this can be explained by recognizing that full individual development (maturity) with adequate separation-individualization is not so frequently encountered. Many individuals, who may appear to be mature in many spheres, do not really feel free to question the nature of their marital relationships. Neurotically-determined fears of being alone are frequently encountered among divorcing individuals. These are undoubtedly reinforced by some of the practical problems of being alone after a long period of living with another person, as well as with children. If dependency of various sorts, guilt, financial reality, loyalty and habit all are on the side of maintaining marriages, why is it that divorces do occur? Is there an answer to this question which makes use of the more intimate data of psychotherapy as well as the more general material of adult life changes?

THE CONDITIONS OF MARRIAGE

Many patients who seek psychiatric treatment in their late thirties, while not necessarily expressing marital concerns, nevertheless convey a sense of not having made a free and active choice of a marriage partner. Individuals in their mid-twenties, a period which has been considered by upper-middle-class values as the right time for making a marital choice, do not necessarily have the emotional maturity which allows for a decision to marry. Sexual intimacy, attractiveness and a similar class background often are the major factors in making the decision. Love is also involved, but it is often a romantic love, which is not particularly sustained by experiences of living well with another person who is respected as a result of repeatedly experienced mutuality. The idea of marriage or an enduring companionship as enhancing individual development and freedom is certainly a relatively new concept which is far from generally accepted. Marriages casually made, chronologically and socially promoted, are obviously good enough for many, if not most, individuals. Furthermore, once a legal commitment has been made, there is a tendency for the relationship to develop; it is a human characteristic to love those with whom we live, in one way or another. To be mildly in love is in many ways a compatible state of being, enabling one to cope with the demands of a complex life. The problem arises, however, when we begin to experience the ubiquity of neurotic illness in the general population. Living together makes people less lonely; it also offers the increased possibility for effectiveness that any division of labor makes possible. Frequently, however, the scenario does not proceed in this smooth fashion. When lack of satisfaction within a marriage is manifest, whatever the nature of complaints in general, one or both parties feels that they are not happy with their situation or with themselves.

Often the unhappiness that evolves at the mid-life period was evident to one or both parties even in the days of their courtship. This set of incompatibilities may have been accepted by virtue of one of several maneuvers, e.g., denial of its importance, eagerness to be married, failure to anticipate its effect on daily life. Surprisingly, a psychoanalytic investigation of older patients who either are divorced or get divorced in the course of a long-term treatment reveals that the issues underlying a divorce have usually been there in an identical form from the time of the marriage. Furthermore, the initial difficulties, as well as the unconscious underpinning of the choice of marital partner, relate to unresolved issues of the oedipal period. In marriages that dissolve after many years, it can be hypothesized that the elements of incompatibility have been there from the start; they may, in fact, for certain neurotic patients be there in an inevitable fashion, unless some therapeutic intervention makes available to them the insight into unconscious needs for a limited type of object relationship which, while attractive and even necessary to them, has qualities of the proverbial double-edged sword. They can neither live with a choice of a person with that type of limitation nor change the unconscious need for such a person. However, the passage of time, with its general intensification of character limitations and its rational message regarding the limited years available for comfortably living, causes some individuals to fight for a new chance in their personal life. In other cultures, and in other times, such possibilities were extremely limited. While it was possible to conduct extramarital relationships in secrecy, divorce and remarriage extracted too high a price for many. Some societies and religions felt entitled to rule out such possibilities entirely for all their members.

In summary, it should be apparent that divorce does not come easily to those who have endured a relationship into their mid-life. Divorce in mid-life is less frequent than the continued unhappy marriage where difficulties are ignored through withdrawal into the self, work or extramarital relationships.

MARRIAGE, PURPOSEFULNESS AND HEALTH

With good reason we view relationships as essential to the gratifications required by individuals. The problem facing an individual with many years devoted to a relationship (even where the devotion does not reflect a deep commitment) is that a sense of purpose has been integrated into that relationship. Two people think of the meaning of their individual lives in terms of shared achievements and aspirations. One of the most formidable resistances to making a change in marital status involves the fear of losing this sense of purposefulness, not only in terms of pursuing an independent future, but also in the sense of acknowledging that the past energies were misdirected with an inadequate partner. Many people, although otherwise well integrated, have never really thought of themselves as having meaning as separate individuals. Existence for them has always been in some connection to others. They are sons-daughters, husbands-wives, fathers-mothers who are important as child, spouse, parent. Can a person who has lived with such an orientation really feel it is important to think of a purpose for him/herself outside the frame of reference of being in a relationship with others?

Clinically we see many adolescents who, while not suffering from severe symptomatology, are unable to embrace goals for themselves that are beyond the scope of peer group importance. These individuals, while bright and often energetic, seem confused about how to plan for the future. In particular, the centrality of meaningful work seems absent in them. Their parents, though concerned and present, are often unable to communicate the importance of work, purpose and achievement in life. The purposeful elements in these adolescents' lives are then appropriated from their peer group or even from the less serious visual picture of life that is made available to them through the popular media.

Single individuals who enter mid-life with no major commitments to a relationship or to work may develop some of the same regressive manifestations in the face of their aimless lives, even when their abilities to achieve gratification of sexual and monetary nature are present.

THE RELUCTANT MIDDLE-AGED DIVORCED

Most people who remain in marriages into the mid-life period leave those relationships with great reluctance. Actual separation often follows years of stable dissatisfaction. In psychotherapy it is noted that progress for an individual in understanding neurotic conflict can occur, with resultant improvement in many spheres of life—except that of the marriage. Even there, improvements may occur in the sense of decreased overt conflict without any ability to better the relationship in a deeper sense. Both men and women fear that they will fail to find another relationship; this is far from an irrational fear. There is some truth to the assertion of women in their thirties and forties that they are unable to locate suitable men for companionship or marriage. While the situation is somewhat better for men statistically speaking and while it is socially more permissible for men to freely date women from 22 to 50, it is not unusual for men to experience difficulty in finding a female companion who both wants a relationship and is desirable to them. The theme, a ubiquitous one, is that all the good ones, men and women, are married to someone else.

The problem of meeting others for serious relationships is common to both men and women. Clinically, the situation of a man who has been in an overtly unhappy relationship for 10 to 15 years and has an extramarital affair as the first important step in leaving his wife is not uncommon. One special fact of the mid-life marriage (unless either party has been successful in having good affairs) is that its participants feel uncertain about how these things are done nowadays. In fact, at this time in our society many, if not most, individuals never did know "how these things were done" because they married from a position of minimal experience. So, for many, the continuation of a marriage, regardless of the conditions, is a necessity. There are individuals who leave chronically stressful relationships without the benefit of trial relationships or expectations for future relationships. One patient, for instance, felt only resignation when he left a wife of 18 years. Their sexual life had been marginal for several years; he had decided that he could tolerate the absence of a sexual life because he was quite certain he would not try for any more relationships in his life. He was surprised to find that there were woman partners who wanted intimacy without demanding the commitments he was not ready to make.

The concept that any middle-aged person who gets divorced is seeking a change to deal with his or her mid-life crisis or because he or she has grown bored is a hard one to dispel. Since, in adjusting to single life, divorced persons usually do continue to be involved in sexual relationships, it often looks like this is the basis for the change. This conviction is particularly strong regarding men who leave a wife of many years and eventually remarry a younger woman. The fact that many men obtain divorces and then remarry a similarly aged woman or even one who is older is often not noticed or publicized.

ON BEING MIDDLE-AGED AND DIVORCED

Patients who either are divorced and enter therapy for problems superficially related to that status or join the ranks of the divorced in the course of psychotherapy notice immediately that several things are true. First, it is not as bad as they had anticipated. Life indeed goes on, is even more peaceful, and may be interesting in new ways. The more that fundamental developmental issues around being an independent person had been hidden within the marriage status, the rougher the post-separation period will be. In fact, those who feel complete in themselves may experience intense feelings of sadness; they grieve the lifetime that they have given to something far from satisfactory. However, life is different for the single—particularly for the mid-life single. Everyone else may not, in fact, be married, but it seems that way to the newly separated. Worse still is the fact that those single people around them are often in a very different position—well established in their single lives, whatever the pattern of these may be. A divorced woman in her forties with three children of varying ages is indeed single, but not in a way that makes her companionable with an unmarried 40-year-old woman who finds the acceptable single life to include long periods of time without male companionship and free from the obligations of child care.

In addition, a new single status at mid-life challenges all assumptions of what the person has placed central in his or her emotional life. Some of this questioning will be part of mid-life development for all sensitive adults. For instance, the mother-housewife who is an alert, entertaining woman may have to find ways to utilize her energies as children become more self-sufficient and the opportunities for entertainment seem limited and less gratifying. When this kind of reassessment in mid-life also involves divorce, the situation is more complex.

Indeed, one of the strongest justifications for discouraging women from developing a so-called feminine identification based on culturally determined, infantile hysterical characteristics has to do with the increasing evidence that such an identity is no longer adaptive. This is a point which needs to be stressed beyond the issues raised by feminists. Many intellectuals who reflect upon such issues as woman's role seem to forget that some determinations may not be best left to the choice of the individual woman. Allies of change for women have often felt it necessary to add the provision that they approve increased freedom of action and role for women, so long as it is accepted that some women will continue to choose a restricted housewife role. The mid-life period of these women has always been vulnerable; the "empty nest" syndrome and other terms have pointed out that somehow these women were liable to spend a good deal of the mid-life in states of varying degrees of depression and emptiness. A woman without training and an ongoing career is in a similar situation as the man who works in a demanding field where, unbeknownst to him, retirement will come suddenly between 40 and 45.

Both men and women who terminate their marital status share the risk of aimlessness. Men who have invested much energy in their work lives may well feel that the efforts they have made in behalf of family object relationships have been made in vain; women may concentrate on all that they have sacrificed for the man in their life, who has now either left them or been left by them.

The issue of time becomes crucially important for most individuals who divorce in mid-life. How much time do they have left to reestablish and build a life with a significant other? For women in our culture this may be particularly urgent. Women do not feel that their options are as great as men. Although increasing numbers of women from 35 to 50 do find companionship with younger men, this is still far from a popularly entertained notion. While a middle-aged man may actively fantasize about meeting, sexually enjoying and even remarrying a much younger woman, it is rare to encounter a woman who feels this same expansiveness and freedom of range in prospects for companionship. Men at this point may enter a series of sexually-oriented relationships, which may, in some instances, gradually become transformed into a way of life. One relationship of apparent depth follows another similar relationship, with the basic unwillingness to make a commitment remaining outside of the man's awareness. Women in mid-life do not tend to stand the same "risk" of becoming permanently fixed in a pattern of relationships without definite commitment. The danger facing them is of isolation and sexual deprivation, which either become accepted with resignation or are completely avoided by their intense involvement in work, children or retraining for further work.

WHO DIVORCES WHOM AND WHY?

Divorce in mid-life is unlikely. Despite the insistence in the popular literature that mid-life is a time for reappraisal, the fact remains that this idea is more the product of literary imagination and adolescent values than of reality. A mid-life reappraisal may be a luxury available for few or it may be the product of circumstance for those unfortunate enough to precipitate one or be caught in its pathway. Good adjustments tend to "hold" through mid-life, and naturally enough, for this is the period in which hard-won achievements can be enjoyed. A good marriage improves with the freedom of economic security or children's increasing self-sufficiency. A professional person can now reap some of the rewards of building a meaningful work life. Longer periods of vacation, increased leisure, more help from younger colleagues and children help. Major changes in relationships or occupation are unlikely to occur under these circumstances. Those who divorce in mid-life do not do so lightly. The most cogent generalization about mid-life divorces would be that they most frequently follow premature marriages.

Prior to the recent trend of chronologically delayed marriage, there was ample opportunity for premature marriage. By premature I refer now to permanent alliances which are made without an intense meshing of psychological factors, including psychological compatibility at a variety of levels. Individuals who cannot integrate their marital choice with the achievement of adequate happiness in reality have chosen for neurotic reasons and under pressure from external circumstances. The ubiquitous influence of the oedipal picture can be seen in the selection of partners with negative but powerful characteristics resembling the parent of the opposite sex. In conditioning terms, one sees an object choice which carries with it the obligation of continuing a neurotic, non-gratifying form of object relationship. Hence, individuals are often seen in clinical practice who clearly have capacities for relationships of a healthier level but who cling to a spouse who seems to offer nothing more than the burden of care or, worse still, the source of complaints and bitterness. If good marriages are based on the choice of compatible individuals who resemble a loved mother or father, then bad marriages can be said to repeat negative aspects of an unconsciously loved but inadequate parent.

Marriages based on such unconscious bases may well tend to survive and, despite the rising divorce rates, many difficult marriages do not terminate. Divorces occurring in mid-life may result from deep-seated attachment processes; these are marriages that have lasted from seven to 20 years, so that the complexity of the attachment-repulsion phenomenon should not be underestimated. The attachment side of such relationships may be based on masochistic surrender, i.e., the need to take care of another person without deriving an adequate amount of realistic gratification from the relationship. When divorce does finally occur, it is usually based upon a shift in an individual's assessment of personal needs, often in the course of an analysis or psychotherapy, but occasionally without the benefit of such treatment. In the latter case, it is frequently a more dislocating process, with considerable ambivalence and confusion as to the cause of the split. Unexamined divorce, like many other processes proceeding without insight, is the source of much suffering. When a patient enters psychiatric treatment with any marital complaints and a partner with a prejudiced attitude towards therapy, it offers a clue to the fact that divorce may result in the course of the treatment.

WHO IS TO BLAME?

Surprising as this may seem, there usually is someone to whom one can assign more prominent responsibility for the failure of a marriage of long duration. The prominence of significant and inflexible psychopathology in one individual appears to be the cause. Usually this involves the presence of a narcissism which precludes the understanding of the other partner's needs and rights. This may be subtle and hard to define, particularly in those cases where one of the partners is chronically depressive in outlook and feels that the need to express suffering and despair is not burdensome to the other person. This factor does seem to vary on the basis of sex. Culturally it is more acceptable and therefore more common to find obsessive, self-need negligent men married to infantile hysterical women. These marriages have often occurred prematurely in the man's life as a result of his orientation towards work as being of central importance. Characterologically, such men have not been able to explore and experiment with a variety of women. Rather, they are driven by an overly demanding superego to feel committed to a woman on the basis of her helplessness. The early years of these marriages may be stormy. The survival of the relationship relies upon the male's misdirected equation of strength with not needing adequate help with family burdens from a companion. Being the person who takes care of an infantile wife duplicates the past fantasy of being the person upon whom mother depends. The persistence of such marriages is often amazing; even the clarification and insight of an analytic treatment may not lead to change or liberation. These are relationships which on occasion will change when, after what seems like an interminable period, the male has a relationship with another woman. The discovery through action that all women are not the same can have more impact than the insight of the best interpretations. These new relationships are often imperfect and impermanent in nature, but their importance as catalysts for change cannot be ignored.

When the marital imbalance involves a woman of greater flexibility and emotional health, the pattern appears to be somewhat different. Women of considerable emotional capacities are often masochistic in their orientation towards men and tend to overlook their spouse's emotional shallowness under the misconception that the mental and emotional life of males differs from their own. Thus, they excuse rather severe deviations from emotional maturity on the conscious grounds that their husbands care but, being male, are unable to show it. The less acceptable fact of a deficiency of caring capacity is often denied until even the most efficient of avoiders is overwhelmed by contrary evidence.

The process of the earlier years of marriage may help obscure the emotional dissatisfactions in marital relationships. The demands of training and career or of child-rearing may blind partners to the suffering involved in their enduring marriage. While I have maintained that divorce in mid-life does not easily occur, the continuation of the marriage may be based on resignation and distancing within the framework of an unsatisfying relationship. Many marriages which survive beyond mid-life leave much to be desired by any reasonable standard of complementarity in marriage.

RISKING THE CHANGE VS. ENDURING THE STATUS QUO

Both men and women may live with their mistakes, hoping that there will be change or attempting to effectively minimize an awareness of their dissatisfactions. The concept that people should be free to change and not be legally and morally bound to an ungratifying relationship is socially a new one. Assuming that there is a choice for the middle-aged about the continuation of an unsatisfactory marriage, then the greater possibilities for positive adaptation lie with those willing to risk change. Basically this follows the general rules of healthy human development in which change towards autonomy and the ability to find sources of constructive gratification are recurring crucial elements. Unfortunately, even in psychiatry there remains a tendency to view the termination of a marriage with distress. It is not uncommon to see patients in consultation who have been warned by another professional that it is a failure to separate and important for them to stay together for the children's sake or out of loyalty to a commitment.

In my clinical practice, where divorce in mid-life has resulted from an insight-directed decision, the outcome has been highly positive. The persistence of a therapeutic relationship can be critical in helping the individual make a transition away from a relationship that is ungratifying and painful. Certainly, by mid-life an individual deserves to find in an intimate relationship the support, ease and tenderness which a good marriage offers. Life experiences help in the selection process of another partner. A decision to forego any further committed relationships may be necessary in some instances, but it is possible that work, friends or travel may be sufficient to sustain an existentially viable life without a pattern of companionship. The mature, divorced individual, however, like a well-tested house, is a good risk for the future. This, of course, is an area of expertise which has just begun to establish itself in our culture. The predominant fear from traditional conservative elements of our culture is that, without constraint, marriage will fail to continue as the predominant mode of living. In some sense this may be true. When people divorce in mid-life, they may hesitate to try again; their relationships with the opposite sex, although pleasurable, may not lead to marriage in the legal sense, but it is unlikely that most divorced men and women in mid-life will not form some form of stable heterosexual relationship. Despite the trauma associated with divorce, the predominant need for a shared adult relationship undoubtedly will survive the liberalization of attitudes towards divorce. Increasing numbers of divorces will lead most probably to increased remarriages or satisfactory realignments of living situations, perhaps without the benefit of marriage, but with the stability of a committed couple interaction.

REFERENCES

1. BAGUEDOR, E. (1972). *Separation: Journal of a Marriage*. New York: Simon and Schuster.
2. CLAUSEN, J. A. (1967). Glimpses into the social world of middle age. *Int. J. Aging and Human Development, 7*, 99.
3. EPSTEIN, J. (1974). *Divorce in America*. New York: Dutton.
4. FELDER, R. L. (1971). *Divorce*. New York: World.
5. LEVINSON, D. J. et al. (1978). *The Seasons of a Man's Life*. New York: Knopf.
6. MANNES, M. & SHERISKY, N. (1972). *Uncoupling*. New York: Lippincott.
7. MAYER, Nancy. (1979). *The Male Mid-Life Crisis: Fresh Starts After 40*. New York: Synet Books.
8. NEUGARTEN, B. (1968). *Middle Age and Aging*. Chicago: University of Chicago Press.
9. NEUGARTEN, B. (1979). Time, Age and the Life Cycle. *Am. J. Psychiat., 7*, 136.
10. NYDEGGER, C. N. (1976). Middle Age: Some Early Returns—A Commentary. *Int. J. Aging and Human Development, 7*, 137.
11. SHEEHY, G. (1976). *Passages: Predictable Crises of Adult Life*. New York: Bantam.
12. THURNHER, M. (1976). Mid-Life Marriage: Sex Differences in Evaluation and Perspectives. *Int. J. Aging and Human Development, 7*, 129.
13. WEISS, R. S. (1975). *Marital Separation*. New York: Basic Books.

8

THE MIDDLE-AGED MALE
AND FEMALE HOMOSEXUAL

NORMAN J. LEVY, M.D.

Faculty, Postgraduate Center for Mental Health
New York City

INTRODUCTION

Despite the recent spate of publications on homosexuality, male and female, there is little factual information available regarding the life-styles, pleasures and problems of those who have reached their middle years. Bell and Weinberg (2), Jay and Young (6), Kimmel (8), Levy (13), and Marmor (15, 16) have reported on the variety of social, sexual, and psychological life-styles of homosexuals in this age group. Clearly, however, there is a need for more systematic and detailed studies to understand the different needs, sensitivities, and values of the various individuals between the ages of 40 and 60 whose ways of relating sexually are totally or predominantly homosexual.

For the psychotherapist it is especially important to free oneself from stereotypic attitudes or psychodynamic concepts based on a limited number or skewed sampling of patients. As Marmor (15) has written, "There is as yet no single constellation of factors that can adequately explain homosexual deviations." Arieti (1) has noted, "A homosexual orientation is compatible with a rich life, although in its pure forms it is not compatible with reproduction. It is also compatible with pleasure achievement and with the fulfillment of the fundamental human potentialities. Many of the problems connected with homosexuality are derived from the fact that the patient must live in a heterosexual society." Salzman (18) has stated that "homosexual activity is no single discrete symptom, syndrome, or disease. It is a form of behavior which derives from a spectrum of causes."

116

PATTERNS OF RELATING

This chapter will first consider some of the ways the patterns of homosexual relating have been grouped. Kimmel (8) has listed at least six socio-sexual patterns a gay person may follow for varying lengths of time during adulthood: a) a heterosexual marriage with or without periodic homosexual relations following or followed by a gay life-style; b) celibacy without homosexual affectional orientation; c) raising children, including adopted children, d) long-term gay friend/lover relationships; e) gay life-style with no long-term sexual relationship; and f) bisexual life-style without marriage.

Lehman (10) stresses the fact that lesbianism, for which there are many different life-styles, is a very complex behavior pattern not readily accessible to simplistic analysis. She lists some of the common types of relationships as the monogamous, the non-monogamous, the affair, the friendships, and the groups.

The five categories described by Bell and Weinberg (2) have provided us with an effective framework when discussing the characteristics one can observe in studying the life-styles of homosexual men and women. These categories are the *close-coupled*, the *open-coupled*, the *functional*, the *dysfunctional*, and the *asexual*. Some of the main characteristics of each group will now be presented.

Patterns Among Men

Among the men one finds that the close-coupled, essentially, tend to look to each other rather than others for sexual and interpersonal gratification. I find them to be warmer and more open to their feelings. They want to and are able to share intimately with a particular partner. They are able to communicate on an honest level, and when they have differences, they can discuss the problems more productively. Considering their partners as good friends, they are aware of more mutuality and sharing and less struggling for power between themselves. For them, being able to give and take, share interests, and also have separate interests are all vital to a good relationship. They seem to have fewer sexual problems and less regret over being homosexual than those of the other groups. They have less need to seek sexual or social gratification in bars or baths, and they rarely have difficulties with the police, at work, or with assaults or robberies. They seem less tense or paranoid than the other groups.

Among the open-coupled there is evidence of greater conflict and dissatisfaction. Although living with men who are their primary sexual partners, they seem unable and unwilling to relate in a monogamous manner and seek outside partners with and without the knowledge of their lover. They tend to focus more on technique than on relating and feel frustrated when they cannot get their partners to meet their sexual requests. They frequently need the presence of a third person in the act and use him in a functional rather than a relational way. Eventually, they may live together like close roommates, sharing and fulfilling nonsexual needs. They need a larger circle of friends and outlets than close-coupled partners. They also seem lonelier, and less happy, self-accepting and relaxed than the previous group.

Functional men, like the "swinging" heterosexual singles, organize their lives around their many sexual experiences and their involvement in the gay world. Their overtness and possible recklessness expose them to greater chances of having trouble with the law and unsavory situations. Although it is probably among this group that the term "gay" originated, and they are described as energetic, self-reliant, cheerful and optimistic, unrestricted by convention, they are also described as more tense, unhappy, and lonely than their close-coupled counterparts, a state they seek to conceal from most of the world.

Dysfunctionals are described as the "stereotype of the tormented homosexual." The members of this category most often come for therapy because for them life seems to offer little hope for gratification. They have great difficulty in managing their existence in all areas of their lives—sexual, social, and psychological. Experiencing much self-hate affects the way they relate to others and invites rejection from potential partners. Since they believe they are going to be rejected, they very often reject first. They believe that the interest another shows in them is insincere. They are convinced that the other wants them for ulterior motives. Various men have said that those who show interest probably are interested in being paid for sex or in some sort of "kinky" sex, or because no one else wanted them. Being essentially detached and alienated from their feelings, they use sex as a means of reducing, for the moment, sexual tensions and the feeling of loneliness. Having difficulty in allowing others to touch them emotionally in depth or continuity, they most often have impersonal sex and quickly withdraw (13). Many need alcohol or drugs before searching for a contact. I find that even their fantasy life is relatively barren and devoid of hope. They often show poor judgment, act impulsively, and repeatedly get into trouble. Some have been arrested, robbed, beaten up, and even murdered when they have picked up "hustlers" or "rough trade," so-called heterosexual men who act out their perverse psychopathology after they have had sex with a gay man. None has ever had a long-term ongoing sexual-social relationship. Following each "quickie" experience, the person may resolve never again to give in to his urges, while knowing that soon he will again be compulsively driven to repeat the experience.

Asexuals are noted for their lack of involvement with others in all areas. They are often schizoid, if not borderline or psychotic, and live more in fantasy than reality. As a group they can be described as persistently resigned individuals who feel there is nothing they can do about their life-style (5). Their past empty of meaningful experiences, their future looking bleak, they are the loners who exist on the fringes of social and sexual activities. They have trouble both in making friends and in finding sexual partners. Their quietness, unhappy flat demeanor, and remoteness do not encourage others to approach them. They may be aware of occasional upsurges of great anger and pain about their unhappiness, but these are quickly followed by a squelching of the feeling through resignation to their fate.

Patterns Among Women

Among homosexual women, the findings are similar; there are, however, certain differences. There are more women who live in close-coupled relationships than any other group. They exhibit a high degree of sexual fidelity. In fact, "the most viable option for most lesbians may be that of a fulfilling and relatively monogamous 'marital' relationship with another woman" (2). They are the least likely to seek professional help because of their concern about their sexual orientation. Open-coupled lesbians tend to be younger and more sexually active, to have more sexual problems, to be more exclusively homosexual, and to have more regret over their homosexuality. Functionals score low on regret over being homosexual and on sexual problems and high on sexual activity and cruising. Dysfunctional and Asexual women are essentially similar to the men. Asexual women are more apt to rate themselves toward the bisexual direction of the homosexual-heterosexual continuum. They also are most apt to have sought professional help about their sexual orientation, to have given up therapy quickly, and to have had the highest incidence of suicidal thoughts.

PROBLEMS OF MIDDLE ADULTHOOD

In reviewing these groupings, one can see that attention should be paid less to the sexual orientation and more to the problems in developing and maintaining a loving relationship. Fromm (3) described these qualities as the capacity to care for, respond to, respect, and know one's beloved. By the time someone is in the middle years, the difficulties to be dealt with are those related to the uses and abuses of love and sex in an ongoing intimate relationship or an occasional short-term one, the forming of morbidly dependent relationships, the power struggles and the demands for exclusivity, with the concomitant possessiveness and resultant anger, hate and jealousy (12), the difficulties in communicating thoughts and feelings, and problems in resolving differences between the two individuals involved. One very important issue that must be worked through is the compulsive need for one person to make a fetish of the partner. Hoffman (4) describes it as "the narrowing down of one's range of activity from a rich or full existential encounter to a narrow segmental experience."

For a fuller understanding of middle adulthood in the male generally, the findings of Levinson et al. (11) are most informative. They discuss the midlife transition when a man (although these days it is becoming equally applicable to a woman) must come to terms with the past and prepare for the future. He must review and reappraise what he has done with his life. He must, to the extent he is open and flexible, modify the negative elements and test new choices. Finally, he must deal with the polarities, including among them one of masculinity/femininity, that are the sources of deep division in his life. In so doing he must take time to reexamine long-held assumptions and beliefs about himself and the world and attempt to resolve the process of compulsively driving himself to fulfill the impossible demands of what Horney (5) called one's idealized image. Levinson et al. note that "many homosexuals have strong masculine identifications and personal qualities and many men who are strongly heterosexual in their lives have intense interests, traits, and feelings deriving from the feminine aspect of the self." They further observe that during this reconciliation the neglected part of the self often urgently seeks expression, and the intense voices, muted for years, now clamor to be heard. Levy (12) has found that "middle-aged men who have dimly or clearly known, but have for years suppressed, rationalized, or denied their homosexual feelings have "come out" and acknowledged these feelings to themselves and others."

WAYS OF RELATING TO OTHERS AND SOCIETY

It must be stressed that many intrapsychic and social factors will determine the extent to which homosexual men and women will reveal their sexual orientation and the quality of their relationship with significant or casual partners. In some few communities throughout the world, being "out of the closet" is to a great extent acceptable. However, even in these places, there are many who believe it to be wise for political and professional reasons to keep a low profile, since they have seen the winds of fortune change direction from time to time at the polls, in the laws, and in public opinion. Thus, while many do not socialize exclusively in a homosexual environment, they do often live a double existence. In the past, the opportunities to meet new homosexual partners were limited to bars, baths, and other public places, for men, and almost exclusively to bars for women. Today, there are more middle-aged persons, both men and women, who not only openly acknowledge their sexual preferences but also attend and participate in such activities as consciousness-raising groups and conference workshops. Clearly, in the last decade the number of people working actively and openly for the rights of the gay and lesbian community has brought about much change. Politically and behaviorally, there is a whole range of positions from the ultra-conservative and less organized to the militant, radical gay and lesbian activist groups.

Among the problems that have to be dealt with among the coupled and single homosexuals are those of how to relate to family, non-homosexual friends, acquaintances, and business associates. For many who have lived in long-term relationships, there seems to be some degree of acceptance by some or all members of the family. At one end of the continuum there has been outright rejection of the individual, coupled or non-coupled. At the other there is open acknowledgment of the homosexuality with acceptance of it. In many, however, there is open acknowledgment and acceptance of the relationship, but with an elaborate system of defenses to avoid direct revelation or verbalization of the specifically sexual aspects of it, even after the homosexual partners have lived together for many years. In these situations such terms as "best friends," "roommates," "sharing an apartment" are used by both the couple and the families. Families of middle-aged close- or open-coupled homosexuals seem to be more accepting if there is evidence of some stability and continuity in the relationship. In such cases the partner is often accepted as a member of the family. Unfortunately, this attitude may change in the event of such legal matters as division of an estate in the event of the death of one of the couple. When there is a great discrepancy in the age of the partners or a rapid turnover in partners being introduced to the family, one can often observe in the family a rise in the level of anxiety and hostility and a difficulty in accepting the person with the "current lover." Whether the adverse feeling is overtly or covertly expressed depends on the quality of the relationship. Those who are more conservative tend to believe that as long as they have not flaunted the sexual aspects of their relationship or behaved indiscreetly or "outrageously" they have been accepted for themselves without apparent adverse judgments. There are those, of course, who project a stereotypic image and who attract or repel heterosexuals, as well as other homosexuals, for a variety of reasons.

Regarding choice of work and relationships with fellow employees, many homosexuals select fields where their sexual preferences and their social behavior are acceptable. Others work in a wide range of professions and areas, such as executive positions in corporations, government agencies, the military and such city jobs as teaching or working for the police or fire department, where it was and still is considered wiser not to reveal their sexual preference. Often such people will have available several friends of the opposite sex who will attend social functions with them and provide the proper cover. In some ways lesbian women seem to have greater problems than the men. As one patient put it, "The world is set for married couples. The single middle-aged man can still be considered an eligible bachelor, but the woman who is alone is considered unsuccessful. She can't really go some places and feel comfortable even when it's not required to have a man. Some of my friends fool themselves when they think straight people don't care. If they know we are lesbians they look at us as social curiosities or outcasts. They have a morbid curiosity about what we do and interpret everything in terms of sexual behavior. My straight friends pretend it doesn't exist. They don't want to talk or know about it." Another woman, in an executive position, said that even at age 44 she finds that she not only has all of the problems of a woman, but also the problems that arise when a man knows she is a lesbian. "They all seem to believe that if I had gone to bed with the right man (namely themselves) I wouldn't be gay; I'd 'straighten out.' Many of them believe I can't go to bed with a man, even though I had been married for many years. They can't believe I really prefer to be with a woman—that's where all my feelings are."

HOMOSEXUALS IN HETEROSEXUAL MARRIAGES

In comparing their findings, Bell and Weinberg (2) have reported that one-fifth of the white homosexual males and a slight number of black homosexual males have been married at least once, while more than one-third of white homosexual females and almost one-half of black homosexual females in their study have been married at least once. The greatest number of all groups had married before age 25. Jay and Young (6) have indicated that about 83% of the women and 66% of the men in their study had had heterosexual relationships at least once. In Puerto Rico, informants have advised me that almost 95% of the lesbians conform to the Spanish tradition of getting married, with most of them having children. Among the close-coupled male pairs with whom I have worked and who have lived together from 19 to 42 years, at least one member and in some cases both members of 23 pairs have been married before and are fathers of from one to five children. In fact, several are grandfathers. Among those who can perform with both sexes, many report that, although they function successfully, they do not *feel* the same emotionally or physically with those of the opposite sex.

ROLE-PLAYING

By the middle years, although some homosexuals and lesbians have, in terms of sexual and domestic activities, become aware of role preferences, Saghir and Robins (17) report, "There are usually no strict husband and wife roles in the relationship of male and female homosexuals." In fact, they note that "at age 40 and later . . . a majority of the homosexual men (59%) were interchanging sex roles." Among the women, Jay and Young (6) find that the majority of the lesbians do not role-play either sexually or other than sexually, although they acknowledge that about 19% play sexual roles with any frequency, and only a little over 9% play nonsexual roles. In Puerto Rico, the younger people more actively reject role-playing, although the middle-aged group still seems to have strong role preferences. In my work I also find, among the middle-age group, that, while some seem to be rigidly bound into some particular posture or technique which alone can "turn them on," many more seem to be able to employ a variety of techniques depending on mood and mutual preference of the moment. In the nonsexual area I also find that psychologically and functionally some seem more comfortable in one of the roles (conventionally called masculine or feminine, butch or femme) than in the other. Occasionally, fights have arisen over the division of labor as the pair has worked out "who does what." Among those active in gay libertarian groups, there is an attempt to eradicate sex roles and there is evidence that there is a significant change occurring, with more people striving for a more flexible sharing of activities. In such cases, the pair may role-play in certain areas of their life as it suits their mood.

Quality of Relationships Among Men

Following the model of Bell and Weinberg (2), we can see that the shift from close-coupled to asexual is from the ability to achieve sexual and interpersonal satisfaction predominantly, although not necessarily exclusively, with a single significant person with a pooling of resources, a series of common goals, a wanting to settle down, and a working-through of problems as they arise, through to those who are most uninvolved, fearful of relating, often schizoid or psychotic, living more in fantasy than reality and involved in brief, impersonal and unsatisfactory sexual contacts, self-contained autoerotic experiences or even abstinence.

Among the intermediate groups, the open-coupled tend to deal with their conflicts in the relationship by making claims on their partners for special considerations and license, having excessive expectations, engaging in power struggles, and rigidly demanding gratification of their own needs. They frequently rationalize their own behavior and hold the partner responsible for failing to measure up to the expectations. Functionals very often live a life-style Horney (5) called "the shallow living" form of resignation, with its emphasis on fun, sex, games, conquests, techniques, and a clinging to the youth culture ideals, especially among the men. Signs of aging generate much anxiety. Aging functionals often resort to plastic surgery, hair transplants, rigorous diets, and workouts at a gym to retain the illusion of youthfulness. Evidences of aging are experienced as severe narcissistic blows. Some may become depressed, go to pieces, and be filled with self-hate. They may drive themsevles to greater sexual acting-out, pay for sexual encounters or engage in anonymous sex. Others, particularly among the close- and open-coupled and the functionals, however, who have developed their interests as they have grown older, may become interested in creative activities, sports, hobbies, and organizational pursuits both within and outside of the gay community, including gay activist groups, panel discussions, seminars, and rap sessions, and religious, cultural, environmental, and civic functions. All of these activities serve to extend their horizons and bring additional meaning to their lives.

Dysfunctional homosexuals have difficulty in dealing with interpersonal relationships because they often are stiff, obsessive, cynical and resigned. Working with them in therapy requires much patience and understanding of the role of self-hate and hopelessness that pervades much of their life, and which accounts for their apparent resistance to change.

Quality of Relationships Among Women

Among the women, the middle-aged close-coupled relationships are characterized by the expectation of fidelity. Most lesbians (6) approve of relationships and/or commitment to them. I have worked with couples who have lived together for from 10 to over 25 years. While the sexual aspect of the relationship is considered important, emotional involvement is held to be even more important. Love, affection, liking and working to please the partner are significant features in most lesbian relationships. There is also stress on respecting individual interests and sharing mutually enjoyed activities.

Among this group, one-night stands, cruising, and sex orgies are very uncommon. Tripp (19) notes that "the lesbian couples frequently achieve what virtually no relationship involving a young homosexual can: It can continue smoothly and at a high level of intimacy and personal reward following the double event of a hot fire having quickly cooled." He suggests that women have certain "nestbuilding" proclivities which permit them to extract more nonsexual rewards from a close relationship than men can. The lesbian often has a high level of rapport with her partner. Of course, as a result of this closeness, there can arise an intense jealousy whenever the relationship is threatened by other women who might intrude and attempt to disrupt the coupling.

In terms of the phenomenon of fusion, Krestan and Bepko (9) write that many lesbian couples, feeling "two against a threatening world," may tend to become embedded in the relationship without a clear defining of each person's boundaries within the system. The struggle to individuate and become interdependent with rather than fused to the other may frequently evoke resistance to change out of fear that individuation might lead to the dissolution of the relationship. When such a threat occurs, there may be an attempt to reestablish the morbidly dependent fused status quo.

Lehman (10) observes that there is some doubt whether a successful relationship necessarily requires large doses of intimacy: "More probably it requires a proper ratio of personal space and intimacy." Frequently lesbian couples will come for therapy with complaints of sexual dysfunction, alcoholism, imminent dissolution of the partnership, depression, anxiety, and evolving sadomasochistic sexual patterns. An important role for the therapist, according to Krestan and Bepko (9), is to help the couple not only to develop more autonomous positions within the relationship, but also to relinquish the rigid boundaries between themselves and their world. The therapist will work with them toward replacing those fixed positions with strong boundaries which would allow them private space into which outsiders, family and others may enter, but into which they may not trespass. I have found that what is sometimes called fear of fusion is frequently an aspect of fear of emotional closeness and is often an important factor to keep in mind when working with middle-aged couples who are seen in therapy, regardless of their sexual preference.

An important, but little-known, paper by MacKinnon (14), a homosexual woman, should be required reading for those who would care to understand how one woman more than 30 years ago experienced and understood the phenomenon of being homosexual. The following are some quotes from that article, "To those whose sex life is based on heterosexual relationships, the homosexual is a grotesque, shadowy creature—a person spoken of with scorn, pity, or lasciviousness. . . . If you are not one of us, it is impossible to realize our feelings when this occurs. . . . What is it like to be this way? You are always lonely. . . . The inability to present an honest face to those you know eventually develops a certain deviousness which is injurious to whatever basic character you may possess. . . . How do homosexuals feel about one another? One of the saddest facts in this entire picture is that we seldom like one another." This can then be contrasted with such a book as *Our Right to Love, A Lesbian Resource Book* (20). There is no doubt that, for MacKinnon, living in these days, there would be many more options personally, socially, and politically. She concluded her article with the sentence, "There will be fewer homosexual women in mental hospitals if we are recognized as human beings instead of as material for a chapter in a book on abnormal psychopathology."

ACTIVITIES AND SUPPORT SYSTEMS

Many middle-aged homosexuals, with the encouragement and support from the more activist groups, are slowly developing self-respect and evolving more cohesive and supportive organizations to enable them to grow and contribute moral and financial support and expertise, based upon years of training and experience, not only to the total community, but also to the particular community of homosexuals as well.

Two organizations within the homosexual group should be mentioned: 1. the National Gay Task Force (NGTF), a group of about 10,000 members with more than 2,000 local groups throughout America which helps with legal, technical, and strategic information; and 2. the Gay Caucus of Members of the American Psychiatric Association (GCMAPA). The former has through its efforts won antidiscrimination legislation in 39 communities, held an unprecedented meeting in the White House with an official of the Carter Administration, influenced the Internal Revenue Service to reverse its policy against homosexual groups, negotiated to end policies of discrimination against gay people in the Job Corps, Public Health Service, Immigration and Naturalization Service, and Bureau of Prisons, and is lobbying for the first Federal Gay Rights Bill. They have also supported the adoption of the American Psychiatric Association Board of Trustees resolution which reads:

Whereas homosexuality per se implies no impairment in judgment, stability, reliability, or general social or vocational capabilities, therefore, be it resolved that the American Psychiatric Association deplores all public and private discrimination against homosexuals in such areas as employment, housing, public accommodations, and licensing and declares that no burden of proof of such judgment, capacity, or reliability shall be placed upon homosexuals greater than that imposed on any other persons. Further, the American Psychiatric Association supports and urges the enactment of civil rights legislation at the local, state and federal level that would offer homosexual citizens the same protections now guaranteed to others on the basis of race, creed, color, etc. Further, the American Psychiatric Association supports and urges the repeal of all discriminatory legislation singling out homosexual acts by consenting adults in private.

Subsequently, since 1973, the official position of the APA has been that homosexuality is not a mental disorder. The effect of removing homosexuality from the list of sicknesses has been immeasurable. The NGTF also believes that the effect of removing the stigma of being a criminal for having homosexual feelings and performing homosexual acts by consenting adults in private will enable homosexuals to reintegrate into the community with openness and dignity.

The GCMAPA, formed in 1974, with a membership of nearly 150 psychiatrists, but with many other psychiatrists actively supporting it as non-members, has been active in presenting programs to enlighten professionals and the lay public about the homosexual experience and in providing aid for those who seek therapy.

Special reference should be made to the valuable role Alcoholics Anonymous, and in particular the Gay AA groups, plays in enabling its members to recover and maintain their sobriety. Many middle-aged gay alcoholics feel themselves to be "a minority inside a minority." When they appeared at predominantly heterosexual AA meetings, unable or unwilling to risk revealing themselves because they were fearful that their "straight" members might view their sexuality with prejudice and hostility, some had difficulty in telling the complete truth about themselves. This often led to an impasse and endangered their sobriety. With the advent of the Gay AA meetings and the possibility of "double anonymity," the members, for the first time, felt free not only from alcoholism but also from self-hatred, guilt, fear of exposure and rejection. Subsequently, many of them have gone on to become sponsors for new members, which gives their life the additional satisfactions of belonging to a larger social group and of providing useful service to other suffering human beings.

There are many more middle-aged homosexuals and lesbians living full productive lives with an ongoing relationship or alone than most people realize. Not much is heard about them because there is very little about them that would make them newsworthy for prurient or sensational reasons.

While the majority of uncoupled homosexuals, male and female, are not more lonely, frustrated and depressed in their middle years than their counterpart, the uncoupled heterosexual, those who are predominantly dependent or detached often find increasing difficulty as they get older. I have worked with several men who, in their late fifties, are still looking for older men to care for them. Those who are both more self-reliant and able to sustain an interdependent relationship fare better. These men frequently have good peer group relationships within their community of friends. With younger homosexual men, they tend to be effective mentors, resource persons, and good fathering figures.

Toward the end of the middle years, physical illnesses, the death of friends, problems of emotional and financial security, and the occasional breakup of relationships through death of a lover or through untenable psychological factors are all frightening possibilities, especially if the individuals have a paucity of family or friends to turn to for support. For those persons who subscribe to the deeply held belief of some that "no one will love you when you're old and gay," the terror of being older, alone, and not loved can be very threatening. However, Weinberg and Williams (21) note that folk beliefs erroneously attribute to older homosexuals and lesbians the perspectives and expectations of both younger homosexuals and heterosexuals.

THOUGHTS ABOUT THERAPY

In working therapeutically with persons who relate homosexually, I have found that individual, couple, and group psychoanalytically-oriented psychotherapy, augmented at times with chemotherapy, has been frequently effective. Through the use of these techniques we enable our patient to do some stocktaking, to understand the genesis and evolving of the personality, including the way of relating sexually, to become aware of and understand the meanings of the person's needs, demands on self, claims and expectations on others, and values, and to recognize the various solutions he or she has resorted to in order to achieve some sort of psychic harmony.

We are all capable of a wide range of sexual feelings. Among them are those we are told we must not act upon and others we are told we must consider pathological, taboo, wrong even to feel or acknowledge—much less act upon. Some patients blame all of their problems on their homosexual feelings, which clash with their image of how they *should* feel and act. These people come into therapy to be "cured." There are therapists who convey to their patients that homosexual feelings and acts, if not sick or bad, are, at least, undesirable and must be arrested and replaced with heterosexual feelings. The patients feel under a pressure to comply with the therapist's expectations or be considered resistant or hopeless. They have come to my office deeply depressed, feeling they have let their therapist down and have failed themselves. I find that those who do present their homosexuality as their main problem are, in fact, externalizing to their way of relating sexually their various intrapsychic and interpersonal difficulties. I agree with Bieber when he says, "Every human being has a right to live his sexual life as he or she sees fit. It is a private matter" (22).

In fact, very few middle-aged homosexuals come with the express purpose of changing their sexual orientation. Those who do want to change their orientation have the magical belief that if they "went straight" all their problems would be solved. I have learned that those who feel they *should be able to feel and perform* heterosexually and demand of themselves that they suppress their homosexual relating and perform heterosexually have greater problems than those who can be honest about and with their feelings. Several persons have become severely depressed, others have attempted suicide and at least three have committed suicide when they could not measure up to these inner "shoulds." One 45-year-old man announced shortly before he killed himself, "I do not object to others being homosexual, but for me it is unacceptable." Another, age 47, said, "When I married I took an oath before God never to give in to my homosexual feelings again. Now I am caught in an inescapable trap. I cannot make love with my wife anymore because I do not feel sexually towards her and I cannot act on my homosexual feelings because I have taken that oath. My life is untenable now."

Kelman (7) notes that enabling the homosexual patient, male or female, to admit into awareness, contain and own the element of murderous rage has been very valuable. When this happens the individual can become happier and more productive. He discusses some of the motivations for help which every therapist would do well to keep in mind, namely, to get over fear of exposure, to seek relief from the depressions which often cover murderous rages when the patient feels rejected, to be helped in any suicidal phase which may follow rejection, or to be supported through these immediate problems. For Kelman the criterion of having been helpful is not whether the patient becomes heterosexual. Rather, his objective is to help the patient become less crippled in his total functioning and to help him live with himself more happily when he interrupts therapy.

Most homosexuals come to the therapist with problems related to conflicts with partners, loss through separation or death of a partner, depression, loneliness, thoughts of suicide, excessive drinking, anxiety and other neurotic symptoms, problems in relating to others, sexually and otherwise, and difficulties in work or creative activity. They come seeking to achieve greater self-fulfillment and satisfaction in their personal lives, with their families, lovers and friends, in their vocations and avocations. The extent to which they can accept themselves with their assets and limitations will affect their sense of well-being and effectiveness as functioning individuals.

If, in the process of our work, the ability to feel and act on heterosexual feelings emerges, and this is something the patient wishes for, well and good. We cannot order what a person *should* feel. Thus, if this shift does occur, we must encourage him to own and experience as valid the feelings he does have, the feelings he has a right to share with others.

Honest self-scrutiny is essential to raising one's sense of self-worth. A holistic approach which emphasizes the totality of the person rather than his sexual orientation will be invaluable in enabling him to get a new perspective on himself and on himself in the world. He will become more able to be spontaneous, open, wholehearted, responsible, and more willing and able to work not only for changes in himself and in his relationships, but also for changes in his community as well.

CONCLUSION

In this paper I have tried to present a few of the ways of classifying homosexual socio-sexual patterns and to discuss, in particular, the framework provided by Bell and Weinberg. Some remarks about the relationship of homosexuals to the general population, and about the particular problems of relating to family, friends, and acquaintances were presented. The nature of the problems both within the homosexual individual and in homosexual relations was explored, particularly as the middle-aged person became older. Finally, some comments were made regarding some of the aims a therapist should have in mind in working with homosexual patients.

REFERENCES

1. ARIETI, S. (1974) *Interpretation of Schizophrenia*, 2nd Edition New York: Basic Books, p. 610.
2. BELL, A., and WEINBERG, M. (1978) *Homosexualities, A study in diversity among men and women*. New York: Simon and Schuster.
3. FROMM, E. (1956) *The Art of Loving*. Perennial Library. New York: Harper and Row, pp. 22-27.
4. HOFFMAN, M. (1968) *The Gay World. Male Homosexuality and the Social Creation of Evil*. New York: Basic Books, p. 62.
5. HORNEY, K. (1950) *Neurosis and Human Growth*. New York: Norton, p. 281.
6. JAY, K. and YOUNG, A. (1977) *The Gay Report: Lesbians and Gay Men Speak Out about Sexual Experiences and Life Styles*. New York: Summit Books.
7. KELMAN, H. (1971) *Helping People: Karen Horney's Psychoanalytic Approach*. New York: Science House, pp. 306-08.
8. KIMMEL, D. (1978) Adult development and aging: A gay perspective. *J. of Social Issues*, *34*, No. 3, pp. 113-130.
9. KRESTAN, J. and BEPKO, C. (1980) The problem of fusion in the lesbian relationship. *Family Process*, *19*, Sept., 277-289.
10. LEHMAN, J. (1978), What it means to love another woman. In: *Our right to love, A Lesbian Resource Book*. Englewood Cliffs, N.J.: Prentice-Hall, Inc., pp. 21-27.
11. LEVINSON, D. et al. (1978) *The Seasons of a Man's Life*. New York: Knopf.
12. LEVY, N. (1956) *Anger, Hate and Jealousy*. ACAAP Pamphlet. New York: Assn. for Advancement of Psychoanal.
13. LEVY, N. (1979) The middle-aged male homosexual. *J. Am. Acad. Psychoanal.*, 7, No. 3, pp. 405-418.
14. MACKINNON, J. (1947) The homosexual woman. *Am. J. Psychiat.*, *104*, No. 3, pp. 661-64.
15. MARMOR, J. (ed.) (1965) *Sexual Inversion, the Multiple Roots of Homosexuality*. New York: Basic Books.
16. MARMOR, J. (1980) *Homosexual Behavior, A Modern Reappraisal*. New York: Basic Books.
17. SAGHIR, M. and ROBINS, E. (1973) *Male and Female Homosexuality, A Comprehensive Investigation*. Baltimore: Williams and Wilkins.
18. SALZMAN, L. (1977) Elements of free choice in homosexuality. *Medical Aspects of Human Sexuality*, June, p. 119.
19. TRIPP, C. (1975) *The Homosexual Matrix*. New York: McGraw-Hill, p. 164.
20. VIDA, G. (ed.) (1978) *Our Right to Love, A Lesbian Resource Book*. Englewood Cliffs, N.J.: Prentice-Hall, Inc.
21. WEINBERG, M. and WILLIAMS, C. (1974) *Male Homosexuals, their Problems and Adaptations*. New York: Penguin Books.
22. WYKERT, J. (1978) Irving Bieber, An interview. *Psychiatric News*, October 6, p. 19.

9

STUDIES OF A NEW POPULATION: THE LESBIAN MOTHER

MARTHA KIRKPATRICK, M.D.

Associate Clinical Professor,
School of Medicine, University of California
at Los Angeles

RON ROY, M.D.

Private Practice, Los Angeles

and KATHARINE SMITH

Staff Psychologist, Tri-City Mental
Health Clinic, Pomona, Ca.

INTRODUCTION

Maiden ladies, whose childless state was blamed on ill fortune, have long been considered especially suited to instruct and supervise children's development. Thus they are found in large numbers among baby nurses, governesses, nursery teachers, educators and child-care workers of all types. The extended family system regularly made use of maiden aunts as substitute mothers or as adoptive mothers for orphaned children. Neither marriage nor child-bearing was deemed necessary to elicit their maternal interests and capacities.

Lesbian women, on the other hand, were assumed to possess none of these interests or capacities. The social myth asserted that such women's sexual interest in other women resulted from a desire to approximate maleness and eschew any suggestion of feminine interests or traits. This limited view led to an assumption that the categories "lesbian" and "mother" were mutually exclusive. This assumption was further confounded by the tendency to view female sexuality, including homosexuality, as a response to or mirror image of male sexuality. The unique nature of female sexuality was obfuscated by the male model. Lesbianism was assumed to be a permanent state, even more basic than heterosexuality since, once embraced, it was assumed that the capacity to seek out and enjoy men, particularly as sexual partners, was permanently lost. While many of these old assumptions have been questioned by new research, they previously provided a "cover" for mothers whose lesbianism was automatically denied by their state of motherhood. We believe that lesbian mothers are not a new phenomenon. Prior to the current Women's Movement and the Gay Liberation Movement, such women lived in frightened and intended disguise. Not only was lesbianism contradictory to motherhood, but it was also dangerous to children. On this basis even a suspicion of lesbianism was liable to deprive a mother of the custody of her children if contested in a divorce action (2, 12, 14).

The studies of the '60s and '70s comparing nonpatient populations of homosexual and heterosexual women began to erode the myths of significant differences between these groups. Armon (1) found that sophisticated psychologists were unable to distinguish members of one group from the other by the Rorschach Protocols or Draw a Figure responses of 30 lesbian and 30 heterosexual women. Hopkins (8) concluded from comparing the responses of 24 lesbians to those of 24 heterosexual controls on Raymond Cattels N = Personality Factor Test that the difference between the two groups was not in terms of neuroticism, but rather that the lesbian group was "more independent, resilient, reserved, dominant, bohemian, self-sufficient and more composed." Similar findings were revealed by other studies (15, 16, 18, 20).

In custody disputes involving lesbian mothers, judges and attorneys have sought to arrive at decisions which would protect the best interests of the child, but they have been required to do so without precedent, experience, or research data to assist them. Up until the new visibility of this group of mothers, no data could be collected. The recent studies of nonpatient lesbian populations has freed professional thinking from limited stereotypes, but these studies have not included information on lesbians as mothers nor on children raised by lesbians.

REVIEW OF THE LITERATURE

Early Studies

Very little is currently in print on this subject, although several studies have been completed and a number are in progress at this writing. Goodman (5) reported to the American Orthopsychiatric Association on comparisions made over a two-year period of working with a lesbian mother group and a heterosexual single mother group. She emphasized the similarity of personality types, problems, concerns, and reactions to child-rearing events. She found that there were no distinguishable differences in the expectations of children, knowledge or ignorance about child-rearing, or capacity to respond maternally. A number of studies confirming Goodman's observations were completed in the succeeding few years. Since none of these studies are as yet published, it may be appropriate to briefly review them.

Bryant (4) presented her data as a thesis for a Master of Social Work in 1975. Her study was based on a self-administered 48-item questionnaire. The questionnaire was developed in consultation with lesbian mother groups and her population was contacted through lesbian/feminist periodicals. Her questions were designed to obtain information on the demographic status and backgrounds of the mothers, the social effects of being a lesbian and a mother, the expectations and interactions with their children, and the mothers' perceptions of their children's psychological status. She received responses from 185 women who identified themselves as lesbians and were raising or had raised children. In comparing this group to statistics on the general female population, she found this lesbian group to be less religious, more educated, more often professionally employed and more involved with the Women's Movement. These findings, particularly the last, may be biased by her use of lesbian/feminist periodicals for contacts. From the responses to the questionnaires, she found that the majority of these women had been heterosexually married, had male friends who participated in their children's lives, and had no preference as to their children's eventual sexual object choice. There was no evidence from the responses that these children showed a higher frequency of homosexual interests than other children. Approximately 10% of the mothers considered their children to have some problems in development. In those situations in which the mother's partner shared the home, 9% reported continuing jealousy and/or hostility from the child. Both these figures seem comparable to the non-lesbian population. Bryant concluded that whatever difficulties there may be for lesbian mothers, they were not inherent in the role, but in society's condemnatory attitudes and discriminatory practices.

Additional Studies

In 1976, three additional studies were completed, two of which are still unpublished (17, 19). Pagelow (13) compared a sample of 23 single heterosexual mothers with a total of 51 children with 20 single lesbian mothers with a total of 43 children. To explore her hypothesis that single mothers are discriminated against and Lesbian mothers doubly so, she compared data on child custody, housing and employment. Her research methodology included participant observation in group discussions, in-depth interviews and a questionnaire. She found evidence to support her prediction in that lesbians employed more "coping mechanisms" to deal with additional prejudice, lesbians had more custody problems (five out of 19 lesbian mothers did not have full custody of all their children, compared to three out of 22 heterosexual mothers). However, lesbian mothers showed a higher rate of self-employment and home ownership, which Pagelow interpreted as showing high levels of competent coping mechanisms. Again, mothers in the two samples showed many more features in common than differences and were beset by the same burdens of low wages, lack of adequate child-care facilities, babysitting problems, housing difficulties and concern over children's health. Both also expressed concern over possible social disapproval of their "lovers," whether heterosexual or homosexual.

The two other studies were descriptive in nature. St. Marie (17) studied ten lesbian mothers. She found a large percentage (50%) actively involved, often in leadership positions, in their children's school, club or sports activities. She added several observations: 1. The lesbian mothers had more heterosexual friends than childless lesbians. 2. Several lesbian mothers stated they had more and closer friendships with men now than during their marriages when close relationships with men other than the husband were precluded. Steirn (19) studied eight lesbian family units, four of which contained children. She remarked on the warmth, openness, and nurturance available in her sample. She suggested that this might be a consequence of more active help and participation in parenting by the lesbian partner as compared to the traditional marriage in which the mother often does the major parenting job in relative isolation.

Recent Studies

Presentations at the American Psychiatric Association and American Psychological Association meetings over the last few years of as yet unpublished studies have added additional data to our picture of this group of women. Studies using the most sophisticated research design come from presentations at the 1979 annual meeting of the American Psychological Association.

Since none of these studies are in print, brief descriptions of methodology as well as results will be presented. Lewin and Lyons (11) reported on data collected from interviews with 80 formerly married mothers, 43 lesbian and 37 heterosexuals, who had children ranging in age from one to 20 years. Varying custody arrangements were noted, but only those with at least halftime physical custody of one or more minor children were included. Data were collected by means of an in-depth, semi-structured interview lasting three to six hours with each mother. Questions focused primarily on adaptive strategies pursued by the mothers and the influence of particular sexual orientation on the resources available to mothers and the choices they made with respect to utilization of these resources. Economic issues, interpersonal support systems, institutional support systems, beliefs and values held by informants about their situations as single mothers were stressed.

Results of this study point to dramatic similarities in the organization of family life for lesbian and heterosexual mothers. Both lesbians and heterosexuals place a strong emphasis on the maintenance of ties with kin, often relying upon relatives for day-to-day support. Like heterosexuals, lesbians stress the importance of an ongoing connection for the children with the father, even when failure to pay child support and the threat of a custody challenge present serious problems. Heterosexuals, no less than lesbians, express satisfaction with their lives as single mothers, glorying in their ability to overcome adversity, deriving pride from their independence and autonomy, despite an almost universal need to adapt to a reduced standard of living following divorce. Both groups of mothers also speak of the isolation of heading families on their own, of the pressures which sole responsibility for their children places upon them. Lewin and Lyons (11) found lesbian mothers to experience more difficulties with custody litigation and to feel greater vulnerability to potential social disapproval when a homosexual partner was residing in the home.

Lewin and Lyons concluded that motherhood, especially single motherhood, provides a basic structure within which both lesbian and heterosexual mothers organize their lives. Sexual orientation, far from being a determinant life-style, appears to have no consistent effects on the centrality of kinship relations in the lives of single mothers, nor does it have much impact on the organization of friendship and sexual relations.

Hoeffer (7) studied a sample of 20 single lesbian mothers and 20 single heterosexual mothers and their only or oldest children between ages six and nine. The samples were matched in gender and age of the children and educational background of the mother. Methodology included psychometric measures and interviews with the mother and her child regarding play and activity chores. Data were collected to identify differences in 1. sex-role models presented to the children by the mothers; and 2. reinforcement of specific sex-role traits and behaviors. These two groups of mothers were all white, living in the San Francisco Bay area. Overriding similarities were again noted: The majority of both groups 1. had been married and were currently separated or divorced; 2. held a B.A. or higher degree; 3. worked in a white collar occupation. The mean age for both groups was 33, indicating marriage and child-bearing had taken place during the same age period. The one difference elicited in Hoeffer's study was the high rate of self-reported identification with feminism (95%) of the lesbian mothers, compared to less involvement (55%) of the heterosexual mothers.

The mothers in Hoeffer's study completed the Bem Sex Role Inventory, an instrument consisting of 60 items prejudged as masculine, feminine or neutral on which mothers rated themselves on a seven-point scale. The data were analyzed using Bem's (3) scoring procedure of classifying subjects as androgynous (high masculine/high feminine), sex-typed masculine (high masculine/low feminine), sex-typed feminine (low masculine/high feminine) or undifferentiated (low masculine/low feminine). On this scale there were no statistically significant differences between the two groups of mothers. The mean scores of lesbian and heterosexual mothers were almost equal on femininity, but lesbian mothers had a higher mean score on masculinity than did heterosexual mothers, and a larger portion of heterosexual mothers tended to score as undifferentiated. If lower self-esteem and an undifferentiated sex-role trait profile are linked, as the literature suggests (3), these heterosexual mothers may be at greater risk for problems related to self-esteem. The two groups of mothers were similiar in their self-reports of encouraging sex-role traits and behavior in their children, although some lesbian mothers were more willing than heterosexual mothers to accept some cross-gender sex-role traits and behaviors in their children.

Hotvedt, Green and Mandel (9) studied 51 single lesbian mothers and 34 single heterosexual mothers with children between the ages of three and ten. All families had been living without adult males (18 years or older) in the household for at least two years. Families were matched on age of mother, length of separation from father, circumstances by which mother became a single parent, educational level, income, number, ages and sex of children, race, and, where possible, religion of upbringing.

Each accepted adult volunteer filled out questionnaires and attitude scales pertaining to her parenting experiences, upbringing, marital and relationship patterns, and attitudes toward divorce, sex roles, sex education for children, and discipline. Personality scales, including the Bem Sex Role Inventory and Jackson PRF, were also included. An audiotaped interview with each mother was made, usually in the home, and transcriptions were edited to delete the location and identity of the participant. The interview reviewed the material from the questionnaires, adding depth to several areas, and included a sexual history of the mother.

The differences noted in the two groups were limited to the presence in some of the heterosexual sample of male sexual partners which might lead to sharing a household. Sixty-eight percent of the heterosexual women, compared to 25% of the lesbian sample, would consider remarriage. The reasons for possible remarriage differed, with lesbian mothers citing the children's assumed benefit, economic security, or concealment of homosexuality, while heterosexual mothers cited emotional and sexual needs. Forty percent of the lesbian group and 47% of the heterosexual group sought psychological counseling during the first year as a single parent. Homosexual mothers reported a preponderance of homosexual male and female friends compared to heterosexual mothers.

Kirkpatrick, Roy, and Smith (10) collected data on a nonpatient population of 21 lesbian mothers and 13 heterosexual mothers incidental to a blind evaluation of the psychological status of their 40 children. In-depth, semi-structured interviews lasting two to six hours were conducted with each mother. Mothers also completed MMPI, Tennessee Self-esteem Scale, and the Bem Sex Role Inventory Scale.

Responses to the Bem Scale confirmed Hoeffer's finding to the extent that both groups were found to be equally androgynous, although Kirkpatrick et al. found the mean score on feminity to be slightly higher in the lesbian mothers' group than in the heterosexual group!

Kirkpatrick et al. made an attempt to compare the mother's marital history. It was found that the lesbian mother sample had married slightly later than the heterosexual sample (lesbian mothers average age at marriage—23; heterosexual mothers—20), arguing against the notion that the lesbian mothers had less self-determination in accepting marriage. In fact, the heterosexual sample more frequently gave unexpected pregnancy or a desire to escape home and/or school as an explanation for marriage than did the lesbian mothers (lesbian mothers—2, heterosexual mothers—7).

Among the lesbian mothers, two had planned pregnancies without marriage and one had married briefly to give the child legitimacy. Of the 13 who married, 11 did so out of love for the husband. All of the heterosexual mothers were married at the time of delivery. In the heterosexual sample, nine stated they married out of love for the husband, although three of those married in their teens and felt they were primarily seeking a way out of school and home.

These two studies by Hotvedt et al. (9) and Kirkpatrick et al. (10) were conducted in different areas of the U.S.A. Hotvedt et al. recruited women thoughout the country, both urban and rural, with an emphasis on ten eastern states within reasonable traveling distance of the State University of New York on Long Island. Kirkpatrick et al. confined their study to women living in Los Angeles County. Both samples showed a wide range of economic, educational, and professional status. For example, both samples included women on welfare, students, "pink" and white collar workers and highly educated professional women. The similiarities in the samples collected in such diverse geographic and cultural areas and from varied educational and socioeconomic levels is impressive.

In Hotvedt et al.'s study, the average age of marriage for both groups was 21 and both groups had an average length of marriage of seven to eight years. The Kirkpatrick et al. sample from Southern California, an area with a reputation for high divorce rates, provided remarkably similiar findings. Both lesbian and heterosexual groups in this study showed an average age at marriage of 21 (although the heterosexual group had actually married earlier since two of the marriages producing the subject children were second marriages contracted in the mothers' early thirties) and, more surprisingly, both groups showed an average length of marriage of between seven and eight years. Both Hotvedt et al. and Kirkpatrick et al. found that most women stated they were the initiators of the divorce action. In the Hotvedt et al. study, 30% of the lesbian sample reported homosexual feelings to be an issue in the divorce. In the Kirkpatrick et al. study, half of the lesbian sample had homosexual lovers at the time of the separation. The divorce was felt by the women to result from an increasing loss of intimacy, mutuality or emotional communication with the husband rather than from the homosexual relationship. Disappointment and emotional divorce came first, followed by lesbian relationships in half of the respondents, and eventually divorce. In Kirkpatrick et al.'s heterosexual sample, one-third reported the same complaint of the loss of intimacy, but only two women saw this as contributing to the divorce; the majority (ten) gave as reasons for divorce alcohol and/or drug abuse, psychotic episodes, beatings, gambling, and affairs with other women. One-third of the lesbian sample had these complaints as well.

In both samples loss of sexual interest led to extramarital affairs but not necessarily divorce. An antipathy toward sexual intercourse with a male was reported by only one lesbian mother and was described as dislike of "the male power trip" rather than dislike of the sexual activity. Problems around status, authority and domestic roles were reported in both groups. Both studies showed all mothers had suffered a decrease in standard of living following the divorce and in both studies all samples showed only 50% were receiving regular child support. Both Hotvedt et al. and Kirkpatrick et al. found 50% of the lesbian sample to have partners in or very near the home who share parenting responsibility. Kirkpatrick et al. found that lesbian partners responded as second mothers or big sisters, not as imitation fathers.

While some heterosexual mothers had regular relationships with men, which may lead to domestic sharing, relationships to the children's fathers were reported in both studies to be similar in all groups of single mothers, with a majority complaining of lack of regular visitation and reliable involvement with the children. Kirkpatrick et al. found lesbian mothers to more frequently express concern that the children have regular contact with supportive males and to consciously provide such opportunities with male relations or friends. Heterosexual mothers who were consciously seeking new marriages tended to regard the eventual success of that search as the means of providing children with male figures.

Both Hotvedt et al. and Kirkpatrick et al. looked at pregnancy and infant care histories to obtain suggestive evidence of the psychological reaction to the maternal role. In both studies no significant differences were found in the desire of the mothers to have children. Kirkpatrick et al. found that reports of pregnancy experiences revealed that almost half of each group had had some problems during pregnancy or delivery resulting in two cesarean sections in each group. However, only one lesbian mother and two heterosexual mothers stated they did not enjoy pregnancy. Neither Hotvedt et al. nor Kirkpatrick et al. found differences in reports of physical contact or breast-feeding. There was a trend in the Kirkpatrick et al. study for lesbian mothers to have breast-fed more frequently and over a longer period. Both studies, however, had more only children in the lesbian mother samples. In the Kirkpatrick et al. study there were seven only children in the lesbian mother group, compared to no only children in the heterosexual group. This appeared to be the consequence of more second marriages (and divorces) in the heterosexual group.

Contrary to unexamined assumptions, we see from these studies that the social and marital histories of mothers currently living as lesbians are similar to other single mothers and are organized similarly around child-care responsibilities. The vast majority of both groups desired marriage and pregnancy and are devoted to their children.

Lesbian partners, who were present in about half the samples studied, contributed as second mothers or big sisters, not as substitute fathers. Several studies have examined the consequences of this type of family on the child. As part of child custody litigation, Green (6) examined 21 children being raised in seven lesbian households. In summary, his data showed that 15 children drew a person of their own sex first on the Draw-A-Person test, one did not draw, and five drew a person of the opposite sex. The peer group of 19 of these children was the same sex. The favorite toy of 20 children was consistent with conventional sex-typed toy preferences and the vocational choices for all 21 were within the typical range of sex-types in our culture. The four oldest children reported erotic fantasy of a heterosexual nature. These measures are the most reliable indicators available of sexual identity and object choice. Green concluded that these findings do not differ appreciably from those of children raised in more conventional settings.

Hoeffer's (7) study also included measures of the children on sex-role traits and sex-role behaviors. Sex-role traits were measured by asking the children to rate themselves on five male-valued traits (outgoing, adventuresome, never cries, strong, likes to be the leader) and five female-valued traits (aware of others' feelings, gentle, behaves, neat, quiet) on a four-point scale for ideal and real self and same gender peers (Guttertag and Bray's Sex-Role Self Concept Scale). Sex-role behavior was measured by Block's Toy Preference Test. The sons of lesbian and heterosexual mothers did not vary on sex-role traits or sex-role behavior; further, both groups chose an androgynous sex-role trait profile as their ideal. However, the boys of lesbian mothers rated themselves higher on two female-valued traits—awareness of others' feelings and gentleness—than did the boys of heterosexual mothers. Both groups of boys gave their peers higher scores on male-valued traits than themselves. Girls in the two groups did not differ on sex-role behavior. The daughters of lesbian mothers rated themselves higher on two male-valued traits—adventurous and likes to be leader—than did the daughters of heterosexual mothers. Both groups of girls choose androgynous ideals. Hoeffer felt the mothers were more effective models for daughters than for sons. She also concluded that the trend in boys of rating their peers ahead of themselves in masculine values resulted from father absence, since both groups of boys showed this finding. However, this trend was not compared with responses of boys in families with fathers present.

Hotvedt et al. (9) examined the children on similiar variables. They found that girls of lesbian mothers were slightly more likely to show interest in masculine occupations. Boys in both of their groups were very similiar and conventionally masculine. The majority of children in both groups reported an interest in getting married and having a family. Draw-A-Person Test, toy and activity preferences showed no differences.

Kirkpatrick et al. (10) used similiar measures of the children's sexual identity. The results of the Draw-A-Person Test, reports of toy and activity preferences, peer relationships and future plans were similiar in the two groups. Kirkpatrick et al. included a blind evaluation by a female psychologist and a male child psychiatrist of the child's general psychological functioning, as well as gender identity. Each child was rated on the Rutter Scale following examination. Approximately 10% of each group was rated as severely disturbed. Of the two boys so rated, one from each group, both drew cross-sex figures on the DAP and both had histories of brief periods of feminine behavior, dressing and interests. Both these boys had physiologic defects which had disrupted their early infancy. The severely disturbed girls did not draw cross-sex figures and had no common features on their histories. There were no significant differences on the ratings of the two groups of children in regard to psychological status, nor could any correlations be made between problems presented and the mother's lesbianism.

CONCLUSION

This unusual group of mothers, lesbian mothers, on closer examination appears to be very similiar to single heterosexual mothers. The notion of lesbianism as causing a change in life-style is not supported by these studies. An interest in having children and fulfilling the maternal role is evident and overriding in the lives of both groups of mothers. Such a finding requires us to examine in more detail the multiple roots of maternal desire and to separate parenting impulses from heterosexual object choice. It is also important to consider that women's sexual object choice may be less fixed than men's and less driven by genital pressures.

While we assume that changes in parental behavior always affect children, there is no evidence from the measures we have available that lesbianism in the mother has a specific effect on the child. The studies so far available suggest that lesbian mothers no less than heterosexual mothers can provide good parenting and an environment which supports heterosexual development of children. Role-modeling may be less important than supposed for the child's individual development.

REFERENCES

1. ARMON, V. (1969). Some personality variables in overt female homosexuals. *J. of Project. Techniques, 24* 292.
2. BASILE, R. A. (1974). Lesbian mothers I & II. *Women's Rights Law Reporter, 2* Dec. 3.

3. BEM, S. L. (1975). The measurement of psychological androgeny. *J. Consult. and Clinic. Psycho.*, 42. 155-162.
4. BRYANT, B. (1975). Lesbian mothers. Thesis for Master of Social Work, unpublished—School of Social Work, California State University, Sacramento, California.
5. GOODMAN, B. (1973). Lesbian mothers. Report to the American Orthospsychiatric Association Annual Meeting, New York City. Unpublished. Available from Lymar Associates, 651 Duncan Street, San Francisco, California 94131.
6. GREEN, R. (1978). Thirty five children raised by homosexual or transsexual parents. *Am. J. Psychiat.*, 135: 692-7.
7. HOEFFER, B. (1979). Lesbian and heterosexual mothers' influence on their children's sex-role preferences. Unpublished. Presented at the American Psychological Assoc. Annual Meeting on Sept. 4, 1979, New York.
8. HOPKINS, J. (1969). The lesbian personality. *Brit. J. Psychiat.*, 115, 1433.
9. HOTVEDT, M., GREEN, R., and MANDEL, J. B. (1979). The lesbian parent; comparison of heterosexual and homosexual mothers and children. Unpublished. Presented at the American Psychological Assoc. Annual Meeting on Sept. 4, 1979, New York.
10. KIRKPATRICK, M., ROY, R., and SMITH, K. (1979). Adjustment of sexual identity of children of lesbian and divorced heterosexual mothers. Unpublished. Presented at the American Psychological Assoc. Annual Meeting on Sept. 4, 1979, New York. (A review of this study will be published in the *American Journal of Orthopsychiatry*.)
11. LEWIN, E., and LYONS, T. (1979). Lesbian and heterosexual mothers: Continuity and difference in family organization. Unpublished. Presented at the American Psychological Assoc. Annual Meeting on Sept. 4, 1979, New York.
12. MARTIN, D., and LYON, P. (1972). *Lesbian/Woman*. New York: Bantam.
13. PAGELOW, M. (1980). Lesbian mothers. *Journal of Homosexuality*, 5, 3:189.
14. RILEY, M. (1975). The avowed lesbian mother and her right to child custody; a constitutional challenge that can no longer be denied. *San Diego Law Review*, 12, July, 799.
15. ROSEN, D. (1974). *Lesbianism—A Study of Female Homosexuality*. Springfield, IL: Charles C Thomas.
16. SAGHIR, M. and ROBINS, E. (1973). *Male and Female Homosexuality*. Baltimore; Williams & Wilkins.
17. ST. MARIE, D. (1976). A descriptive study of lesbian mothers. Unpublished. School of Social Work, University of Hawaii, Honolulu.
18. SIEGELMAN, N. (1972). Adjustment of homosexual and heterosexual women. *Brit. J. Psychiat.*, 120: 477-481.
19. STEIRN, C. (1976). We are a family—an exploration of eight lesbian family units. Unpublished. Available from Lymar Assoc., 651 Duncan Street, San Francisco, Ca. 94131.
20. THOMPSON, N.D., McCANDLESS, B. D., and STRICKLAND, B. R. (1971). Personal adjustment of male and female homosexuals. *J. Abnorm. Psychol.*, 78: 237.

10

RETIREMENT

DONALD WASYLENKI, M.D., F.R.C.P.(C)

Staff Psychiatrist, Social and Community Psychiatry Section,
Clarke Institute of Psychiatry

and

ARLENE MACBRIDE, B.A.

Researcher, Social and Community Psychiatry Section,
Clarke Institute of Psychiatry, Toronto

INTRODUCTION

Throughout the world, the elderly population is growing. It will continue to grow for several decades, both in absolute numbers and as a proportion of the total population. In Canada, absolute numbers of people over 65 will double by the turn of the century. The increase will be from 1.7 million in 1971 to 3.3 million in 2001. Today Canadians over 65 represent 8% of the population. By 2001, 12% of the population will be in this age range. By the year 2031, when most of the "baby boom" will be in retirement, 6.1 million will be over 65—20% of the population. By that time there will be more people over 65 than from 0-19 (77).

In the United States, the over-65 population will grow from an estimated 22.9 million in 1976, which was 11% of the population, to 31.8 million in the year 2000, about 12% of the population. By 2031, there will be 55 million elderly Americans—14-22% of the U.S. population—and there will be only three workers for every retired person (at present, the ratio is six to one).

Because of longer life expectancy, the population over 75 will more than

---

Portions of this chapter appeared in: MacBride, A., Retirement as a Life Crisis: Myth or Reality? A Review. *Can. Psychiatr. Assoc. J.*, 21, 1976, and Wasylenki, D., Coping with Change in Retirement. *Can. Fam. Physician*, 24:133-136, 1978.

double by the end of the century. In 1971 there were 529,600 people age 75-84 in Canada; by 2001 there will be 1,130,200. The over-85 group will increase from 137,400 to 352,000 over the same time period. In North America, life expectancy at age 65 has jumped sharply, to 18 years for women and 14 for men. For anyone who lives to retirement age, the post-working years are likely to last as long as childhood and adolescence.

Thus, there will be many more elderly, retired people in the future. For the first time, most people will know their grandparents and even their great-grandparents into adulthood. And so many more people will be involved with the concerns of the elderly, including those related to retirement.

What are the general characteristics of the elderly retired population (77)? Many retired people are poor. In Canada 20 to 30% of those over 65 have incomes which are below the poverty line. The elderly population is largely urbanized; 80% live in cities, and in cities they tend to concentrate in the older, more central areas. Old age is also more of a woman's world. In North America female life expectancy is 76 years, whereas male expectancy is 69 years. The average North American woman can expect a widowhood of about ten years. Two-thirds of people over age 75 are women. The elderly utilize a major and disproportionate amount of health care services, and Canada has one of the highest rates of institutionalization of the elderly in the world. Nine percent of the over-65 population is in institutions, compared with less than 5% in the U.S. and U.K.

The elderly suffer disproportionately from psychiatric disorders (14). In general, the incidence of psychopathology rises with age. Non-organic disorders, especially depressions, increase with each decade, as do organic brain diseases after age 60. Suicide also increases with age. Individuals over 65 are the group most susceptible to mental illness.

Old people are no longer a small, homogeneous group. They can now be divided into the "young old," who are between 65 and 74, and the "old old," who are over 75. The "young old" are relatively well-off physically and economically and in terms of social and psychological resources. They are people who have recently retired, who are still married, who have less chronic illness and who still have friends and relatives around them. The "old old" however are beset by ill health, bereavement, loneliness and poverty. Many are in institutions. People over 75 are three times as likely to be in an institution as those in the 65-74 age group. People over 85 are twice as likely to be in institutions as those over 75.

CURRENT TRENDS

The widespread practice of compulsory retirement at age 65 was originated by German Chancellor Otto Von Bismarck in the late 19th century. He established state pensions at age 65 at a time when life expectancy in Europe was 49. This age was borrowed by other countries, and it is the mostcommon demarcation in pension and retirement plans. Article 15 of the International Labor Organization's Convention No. 128 of 1967 established age 65 as the "normal retirement age," but recognizes that a higher age may be prescribed by competent authority based on demographic, economic or social considerations (94). In a 1974 survey of retirement age in 31 selected industrialized countries, only the four Scandinavian countries offered higher retirement ages than 65 (10). This may relate to the fact that these countries head life expectancy tables, and also to their reputation for advanced social services.

More recently, opposition has developed to the whole concept of a compulsory retirement age. Mandatory retirement is seen as a form of discriminatory "ageism." With longer life expectancy and improved general health, many people feel no loss of ability or capacity at age 65. Proponents of this point of view argue that every worker should be judged individually, and that the right to a job should be determined only by ability—not by color, sex, or age. Another compelling aspect to the argument is that the more people who continue working, the lighter will be the burden on pension plans. How to keep public pension plans solvent in the face of the rapidly expanding elderly population has become a major economic concern.

But will the abolition of compulsory retirement have much economic impact? In the United States, the compulsory retirement age was increased from 65 to 70 and eliminated altogether for employees of the Federal Government, effective January 1, 1979. This provision will affect some 70% of the national labor force. However, estimates are that the number of workers who will choose to work beyond age 65 will be only about 200,000—7% of the workers of that age, and a mere 0.2% of the entire labor force. In Canada, one of the most striking features of the over-65s has been the steady decline in their participation in the labor force (10). In 1953 the participation rate for this group was 19.4%. By 1974, it had fallen to 10.2%. For males, the decline has been from 34.8% to 17.8%, but there has been an increase in participation among females over 65—from 3.6% in 1953 to 4.2% in 1974. Factors which have been thought to contribute to this decline include better pension availability, a greater tendency to retire for health reasons, more widespread compulsory retirement, a greater need for technological education and an increasing general unemployment rate.

Somewhat in opposition to raising the retirement age is the increasing trend to earlier retirement. Before the establishment of old age pensions, there was a deep-seated fear of retirement, which for most equaled dire poverty with, at best, dependence on children, the welfare system or private charity. As the most desperate financial need was relieved, retirement has become possible as an option for many more people. Another important impediment has been the strong work orientation of society. Loss of a place in the labor force was seen as a disaster to be postponed as long as possible. Increasingly, however, this ethic has been challenged and the assumption has arisen that a particular number of years (30-45 years) in the paid labor force is an adequate "tribute" to the work ethic. Compulsory retirement in this context is seen as advantageous, as it offers a clear cutoff point forcing people into thinking about alternate ways of life. People are encouraged to consider the most constructive ways of using their retirement years, and there is some evidence that those who postpone retirement finally retire with their health in such poor shape that they cannot enjoy retirement when it comes. An example of this comes from General Motors, where an assembly-line worker can retire after 30 years of service, irrespective of age. Only 2% of the company's 748,000 employees actually stay on the payroll until 65.

Information available on the views of working people on retirement indicates that retirement as a way of life is being seen as more and more acceptable (10). The most popular period for retirement seems to be between 60 and 64. Studies of retirees also support this pattern. A cross-national study of old people in three countries (78)—Denmark, Great Britain, and the United States—says of the retired:

> It is generally believed that most retired men want to continue at work if a job was available to them. This does not seem to be the case. Only a minority of retired men want to work, one of every ten in Denmark, one in every five in Britain, and one of every four in the U.S.

The study also states:

> An interesting phenomenon in all three countries however is the high proportion of men retired for more than three years who say they stopped work before reaching the age of 65. These early retirees make up 37% of all long-time retirees in Denmark, 27% in Great Britain and 33% in the United States.

What has emerged then is an increased emphasis on the need to ensure the right to work and the right to retire through flexible rather than mandatory approaches. Thus, there is a need to "individualize" retirement policies. At the same time, there is evidence of a trend towards earlier retirement, which appears to be accelerating. Taken in conjunction with population projections, one may safely say that retirement, a major event in the adult life-cycle, will affect many more people in the near future. This transition from worker to retiree may represent one of the most significant changes in the lives of many.

LIFE EVENTS

Adolph Meyer, an outstanding figure in the early development of American psychiatry, stressed the careful study of life events as a means of understanding emotional disorders. He insisted that this study concern itself with the ongoing interaction of the individual with life situations. His development of the "life chart," the basis of modern psychiatric history-taking, reflected his overriding concern with significant events in the life of the patient: "the changes of habitat, of school entrance, graduations or changes, or failures; the various 'jobs'; the dates of possibly important births and deaths in the family, and other fundamentally important environmental incidents" (45). In the Meyerian tradition, certain life events, widely viewed as stressful, have been studied with regard to their effects on individuals. Erich Lindemann's 1944 study of grief in members of Boston families suddenly bereaved after the Coconut Grove nightclub fire provides a classic description of physical and emotional sequelae of a single event (51).

More recently, several groups of investigators have become interested in the additive impact of life events. To provide an index of the amount of change in the life of an individual over a given time period, Thomas Holmes and Richard Rahe (45) developed the Social Readjustment Rating Scale. This is a list of 43 life events, each assigned a value between one and 100, indicating the amount of change from an existing steady state required by each event. Scores on this scale have been used to predict probability of both major and minor physical and psychiatric illnesses (71).

On this scale, the impact of retirement is ranked ninth of 43 events, only two points below "being fired at work." Paykel (67) and his group, who have constructed a scale to measure the amount of "distress" associated with each of 61 life events, rank retirement fortieth, whereas being fired is eighth, as on Holmes and Rahe's list. This divergence highlights a central point of contention in life events research. Holmes and Rahe argue that retirement is a big change likely to produce dysfunction; Paykel's position is that retirement, although a change, is in most cases not distressing and therefore should not result in symptomatology.

Crisis Theory

Many such life events, including retirement, have been conceptualized as normal life crises. Crisis is regarded as a state of temporary disequilibrium, precipitated by inescapable life change events. This disequilibrium is manifested by cognitive uncertainty, psychophysiological symptoms and emotional distress. Crisis theory argues that the temporary disorganization of the personality in such situations provides an opportunity for personality expansion if the crisis is successfully mastered, as well as the danger of constriction, restriction and illness onset when inappropriate defenses such as excessive denial are brought into play.

Hirschowitz (43) has described the phases of crisis. He outlines a sequence of impact, recoil-turmoil, adjustment and reconstruction. Impact is a state of dazed shock accompanying the assimilation of distressing news. Recoil-turmoil is a period of intense negative emotion as the full impact of the inevitable loss involved with every change sinks in. In the phase of adjustment and reconstruction, the individual begins to feel hopeful about the future and ready to make new attachments.

In dealing with a crisis situation, the individual utilizes both external social supports and his own coping skills. Social support refers to the help one receives from family, friends and others which may involve intimacy, interest, nurturance, recognition and assistance. An adequate coping repertoire is both general and specific. Hirschowitz describes individuals with low vulnerability to crisis events as having "the capacity, similar to ego strength, to orient themselves rapidly and plan decisive action in response to change. They can mobilize emergency problem-solving mechanisms and use external resources for assistance." Highly vulnerable individuals, on the other hand, "become rapidly disoriented when confronted with change. They may experience paralysis of thought or will, unable to plan action or seek assistance." Specific coping skills develop from previous experience with similar problems and tend to be largely situation-bound. However, activity and information-gathering have been shown to be useful in dealing with most major change situations.

Adjustment

Central to the concept of crisis is the assumption of change being equal to loss. A given life event will precipitate a crisis in proportion to the degree of loss experienced by the individual. Thus, loss of a spouse, precipitating the crisis of bereavement, is usually ranked highest on life events scales. The nature of the "change" in retirement may also be conceptualized in terms of specific losses. These include loss of income, loss of occupation, loss of status identity and partial loss of opportunities for socialization.

Kuypers and Bengston (50a) have argued that the unique social reorganizations in late life, including retirement, produce a situation characterized by role loss, vague or inappropriate normative information and lack of reference groups. The consequences they predict as arising out of such circumstances are the loss of coping abilities and the development of an internalized sense of incompetence—a social breakdown.

When a person retires, the role of worker is relinquished. For some people, this has been the single most important aspect of their adult identity. In many instances there is no alternate role for the retiree which is valued by him and/or by society, with resulting loss of self-esteem and feelings of usefulness. Attempts to propose new roles for the retired will be dependent upon the extent to which these are legitimized as valid and valued.

Loss of normative guidance refers to the fact that, although there are expectations concerning appropriate behavior as one moves from one age-grade to another, there is a notable absence of norms specifically built around old age. There is very little evidence of clearly defined expectations concerning what the retired person should do during this period of life. Many of the hallmarks of "successful retirement" are really norms pegged to an earlier period in the life-cycle—middle age—in the absence of available middle-aged roles.

One's reference group is the aggregate of individuals to whom a person looks in patterning his behavior. Again, the reference group for the retired seems to remain middle-aged workers. There are no institutional provisions to assist people in adapting to retirement. Retirement ceremonies mark the end rather than the beginning. The way in which the individual copes with these losses will be colored by his adjustment to the aging process per se. The two major theories of adaptation to aging are activity theory and disengagement.

Activity theory, as developed by Friedman and Havighurst (32), has been outlined as follows: (80)

1. Giving up work will involve a sense of loss.
2. The focus of this sense of loss will differ from person to person.

3. For satisfactory adjustment in retirement, the individual must make some substitution for what he has lost in work.
4. This substitution involves replacing one set of activities by another.

Activity theory states that for good adjustment in retirement an individual must substitute for work other activities which will give him the same satisfactions. Research questions raised by this theory have tended to focus upon the issue of the meaning of work and the extent to which non-work activities can replace work values. Proponents of the theory have been criticized as promoting a middle-class "work ethic" view of human experience which contributes to trapping retired people in a vicious cycle of incompetence and feelings of uselessness.

Disengagement theory, on the other hand, holds that retirement is a necessary manifestation of the mutual withdrawal of society and the older individual. Cumming and Henry (20) define disengagement as an "inevitable process in which many of the relationships between a person and other members of society are severed, and those remaining are altered in quality . . .an inevitable mutual withdrawal . . . resulting in decreased interaction between the aging person and others in the social system he belongs to." Disengagement is seen as functional for the individual because it means a realistic acceptance of one's situation, and for society because the disengaged person does not perform any useful maintenance function. Retirement is "society's permission to disengage." This theory has been criticized for making the rejection of older people by society seem "natural" and, therefore, right. However, many people do want to withdraw from energy-sapping full-time jobs, often to redistribute declining energies.

Shanas (80) argues that accommodation rather than activity or disengagement would seem to be the key process in adjustment to retirement. Accommodation theory states that adjustment to retirement is a process which begins when retirement is first considered by the individual and which abates when the individual has achieved a new distribution of his energies in non-work roles and new modes of behavior. Accommodation theory assumes that adjustment to retirement is dependent not upon the causes of retirement, but upon the nature of life changes resulting from this event and that adjustment may vary at different times within the retirement period. Haynes et al. (42) summarize factors which might influence adjustment to various retirement phases as: socialization, occupation and commitment to work, retirement preparation, psychological resources, geographic mobility, income, social support, and health.

Although accommodation theory provides a broader approach than either activity theory or disengagement theory, none of the three should be accepted as universally applicable. Each describes one of a range of possible responses to changes with aging, and disengagement, in particular, may be more relevant to the old old than to the young old and therefore "retiring" population.

Phases

Several investigators have argued that retirement should not be viewed as a single life event precipating a psychosocial crisis. The life change, although very significant, lacks the sudden and intense quality characteristic of some other "crises." Retirement is seen rather as a process which begins long before the individual leaves the work force and continues until death. Atchley (4) has postulated seven phases of retirement:

> The *remote phase* is the recognition of retirement as part of one's occupational career. During this phase retirement is viewed at a reasonable distance into the future.

> The *near phase* is the time, soon before the retirement event, when the individual becomes aware of the realities of the retirement role.

> The *honeymoon phase* gives the individual time to adjust to newly acquired freedom of time and space.

> The *disenchantment phase* occurs as the individual begins to cope with the inevitable losses of old age such as inadequate income, failing health and loss of friends.

> Phases of *reorientation* and *stability* involve acceptance of retirement and the establishment of a routine, stable life.

> The *termination phase* is the period of disabling illness ending in death.

Haynes et al. (42) suggest that the "near" and "disenchantment" phases in particular call for considerable adjustment by the individual, and are therefore appropriate foci for stress research. They also point out that specific intervals of time for each phase, if each does indeed occur, cannot as yet be designated in the absence of empirical, longitudinal research.

In terms of the so-called "near" or "anticipatory" phase, Dressler (24) has emphasized the importance of appraisal in a general model of stress. Appraisal may indicate to an individual that he cannot respond to an inevitable occurrence by customary methods of problem-solving or defense. Frequent appraisals are a sense of loss, of threat or of attack. Accompanying the appraisal is an affect reflecting the nature of the perception; thus, loss is associated with a feeling of sadness, threat with anxiety and attack with anger. These affects, along with their cognitive elaborations, may be dealt with via healthy coping mechanisms and the utilization of social supports, or they may be denied, projected or expressed destructively in less flexible individuals. Previous experiences with life stress are a powerful intervening variable mediating the responses.

It seems that the delineation of a process involving anticipation-disenchantment-reorientation is not substantially at odds with the crisis model of anticipation-impact-turmoil-readjustment. Individual coping mechanisms and the use of social supports by flexible individuals counterbalance the disruption in both models, and in the case of retirement, the crisis phases may simply be extended in time and so somewhat ameliorated in intensity of effect. However, knowledge of a retirement "process," if one is empirically outlined, should be helpful to professionals dealing with the problems of the elderly.

RESEARCH FINDINGS

There is very little evidence for the commonly held view that retirement leads to serious physical and/or psychological deterioration. Dysfunction, if it does occur, is reflected in more subtle psychosocial alterations.

Negative Stereotype

Most sources of the most dismal view of retirement are "think papers" which contain no empirical data or even systematic clinical observations. These articles usually discuss the "widely acknowledged" physical, psychological and social problems of adjustment to retirement, emphasizing the need for retirement research (66) and intervention programs (21). Support for the arguments presented in these articles ranges from the Bible to Freud. For instance, Hochman (44) refers to Freud's statement in *Civilization and Its Discontents*:

> Laying stress upon the importance of work has a greater effect than any other technique of living in the direction of binding the individual more closely to reality; in his work, he is at least securely attached to a part of reality, to the human community.

On the basis of this statement, Hochman argues that rupture of the work pattern through retirement precipitates a severe emotional reaction. While such articles sometimes present reasonable and even powerful arguments to support the negative retirement stereotype, they cannot be regarded or cited as proof of its accuracy.

Further examination of original sources reveals that other articles frequently cited in relation to the retirement stereotype do not even study retirement itself. For instance, Pearson's examination of workers in Scotland studies the anticipation of retirement, rather than actual retirement (68, 69). However, the greatest confusion appears to derive from studies which purport to examine retirement but which, in fact, study aging. For example, Nadelson (65), in his review of the literature on the adjustment of the aged to retirement, states that Granick (39) and Blake (9) have demonstrated the detrimental effect of retirement on adjustment. However, Granick's article is a survey of the literature on psychopathology of later maturity which does not "demonstrate" that increases in emotional disorders beyond age 65 are linked specifically to retirement rather than to the aging process. Similarly, Blake examines adjustment problems of residents in a home for the aged, but does not demonstrate that maladjustment can be directly attributed to retirement rather than to the aging or institutionalization of his subjects.

Still other studies cited as support for the negative retirement stereotype are often considerably more impressionistic than scientific. Tyhurst et al. (93) point out that assumptions about retirement seem to have sprung mainly from "isolated impressions" which have been generalized extensively but seldom investigated scientifically. For example, Fried (31) is cited as having demonstrated the detrimental effects of retirement—yet only 24 of Fried's 75 subjects were retired and the investigation was in the form of a subjective analysis of case histories; no attempt was made to objectify the criteria for maladjustment or to examine the retired subjects against any matched control group of subjects still working. Another example of unwarranted overgeneralization is the frequent citing of a statement by Wolff (95) that retirement is the principal cause of maladjustment among the aged. Wolff's statement was not a finding based on any systematic study of the causes of maladjustment in the aged, but was an opinion based on his personal experience in the field of geriatric psychiatry. He and others are not to be criticized for drawing conclusions from their clinical experience, but, unfortunately, subsequent authors have often bestowed upon these conclusions an unjustified aura of empirical authority.

An added danger in basing an overall opinion of the effects of a normal life transition, such as retirement, on isolated clinical impressions is that these cases are often drawn from a psychiatric or an institutionalized population (e.g. 9, 95). Tyhurst (92), in his study of transition states, underlines the obvious fact that the person who comes to the attention of a psychiatrist or of a helping institution is not necessarily typical of the majority of people who go through the same transition.

Thus, it appears that many of the references found in the retirement literature have been passed from bibliography to bibliography without examination of the original sources to ascertain whether any data are presented, whether these data pertain to retirement, and if so, whether they meet any reasonable standards of scientific or statistical validity. In its present state, it must be concluded that the retirement literature provides little support for the negative retirement stereotype.

Mortality statistics have also been considered as support for the argument that retirement increases the likelihood of dying, since death rates are higher among retirees than among men of comparable age who are still working. However, Meyers (64) has pointed out that when findings are subdivided according to those who retired voluntarily versus those who were retired because of an automatic or compulsory retirement schedule, it is only among those who retire voluntarily that death rates are elevated. This finding has been explained by the fact that there is a disproportionately high percentage of persons already in poor health among those who retire voluntarily (12, 23, 79, 84).

Considerable attention have been focused on military retirement and the unique problems it presents—such as need for a second career, loss of military status and prestige, and lack of community roots (7, 8, 25, 35). Constellations of psychosomatic symptoms following military retirement have been grouped by clinicians under the label "Retirement Syndrome" (60). However, like much of the civilian data, the military data have been based almost exclusively on case histories of severely maladjusted persons. Greenberg (40) points out that the vast majority of military personnel (who are not reflected in the literature) survive the transition of military retirement without major adjustment problems. Moreover, those who do exhibit disturbances often have had histories of deeply rooted personality problems (61, 63). Thus, it is dangerous to generalize the military findings to the entire military population, let alone to the entire civilian population.

Effects on Physical Health

The prevailing opinion among professional and lay people alike has been that retirement frequently leads to physical deterioration (23). However, research findings, if anything, have tended to support the opposing view that retirement might actually improve physical health. As in the interpretation of mortality statistics, failure to distinguish between voluntary and compulsory retirement in early studies may account for the contradiction between popular belief and actual findings. Closer examination of the data reveals that poor health is a major cause, rather than effect, of retirement (12, 76, 79, 88, 90). In a recent study conducted by Health and Welfare Canada, poor health was found to be the leading cause of retirement among males and the second leading cause among females (18). These studies emphasize the importance of longitudinal investigations which examine the temporal relationship between retirement and health decline.

One of the best-known and most comprehensive of the longitudinal studies of retirement is the Cornell Study of Occupational Retirement conducted between 1952 and 1959 and reported by Streib and Schneider in 1971 (86). This study followed 1,486 urban males and 483 urban females through the ages 65 to 70. The moderate decline in subjectively reported health over this age span could *not* be attributed to retirement itself since those who did not retire showed a similar decline. Furthermore, those who did report a health decline after retirement did not regard retirement as the cause of the deterioration. On a smaller scale, Emerson (27) followed 124 Englishmen for one year from their 65th birthdays and compared those who were still working with those who had retired. On several indices of physical health, mental health, and general attitudes, he found no evidence of health decline following retirement.

Other comprehensive studies of varied experimental design actually show health improvement following retirement. Tyhurst et al. (93) used various indices to investigate mortality and morbidity rates of workers who retired from a Canadian communications industry between 1917 and 1954. Examination of death rates and life expectancy data provided no support for the negative retirement stereotype and examination of survival rates showed a higher survival rate immediately following retirement when age was held constant. They also found a tendency toward either no change or an improvement in health in the period following retirement. For example, medical records show that the health of 37% of the pensioners remained unchanged from before to after retirement, and 40% of the pensioners improved in health status. Similarly, Ryser and Sheldon (75) used both objective and subjective health indices in studying 500 men and women between the ages of 60 and 70. The subjects were interviewed three months after and four years after retirement and were found to be in good or even improved health following retirement. Persons who retired because of ill health were excluded from the study. Only 10.4% of the subjects felt their health had worsened after retirement, while 24.1% felt it had improved. Thompson and

Streib (88) contacted 1,260 males between the ages of 68 and 70 who were still working, and again two years later when 477 had retired. Subjective and objective examinations comparing health changes of retirees with health changes of those still working showed an improvement in health with retirement. Other studies support this trend in research findings toward improvement in physical health following retirement (27, 59, 76, 91).

Effects on Mental Health

Very little research has been conducted specifically to investigate the effects of retirement on mental health, and few, if any, studies have produced conclusive findings. In a study of 1,200 old people conducted by the Langley Porter Neuropsychiatric Institute in San Francisco, evidence was not found to support the assumption that retirement precipitates mental illness in the elderly (83). Lowenthal and Berkman (55) found a 19% rate of psychiatric impairment among retired and unemployed subjects, which was more than twice the rate among the employed. However, psychiatric impairment was found to be a function of several "deprivation factors," such as low socioeconomic status and poor physical health, rather than of retirement *per se*. In particular, poor physical health itself (or in some cases the perception of poor health) (87), rather than retirement, appears to be an important, if not a major, factor in the development of psychological maladjustment (58, 75, 86, 91) and psychiatric impairment (54, 82, 83) in retirement. Other often age-linked factors, such as low income and isolation, also appear critical (54, 55, 65, 83). It is extremely difficult to synthesize conclusions from these studies since indices of "mental health" have varied widely, from indicators of lowered morale (which will be discussed in the following section) to evidence of major psychiatric disorder (26, 82, 83).

In their 1974 review article on adjustment to retirement, Friedmann and Orbach (33) cite 210 references, but only two of these references pertain to their discussion of the effect of retirement on mental health and one of these two articles does not deal specifically with retirement, but only with isolation in old age (53). Clearly there is a need for more careful research regarding possible effects of retirement on mental health and distinctions must be made between the interrelated but separate concepts of aging and retirement.

Effects on General Satisfaction

"General satisfaction" or "adjustment to retirement" is perhaps the most loosely defined and yet the most commonly investigated dependent variable in examinations of the effects of retirement. Friedman and Orbach (33) present a lengthy discussion of the various conceptions of and criteria for adjustment, examining the widely differing theoretical bases for these conceptions and the extreme difficulty in trying to examine and compare adjustment to retirement scientifically across studies. They point out, among other factors, the lack of agreement as to what constitutes "good adjustment," the inconsistency on the scaling of items on adjustment measures and the social and cultural biases of some retirement morale scales. With these warnings in mind, interpretation of "trends" in research findings in this field must necessarily be cautious. The findings are conflicting, but again a pattern of satisfactory adjustment in retirement tentatively emerges.

As part of their comprehensive examination of the needs of the aged in New York City, Kutner et al. (50) found the 149 retirees studied to have a low level of adjustment in retirement—41% were classified as having low morale and 32% as having medium morale. As in many of the earlier retirement studies, however, these retirees were not examined before retirement to determine if retirement had brought about any change in morale level, nor were they compared to any matched group of working subjects. Kutner et al. also pointed out that physical health and pre-retirement attitudes had a significant influence on adjustment to retirement, an observation which has since been supported by the findings of Kimmel et al. (49) in their questionnaire survey of 1486 voluntary and non-voluntary retirees.

Streib and Schneider (86), in their large-scale longitudinal study, found that retirement did not bring about a decrease in "general life satisfaction." Again, prior attitude (i.e., willingness to retire) was cited as one of the most important factors influencing retirement satisfaction. Barfield and Morgan (5) found that three-quarters of their retired respondents reported themselves as being either "satisfied" or "very satisfied" in retirement and that situational factors such as retirement income and health were positively correlated with retirement satisfaction.

Almost a decade later, in a national interview survey, Barfield and Morgan repeated some of the questions asked in their earlier study and found that current retirees appear to be somewhat less satisfied with life after retirement. However, retirement satisfaction was again found to be strongly related to economic and health factors and the authors pointed out the need for attention to overall economic trends (e.g., inflation rates, etc.), as well as individual income levels, in understanding changing attitudes towards retirement (6). Thus, attempts to generalize about the impact of retirement without attention to pre-retirement attitude and situational aspects of the specific retirement experience can never be entirely accurate or comprehensive.

Important Variables

Adams outlines over 50 interrelated variables which have been found to influence retirement satisfaction (1). As pointed out in the previous section, *health status, income level,* and *pre-retirement attitudes* have been found to be key variables which can influence the effects of retirement (5, 6, 36, 48, 49, 50, 80). (In his examination of the relative importance of income, health status, the worker role, and family setting in the life satisfaction of the aged, Chatfield (17) points out the interrelationship between income and health variables, in that higher income can reduce the impact of health problems on life satisfaction.)

Socioeconomic or occupational status appears to be another crucial variable in retirement adjustment. Lundgren (56) studied 404 retired men from 13 companies and found that the former salaried workers exhibited a significantly greater degree of retirement satisfaction than did the former hourly workers. In their cross-national study of retired teachers and steelworkers, Havighurst and deVries (41) found that these two occupational groups differed qualitatively in their modes of adjustment to retirement when grouped according to characteristic life-styles and behavior patterns after retirement. For example, the teachers demonstrated greater activity and variety of interests in retirement and remained more engaged in work and formal associational roles than did the steelworkers. Burgess et al. (11) found that, of their 301 subjects, those at a managerial level seemed better prepared for retirement than did manual workers. Similarly, based on their experiences with a specific large-scale retirement counseling program, Davidson and Kunze (22) observed that retirement is often less of a disruption of activities among white collar workers than among blue collar workers. A study by Stokes and Maddox (85) followed 138 workers six years into retirement and found that, while the blue collar workers appeared to adjust more successfully than white collar workers in the short run, they were less successful in the long run. Thus the *time factor* is another important variable, since "adjustment" to retirement depends on how soon after retirement an individual is observed (42, 57).

Job satisfaction has also been studied in relation to retirement adjustment. Maddox (57) has suggested that men with higher job satisfaction resent retirement at first but later enjoy it. Stokes and Maddox (85) support this notion but only among white collar workers. However, other researchers have found no clear relationship between job satisfaction and retirement satisfaction (29, 47, 70). Goudy et al.(38), in their study of 1,922 men 50 years of age or over, attempted to clarify the controversy over the relationship between work satisfaction and retirement attitude. They found that an inverse relationship existed between these two variables only when work acted as a key organizing factor in the worker's life. They contend that the failure of previous studies to investigate the degree to which this is so has resulted in the existing contradictory findings. From a theoretical perspective, Atchley (3) also stresses that the level of importance of job satisfaction in the individual's hierarchy of personal goals influences the impact of retirement on that individual.

Cultural or national differences in the effects of retirement—reflecting, perhaps, more or less emphasis on the work role in different cultures—are of possible importance as well. For example, findings from several British studies were in dramatic conflict with the North American negative retirement stereotype (19, 59). This has also been true of much of the recent North American research, but the possibility of national differences in attitudes and reactions to retirement still cannot be discounted without further investigation (26, 33).

Possible *differences between men and women* in adjustment to retirement are also yet to be established, since until recently few studies have focused on women in retirement. Fox (30) contends that the lack of empirical attention toward female retirees is a function of outdated attitudes among researchers that the work role is central to males but only "secondary" for females and that work imparts status for men, whereas women derive their status from their husbands! As a result of this assumption that work has negligible psychosocial importance among females, most retirement studies have either excluded females, included small, unrepresentative samples of women, or failed to analyze the data by sex (46). There is clearly a need for systematic research on the direct impact of retirement on women and also of the indirect impact on women of their husband's retirement (28).

Perhaps the group of variables which have been most notably neglected in retirement research designs have been those related to the individual *personality structures and life histories* of the retirees (13, 57, 72, 81, 89). It is quite possible that various personality types are differentially prone to retirement maladjustment. Adjustment problems in retirement should therefore be examined in light of earlier adjustment problems, of the specific details of the retirement situation and of one's life history of social integration, achievements, income, health, etc.

Implications

Examination of the retirement stereotype and the relevant literature raises several fundamental questions which cannot be ignored in future research and intervention programs. Is retirement a stressful transition which justifies attempts at preventive intervention? Before this question can be answered with any degree of confidence, there is a need for further research characterized by far more rigorous attention to experimental detail and to the situational (health, financial, etc.) aspects of retirement which have been shown to be so critical (34, 57, 89). If such research substantiates the present trend in findings it would appear that, although the majority of retirees adjust well physically, mentally and socially, intervention *is* justified for those exceptions who do experience severe maladjustment in retirement.

Atchley (3) has estimated that approximately 30% of retirees encounter difficulty in adjusting to retirement, but points out that their adjustment problems are not always directly related to the retirement process, but often to other factors, such as death of a spouse or declining health, which can influence the situation in which retirement adjustment must be carried out. In general, he suggests that there are various "situational prerequisites" which are often necessary to a good retirement adjustment.

Who needs help adjusting to retirement? If people are differentially prone to maladjustment in retirement, what is it that makes them so? In what ways are successful retirees different from those who experience difficulty in retirement? Systematic comparison of these two types of retirees in terms of situational variables, pre-retirement attitudes and personality factors is a necessary first step. If, as many authors contend, satisfaction in retirement can be related to the retiree's personality type and earlier history of social interaction and community involvement, it would be worthwhile to direct attention to developing measures of personal adjustment and social integration which might permit the identification of a high-risk retirement group, towards whom intervention could be aimed.

When should intervention be initiated? If retirement adjustment is related to earlier adjustment, many authors have argued that patterns of social interaction and attitudes which might ease the transition to retirement cannot be taught within the bounds of conventional counseling programs initiated six months to a year prior to retirement, but must be cultivated early in the working life (57, 66, 72, 83). Tyhurst (92) has even suggested that the period just prior to retirement is a particularly poor time for intervention, due to strong denial of the impending transition. Lifelong social engineering of attitudes and actions is hardly a feasible or acceptable solution to the "problem" of retirement, and yet, simply to say that it is "too late" to help those individuals for whom retirement is a crisis is no answer. Research should be aimed at determining not only the most appropriate form, but also the optimal timing for concentrated intervention for those concerned.

What form should intervention take? Until the characteristics and needs of retirees have been more thoroughly researched, little of a concrete nature can be said about the most suitable form of intervention. However, once these varying needs are more accurately assessed, the most important guideline would seem to be to gear intervention programs to the specific needs of the specific retirement group or individual involved (6, 11, 52, 56).

The one guideline for intervention that is supported by the present literature is that preparation for retirement need not be directed solely toward psychological factors (i.e., loss of the work role). Improved economic planning for retirement and more comprehensive health care for the aged, by lessening the economic and health worries of retirees, can be a major step toward reducing the overall stress of retirement (17). It should be noted that much of the retirement research has been conducted in the United States where health care plans for the aged are often considerably less comprehensive than comparable plans in Canada and other countries. It is yet to be clearly established whether there is a significant difference between nationalities in the nature or intensity of the retirement stress experienced, and in the nature of the most appropriate form of intervention.

A final observation is the need for an educational component in intervention. Although old age and leisure are becoming more socially accepted (2, 22, 73, 74), the need for the retiree to accurately perceive society's attitudes towards retirement is as important as the attitudes themselves (56). As early as 1959, Emerson (27) suggested that continued research emphasis on the retirement "problem" might be doing more harm than good, by increasing the anticipatory, and often unwarranted, fears of retirees. Thus, in future research, care should be taken not to inadvertently convey (to subjects) the impression that retirement is being studied as an already acknowledged catastrophe, thereby helping to perpetuate the retirement stereotype and possibly influencing the outcome of the research. Similarly, intervention programs should make positive efforts to promote individual awareness of decreasing societal emphasis on the work role and of increasing focus on such factors as community integration and ability to find fulfillment in leisure activities.

REFERENCES

1. ADAMS, L. (1971). Correlates of satisfaction among the elderly. *Gerontologist, 11,* 64-68.
2. ATCHLEY, R. C. (1971). Retirement and leisure activity: Continuity of crisis? *Gerontologist, 11,* 13-17.
3. ATCHLEY, R. C. (1975). Adjustment to loss of job at retirement. *Int. J. Hum. Dev.,* 6, 17.
4. ATCHLEY, R. C. (1976). *The Sociology of Retirement.* Toronto: John Wiley and Sons, 60.
5. BARFIELD, R. E. and MORGAN, J. N. (1969). *Early Retirement: The Decision and the*

Experience. Institute for Social Research, University of Michigan, Ann Arbor, Michigan.
6. BARFIELD, R. E. and MORGAN, J. N. (1978). Trends in satisfaction with retirement. *Gerontologist*, *18*, 19.
7. BELLINO, R. (1970). Perspectives of military and civilian retirement. *Ment. Hyg.*, *54*, 580.
8. BERKELEY, B. R. and STOEBNER, J. B. (1968). The retirement syndrome: A previously unreported variant. *Milit. Med.*, *133*, 5-8.
9. BLAKE, W. D. (1952). The adjustment of residents of a home for the aged. *J. Gerontol.*, *7*, 474.
10. BROWN, J. C. (1975). *Retirement Policies in Canada*. Canadian Council on Social Development. p. xxvi.
11. BURGESS, E. W., COREY, L. G., PINEO, P. C. and THORNBURY, R. T. (1958). Occupational differences in attitudes toward aging and retirement. *J. Gerontol.*, *13*, 203-206.
12. BUSSE, E. W. (1967). Geriatrics today—an overview. *Am. J. Psychiat.*, *123*, 1226-33.
13. BUTLER, R. N. (Dec. 1966). Patterns of Psychological Health and Psychiatric Illness in Retirement. In: Carp, F. M. (ed.) *The Retirement Process*. Public Health Service Publ. No. 1778, U. S. Dept. of Health, Education and Welfare, National Institute of Child Health and Human Development, Washington, D.C., pp. 27f.
14. BUTLER, R. N. (1975). Psychiatry and the elderly. *Am. J. Psychiat.*, *132*, 893.
15. CARP, F. M. (1967). Retirement crisis. *Science*, *157*, 102-3.
16. CAVAN, R. S. (1962). Self and Role Adjustment During Old Age. In: Rose, A. M. (ed.) *Human Behaviour and Social Processes*. Boston, Houghton-Mifflin.
17. CHATFIELD, W. F. (1977). Economic and sociological factors influencing life satisfaction of the aged. *J. Gerontol.*, *32*, 593.
18. CIFFEN, S. and MARTIN, J. (1977). *Retirement in Canada. Vol. I. When and Why People Retire*. Ottawa: Health and Welfare Canada.
19. CRAWFORD, M. P. (1972). Retirement as a psychosocial crisis. *J. Psychosom. Res.*, *17*, 375-380.
20. CUMMING, E. and HENRY, W. E. (1961). *Growing Old: The Process of Disengagement*. New York: Basic Books.
21. CUSHING, J. G. N. (1952). Problems of retirement. *Ment. Hyg.*, *36*, 449-455.
22. DAVIDSON, W. R. and KUNZE, K. R. (1965). Psychological, social and economic meanings of work in modern society: Their effects on the worker facing retirement. *Gerontologist*, *5*, 129-33.
23. DONAHUE, W., ORBACH, H. L. and POLLAK, O. (1960). Retirement: The Emerging Social Pattern. In: Tibbits, C., (ed.) *Handbook of Social Gerontology*. Chicago, University of Chicago Press.
24. DRESSLER, D. H. (1976). Life stress and emotional crisis: The idiosyncratic interpretation of life events. *Comprehens. Psychiat.*, *17*, 549.
25. DRUSS, R. G. (1965). Problems associated with retirement from military service. *Milit. Med.*, *130*, 382-385.
26. EMERSON, A. R. (1962). Retirement reconsidered: A review. *Br. J. Ind. Med.*, *19*, 105-109.
27. EMERSON, A. R. (1959). The first year of retirement. *Occupational Psychol.*, *33*, 197-208.
28. FENGLER, A. P. (1975). Attitudinal orientations of wives toward their husbands' retirement. *Int. J. Aging Hum. Dev.*, *6*, 139.
29. FILLENBAUM, G. G. (1971). On the relation between attitude to work and attitude to retirement. *J. Gerontol.*, *26*, 244-248.
30. FOX, J. H. (1977). Effects of retirement and former work life on women's adaptation in old age. *J. Gerontol.*, *32*, 196.
31. FRIED, E. (1949). Attitudes of the older population groups toward activity and inactivity. *J. Gerontol.*, *4*, 141-151.
32. FRIEDMAN, E. A. and HAVIGHURST, R. J. (1954). *The Meaning of Work and Retirement*, Chicago: University of Chicago Press.

33. FRIEDMAN, E. A. and ORBACH, H. L. (1974). Adjustment to Retirement. In: Arieti, S. (ed.) *American Handbook of Psychiatry*, Vol. I. The Foundations of Psychiatry, New York: Basic Books pp. 609-645.

34. GEORGE, L. K. and MADDOX, G. L. (1977). Subjective adaptation to loss of the work role: A longitudinal study. *J. Gerontol.*, *32*, 456.

35. GIFFEN, M. B. and MCNEIL, J. S. (1967). Effect of military retirement on dependents. *Arch. Gen. Psychiat.*, *17*, 717-722.

36. GLAMSER, F. F. (1976). Determinants of a positive attitude toward retirement. *J. Gerontol.*, *31*, 104.

37. GOODSTEIN, L. D. (1962). Personal adjustment factors and retirement. *Geriatrics*, *17*, 41-5.

38. GOUDY, W. J. et al. (1975). Work and retirement: A test of attitudinal relationships. *J. Gerontol.*, *3*, 193.

39. GRANICK, S. (1950). Studies of psychopathology in later maturity: A review. *J. Gerontol.*, *5*, 361-369.

40. GREENBERG, H. R. (1965). Depressive equivalent in pre-retirement years: "The old soldier syndrome". *Milit. Med.*, *130*, 251-255.

41. HAVIGHURST, R. H. and DEVRIES, A. (1969). Life styles and free time activities of retired men. *Hum. Dev.*, *12*, 34-54.

42. HAYNES, S. G. et al. (1977). The relationship of normal, involuntary retirement to early mortality among U. S. rubber workers. *Soc. Sci. and Med.*, *11*, 105.

43. HIRSCHOWITZ, R. G. (1973). Crisis Theory: A Formulation. *Psychiatric Annals*, *3*, 36.

44. HOCHMAN, J. (1960). The Retirement Myth. In: Tibbitts, C. and Donahue, W. (eds.) *Aging in Today's Society*. Englewood Cliffs: Prentice-Hall pp. 366-368.

45. HOLMES, T. H. and RAHE, R. H. (1967). The social readjustment rating scale. *J. Psychosom. Res.*, *1*, 213.

46. JASLOW, P. (1976). Employment, retirement and morale among older women. *J. Gerontol.*, *31*, 212.

47. JOHNSON, J. and STROTHER, G. B. (1962). Job expectations and retirement planning. *J. Gerontol.*, *17*, 418-423.

48. KATONA, G. and MORGAN, J. N. (1967). Retirement in retrospect and prospect. In: *Retirement and the Individual Hearings before the Subcommittee on Retirement and the Individual of the Special Committee on Aging*, U. S. Senate, 90th Congress, Washington.

49. KIMMEL, D. C., PRICE, K. F. and WALKER, J. W. (1978). *J. Gerontol.*, *33*, 575.

50. KUTNER, B., FANSHEL, D., TOGO, A. M. and LANGNER, T. S. (1956). *Five Hundred Over Sixty*. New York: Russell Sage Foundation.

50a. KUYPERS, J. and BENGSTON, V. (1973). Social breakdowns and competence. *Human Devel.*, 16: 181-201.

51. LINDEMANN, E. (1944). Symptomatology and management of acute grief. *Am. J. Psychiat.*, *101*, 141.

52. LIVSON, F. and PETERSEN, P. G. (1962). Adjustment to Retirement. In: Richard, S., Livson, F. and Petersen, P. G. (eds.) *Aging and Personality*. New York: John Wiley and Sons.

53. LOWENTHAL, M. F. (1964). Social isolation and mental illness in old age. *Am. Sociol. Rev.*, *29*, 54-70.

54. LOWENTHAL, M. F. (1963). Some Social Dimensions of Psychiatric Disorders in Old Age. In: Williams, R. H., Tibbits, C. and Donahue, W. (eds.) *Processes of Aging: Social and Psychological Perspectives*. Volume 2, New York: Atherton Press.

55. LOWENTHAL, M. F. and BERKMAN, P. L. (1967). *Aging and Mental Disorder in San Francisco*. San Francisco: Jossey-Bass.

56. LUNDGREN, E. F. (1966). Compatibility of a successful work experience with retirement. *Ment. Hyg.*, *50*, 463.

57. MADDOX, G. L. (1970). Adaptation to retirement. *Gerontologist*, *10*, 14-18.

58. MARSHALL, D. and ETENG, W. (1970). *Retirement and Migration in the North Central States: A Comparative Analysis—Wisconsin, Florida, Arizona.* Population Series #20, Dept. of Rural Sociology, University of Wisconsin.

59. MARTIN, J. and DORAN, A. (1966). Evidence concerning the relationship between health and retirement. *Sociol. Rev., 14,* 329-343.

60. MCNEIL, J. S. and GIFFEN, M. B. (1965). Military retirement: Some observations and concepts. *Aerosp. Med., 36,* 25-29.

61. MCNEIL, J. S. and GIFFEN, M. B. (1967). Military retirement: The retirement syndrome. *Am. J. Psychiat., 123,* 848-854.

62. MILLER, S. J. (1965). The Social Dilemma of the Aging Leisure Participant. In: Rose, A. M. and Peterson, W. A. (eds.) *Older People and Their Social World.* Philadelphia: F. A. Davis Co.

63. MILOWE, I. D. (1964). A study in role diffusion: The chief and sergeant face retirement. *Ment. Hyg., 48,* 101-107.

64. MEYERS, R. J. (1954). Factors in interpreting mortality after retirement. *J. Am. Statistical A., 49,* 479-509.

65. NADELSON, T. (1969). A survey of the literature on the adjustment of the aged to retirement. *J. Geriatr. Psychiat., 3,* 3.

66. PAN, JU-SHU (1951). Problems and adjustment of retired persons. *Sociology Soc. Res., 35,* 422-424.

67. PAYKEL, E. G. (1971). Scaling of life events. *Arch. Gen. Psychiat., 25,* 340.

68. PEARSON, M. (1957). The transition from work to retirement: I. *Occupational Psychol., 31,* 80-88.

69. PEARSON, M. (1957). The transition from work to retirement: II. *Occupational Psychology., 31,* 139-149.

70. POLLMAN, A. W. (1971). Early retirement: A comparison of poor health to other retirement factors, *J. Gerontol., 26,* 41-45.

71. RABKIN, J. and STRUENIG, E. (1976). Life events, stress and illness. *Science, 194,* 1013.

72. ROBSON, R. B. (1950). What the general practitioner and the industrial physician should know regarding the problems of retirement. *Can. Med. Assoc. J., 63,* 457.

73. ROSE, A. M. (1962). The subculture of the aging: A topic for sociological research. *Gerontologist, 2,* 123-127.

74. ROSE, A. M. (1964). A current theoretical issue in social gerontology. *Gerontologist,* 46-50.

75. RYSER, C. and SHELDON, A. (1969). Retirement and health. *J. Am. Geriatr. Soc., 17,* 180-190.

76. SCHEFFMAN, J. H. and SCHNORE, M. M. (1978). Retirement and health. In: Pablo, R. Y. (ed), *Psychogeriatric Care in Institutions and in the Community.* London, Ontario: Ontario Psychogeriatric Association.

77. SCHWENGER, C. W. (1977). Health care for aging Canadians. *Canadian Welfare, 52,* 9.

78. SHANAS, E. (1970). Health and adjustment in retirement. *Gerontologist, 10,* 19.

79. SHANAS, E., TOWNSEND P., WEDDERBURN, D., FRIIS, H., MILHJ, P & STEHOUWER, J. (eds.) (1968). *Old People in Three Industrial Societies.* New York: Atherton Press.

80. SHANAS, E. (1972). Adjustment to Retirement: Substitution or Accommodation. In: Carp, F. M. (ed.) *Retirement.* New York: Behavioral Publications.

81. SHEPPARD, H. L. and PHILIBERT, M. (1972). Employment and retirement: Roles and activities. *Gerontologist, 12,* 29-35.

82. SHERMAN, D. E. (1970). Retirement. *J. Am. Geriatr. Soc., 18,* 780-791.

83. SPENCE, D. L. (Dec. 1966). Patterns of Retirement in San Francisco. In: Carp, F. M. (ed.) *The Retirement Process.* Public Health Service Publ. No. 1778, U. S. Dept, of Health, Education and Welfare, National Institute of Child Health and Human Development, Washington, D.C.

84. STEINER, P. and DORFMAN, R. (1957). *The Economic Status of the Aged.* Berkeley, Calif.:

University of California Press.

85. STOKES, R. G. and MADDOX, G. L. (1967). Some social factors on retirement adaptation. *J. Gerontol.*, *22*, 329-333.

86. STREIB, G. F. and SCHNEIDER, S. J. (1971). *Retirement in American Society*. Ithaca: Cornell University Press.

87. THOMPSON, G. B. (1972). Adjustment in retirement: A causal interpretation of factors influencing the morale of retired men. Dissertation Abstracts International 33, 402.

88. THOMPSON, W. E. and STREIB, G. F. (1958). Situational determinants: Health and economic deprivation in retirement. *J. Soc. Issues*, *14*, 18-34.

89. THOMPSON, W., STREIB, G. F. and KOSA, J. (1960). Effect of retirement on personal adjustment: A panel analysis. *J. Gerontol.*, *15*, 165-169.

90. TIBBITTS, C. (1954). Retirement problems in American society. *Am. J. Sociol.*, *59*, 301-308.

91. TUCKMAN, J. and LORGE, I. (1953). *Retirement and the Industrial Worker: Prospect and Reality*. New York: Columbia University Bureau of Publications, Teachers College.

92. TYHURST, J. S. (1958). The Role of Transition States. In: *Symposium on Preventive and Social Psychiatry*, Walter Reed Army Institute of Research, Washington, D.C. pp. 149-169.

93. TYHURST, J. S., SALK, L. and KENNEDY, M. (1957). Mortality, morbidity and retirement. *Am. J. Public Health*, *47*, 1434-1444.

94. WEISE, R. W. (1972). Early retirement under public pension systems in Latin America. *International Social Security Review*, *25*, 257.

95. WOLFF, K. (1963). *Geriatric Psychiatry*. Springfield, IL.: Charles C Thomas.

11

THE PSYCHOLOGICAL TRANSITION INTO GRANDPARENTHOOD

PAULA GORLITZ, B.A.

and

DAVID GUTMANN, Ph.D.

Northwestern University Medical School, Chicago

Grandparenthood is a major life event which has received little attention from a psychodynamic perspective. In fact, life changes which occur during the latter half of life are just beginning to be researched by psychological investigators in an effort to build a comprehensive data base elucidating the specific shifts, capacities, and stresses which emerge throughout the life-cycle. While adulthood has finally achieved the status of a life stage replete with its own potentialities for growth and conflict (a notion behavioral scientists previously reserved for the stages of childhood and adolescence), research on adulthood has primarily focused on the very young or old. Theorists investigating the crucial life stage of parenthood and its influence on development are noteworthy exceptions. Grandparenthood can be approached as one phase in the parenting process, and may represent an important transition of the post-parental years.

The literature on grandparenthood is sparse and variable in quality. There is uniformity in neither the methodological approach to the phenomena under study, nor in the perspective from which grandparenthood is analyzed. No consensus has been reached concerning the various elements or stages inherent in the role, and thus studies continue to focus on disparate dimensions of grandparenthood. Because of the lack of common terminology and the unsynthesized state of the literature, coherent arguments which can be augmented and modified by further research do not emerge.

The majority of studies appear to be small, correlational in nature, and primarily focused upon the grandchild as referent. In addition, they frequently fail to make gender distinctions or to differentiate lines of filiation (i.e., intergenerational connections). Either of these methodological limitations could confound the data and be misleading.

The literature can be categorized into four major analytic perspectives:

1. The social psychological, in which meaning is ascribed to roles, behaviors, and attitudes within the society (2, 3, 11, 34, 48, 58, 61, 64).
2. The anthropological, emphasizing what grandparenthood symbolizes within a cultural frame of reference (4, 44, 54).
3. The psychoanalytic, which looks at its meaning within an intrapsychic framework (1, 7, 8, 15, 19, 32, 33, 56, 65).
4. The psychological family-oriented theories, which view grandparenthood as one segment of an intergenerational model and examine the meaning of the experience to the family interaction (6, 10, 13, 20, 27, 60, 62, 63).

These various approaches have produced fruitful results relating to the significance of grandparenthood within the particular context under study. Moreover, they provide provocative data which hint at the psychodynamic importance of the experience.

The aim of this chapter is to provide a broad organizational framework for the psychodynamic study of grandparenthood. The existing literature suggests that several factors may coalesce within the experience of grandparenthood to press for a redefinition of three major roles. These are: 1. the role toward one's children, or grandparent as parent; 2. the role toward oneself; and 3. a reassessment of one's place in the life-cycle. Within each of these three aspects of the transition into grandparenthood are many foci for further research.

GRANDPARENT AS PARENT

The transition into grandparenthood involves a new relationship to one's adult child, and thus must be considered a special phase of parenthood; for the first time, one must share the role of parent with one's offspring.

The relationship between middle-aged parents and their adult children is frequently conflictual. In her large correlational study, Albrecht (3) emphasized the difficulty in forming reciprocal and mature patterns of relating with family members distant from one another in age. Part of this difficulty could be the tendency, common in parents, to find distant memories of their offspring as infants and toddlers intruding upon their current conceptions of their now grown children (29).

There is a wealth of data stressing the ambivalence between young mothers and grandmothers (15, 57, 65).* According to Benedek (8), the prospective grandmother preparing her daughter for childbirth affectively recalls her own mother's attitudes and assistance with *her* pregnancy. She also recalls both the pleasurable and frightening experiences she herself had with delivery and lactation. However, in reliving her own pregnancy through a deep unconscious identification with her daughter, it sometimes happens that a woman develops an anxious over-identification, which later interferes with the potential pleasures of grandparenthood.

This identification with her daughter can be a lifelong pattern which characterizes one type of "good grandmother" noted by Deutsch (15). For this type of woman, grandmotherhood is not equated with a continuation of her own motherhood; rather, she experiences a "new edition" of motherhood through identification with her daughter. While portions of her world are reawakening in what Benedek calls the "new lease on life" (8) afforded by grandparenthood, Deutsch maintains that the process of identification involves the dangerous unconscious wish to take someone else's place. Consequently, this type of grandmother may be anxious because, "deep in her psychic life she feels the competing jealousy she wants to avoid" (15).

A second type of grandmother mentioned by Deutsch uses the experience of grandmotherhood to continue her own motherhood, and reacts to her grandchildren just as she did to her own children. In fact, for this type of woman the birth of her grandchild is symbolically equated with the return of her own child, and the return of her role as the indispensable provider to young children. If this type of woman is too actively solicitous, her own daughter may consider her an interference.

Deutsch finds that the most contented grandmothers are those who are free of competitive strivings and, contrary to Benedek (8), need no identifications and seek no repetitions. She depicts a woman who is freer at this stage than at any other because: "she is freed from her own passions . . . free of all human ambivalence" (15). This view of grandmotherhood seems unreal, idealistic, and derived from a sterotyped impression of old age. However, even this "grandmother par excellence," contends Deutsch, risks conflict with her daughter due to the desire to pamper her grandchild.

---

*This grandmother/mother relationship is the only one of four possible gender combinations between grandparents and their adult children which has received adequate study, with a particular dearth of material on grandfatherhood.

The other type of grandmothers, the "wicked" ones, are only briefly described by Deutsch as women who either want to possess their grandchildren or take no interest in them at all. Like Deutsch, DeBeauvoir (quoted in Rheingold, 57) assumes that the feelings of the grandmother toward the grandchild are extensions of those that she feels toward her own daughter. She also mentions the propensity of grandmothers to displace their hostile impulses onto their grandchildren. Rheingold (57) concludes that such transference problems and maternal over-identification are common, and result from unresolved intrapsychic conflicts with the grandmother's own mother.

Cohler and Grunebaum (12) argue that this research has mistakenly ascribed the source of the ambivalence to struggles over control and autonomy. Instead, their findings suggest that the more significant issues revolve around the young mother's increased demands upon her mother for assistance and advice regarding child-care, and the grandmother's resentment of this increased dependency.

This suggestion that grandparents may be unwilling to provide extensive child-care touches on one of the central paradoxes in the grandparenting literature. Earlier studies, which espoused the view that grandparents seek a parental role vis-à-vis the grandchild (15, 57, 65), are in sharp contrast to the viewpoint presented above and corroborated in other studies (2, 27, 48, 58), which indicate that grandparents neither desire nor practice a parental surrogate role. Neugarten and Weinstein (48), for instance, found that the majority of American grandparents adopted a "fun-seeking" style in relationship to their grandchildren, rather than one emphasizing baby-sitting or primary care.

Those studies which reveal a grandparental preference for freedom from their adult children's demands may be better understood in relation to their reactions to children leaving home. Thus, a parallel theme in the literature exists with regard to the "empty nest" syndrome. Here, too, early findings which suggest that women in mid-life react with depression when their youngest child leaves home have been challenged. Neugarten, Wood, Kraines, and Loomis (46) and Deutscher (16) found that, to the contrary, the majority of individuals studied looked forward to the increased leisure time available in the post-parental years.

However, the dialogue concerning parental reactions to growing and separating children bears reexamination. The implicit assumption in the literature that the youngest child's departure from the home marks the event which ushers in the stage of "post-parenthood" needs to be broadened. Depending upon the socioeconomic level and ethnic standards, the timing and impact of a child's separation might vary considerably. Frequently, within white middle-class families, for example, a child's leaving home to enter college merely represents another transitional phase. In such cases the student's sense of "home" has not yet shifted away from the parental home, and while he maintains a separate residence, he remains financially and emotionally dependent upon the family. The specific factors which determine when a parent feels the "nest" is emptying, and in what stages he/she must relinquish parental prerogatives no longer appropriate to the separating adolescent, have yet to be elucidated. The child's marriage and pregnancy may be equally critical life events which signal to the parents that the nuclear family must become dyadic once again.

The task of releasing children may well be a multiphasic one, based upon parental reactions to those critical events which indicate that the child is entering adulthood. The child's transition into parenthood can be thought of as the third and last phase in this separation. In fact, Hill and Aldous (28) argue that in American society it is the transition into parenthood which represents the individual's entrance into adulthood.

If the transition into grandparenthood involves such a separation from one's own offspring, one might expect the derivatives of earlier struggles with dependency, separation, and individuation to be stimulated and to reemerge, providing the opportunity to rework and revise earlier adaptations.

While the movement from what Mahler (42) called a symbiotic all-encompassing tie with the mother toward separation and finally individuation has been primarily discussed as a phase belonging to early childhood, the vicissitudes of this developmental task are manifest throughout the life-cycle (10, 12, 42, 51, 62). According to Mahler:

> As is the case with any intrapsychic process, this one reverberates throughout the life-cycle. It is never finished; it can always become reactivated; new phases of the life-cycle witness new derivatives of the earliest process still at work (42).

If we postulate that grandparenthood may be one such "new phase," perhaps the research indicating a lack of grandparental interest in assuming surrogate parental activities may be re-interpreted. Rather than representing a desire for distance, as has been generally assumed, it may signal a shift toward individuation and an attempt to redefine one's role toward one's children in a different, though not necessarily more distant, manner. Even if some grandparents do manifest defensive distancing mechanisms in response to increased demands for dependence, this could represent the unwillingness to regress to a former stage of ego adaptation, and one step toward a reorientation in object relations and roles.

Further evidence for the likelihood of such reanimated themes in grand-parenthood is found in Benedek's theories about parenthood in general (8, 9). She explores parenthood as a developmental process in which intra-psychic conflicts from childhood are recapitulated in the various phases of parenthood. While Benedek posits the revival of that past developmental conflict in the parent which corresponds to the child's current developmental level, she writes most fully and convincingly about the early years of par-enting and the mother's renewed capacity to identify with her infant's de-pendency. Specifically, the mother's memories of her own infancy are activated in the current emotional interaction with her young child and enable her to empathically respond to the infant in a complex identification. Winnicott (66), too, conceptualizes the source of the mother's ability to adapt to her infant's needs and to provide an atmosphere in which mother/infant mutuality can flourish as reflecting her own experience of infancy and its recrudescence. Perhaps Benedek's concept of this parental tendency can be extended to the latter phases of parenthood and include the grandparents' relationship to the grown child. If so, one could expect the new grandmother, in harmony with her daughter, the new mother, to reexperience her own pregnancy and childbirth as well as the derivatives of infantile dependency.

During the transition into grandparenthood, then, one might expect to see the reemergence of tension involving issues of separation and depen-dency. These issues may have the potential for a healthy resolution in a simultaneous re-identification with the child and grandchild, as well as in increased differentiation from them. We would expect some prospective grandmothers to be especially vulnerable to the temptation to exert control over the pregnant daughter's plans, behaviors, and attitudes. Attempts to restrain such urges, recognizing that they are inappropriate, would also be expected. Rekindled memories of one's own or one's wife's experiences of pregnancy and of early parenthood might also emerge at this time. De-pending upon the individual's intrapsychic constellation and concomitant life circumstances at the time of entry into grandparenthood, such a resurgence has the potential to cause conflict as well as to provide the opportunity for further growth and mastery.

GRANDPARENTHOOD AND THE PSYCHOLOGY OF THE SELF

The stages of middle and late adulthood may be characterized by narcis-sistic vulnerability (8, 26, 51). Therefore, the interaction of the vicissitudes of a person's narcissism (his sense of self) with the life event of grandparenthood bears exploration. It is possible that grandparenthood helps to bring about a late life transformation of narcissism, or, alternatively, fosters the emergence of buried narcissistic fixations.

The term "narcissism," when viewed from the perspective of Heinz Kohut's work (36, 37, 38), refers to his theory that the growth of the self constitutes a separate but parallel developmental line from that of object relations, with phase-appropriate infantile stages as well as the potential for fixation and for later transformation of narcissistic energies with maturity. From his work one can extrapolate the specific characteristics which might be found in an individual suffering from a cohesive but weakened or defective self. Generally, for instance, he would manifest lability of self-esteem and extreme sensitivity to disappointments. Such a disorder in the self reflects a failure during early life of the parental capacity to respond to the appropriate narcissistic requirements of the child—to lovingly "mirror" the child's pride in his achievements and to permit the child to idealize and merge with the calming function and strength of the parent (39).

Just as one can specify the characteristics of an arrested narcissist—a person with major fixations or structural deficiencies in this sphere of his personality—so, too, can the characteristics of transformed narcissism be delimited within this framework. Such transformations are manifested in individuals with a cohesive self, reflecting an optimal early environment in which the parent was responsive to the child's narcissistic needs. In this case, the full maturation of these primitive structures can be seen in such autonomous achievements of the ego as humor, wisdom, empathy, and creativity. The potential interaction of each of these ego functions with grandparenthood can be illustrated with examples from the literature.

The grandparenting literature, though primarily written with the grandchild as referent, extols the unique qualities of grandparental love (49, 67). A panoply of labels is applied in an effort to describe this warmth and understanding, and the qualitative difference between this love and other forms is ascribed to various factors. Robertson (58), for instance, implicates the grandparent's increased leisure time as the critical variable in the special bond, while Albrecht (2) suggests it results from the grandparent's freedom from being reflected upon by the child's failures or misbehaviors. Others, most notably family-oriented theoreticians, emphasize the buffering function grandparents can serve in the family (27, 60). These qualities can perhaps be subsumed under the term "empathy," a capacity thought to reflect the mature expression of narcissistic energies. Empathy, according to Olden (50), is defined as "the capacity of the subject to instinctively and intuitively feel as the object does." An empathic response involves an oscillation between moments of subjective involvement and others in which there is a "detached recognition of shared feeling. Empathy presupposes the existence of the object as a separate individual, entitled to his own feelings" (52).

Thus, the idea that the empathic potential may be released in the relationship between grandparent and grandchild dovetails with the suggestion that increased individuation may be manifest with entry into grandparenthood. It would be important, therefore, to note the matrices in which empathy emerges during grandparenthood and to be sensitive to changes within the new grandparent's capacity for empathy.

Humor, which Kohut also cites as often indicative of a narcissistic transformation, is discussed in an anthropological study by Radcliffe-Brown (54) as the major mode of communication between grandparents and grandchildren within several cultures. There is an almost universal way of organizing the relationships of alternate generations to one another, he maintains, called "the joking relationship." In such a relationship, one member continually teases the other, but the latter must not be offended. One common form of the joke is for a male grandchild to pretend that his grandmother is his wife, or for the grandfather to pretend that his grandchild's wife is his own.*

Radcliffe-Brown's thesis is that such "joking relations" exist in relationships which, by their nature, encompass ambivalence; the humor functions to simultaneously discharge and soften the aggression, thereby preserving the tie. This thesis begins to examine and analyze the complex identification between grandparent and grandchild from a cross-cultural perspective. The symbolic link between the members of this dyad, he contends, includes a

---

*The oedipal implications in this form of the joke are apparent. While the grandchild's occasional displacement of oedipal longings from the parent onto the grandparent has been cited in the psychoanalytic literature (19, 32, 33, 56), the grandparent's revived oedipal longings and jealousies toward the child or grandchild have been relatively unexplored. Rangell (55), however, discusses the persisting unresolved oedipal conflicts which are apt to become reactivated in the fifth decade of life, during grandparenthood, and during various stages of one's child's growth. The residuals of the parent's unresolved oedipal problems may occur in later life, according to Rangell:

> stimulated both by the sense of declining power and by contrast, by the lusty coming of age of our children, . . . but this time with a reversal of the process. The object now is not one's own powerful parent, but one's child, grown to his zenith . . . Moreover, just as in the original oedipal problem the solution was largely effected by identification with the . . . parent . . . so in the reverse process healthy derivatives again ensue by means of a process of identification . . . with the lives and fortunes of one's children. There is even another chance, when, as a grandparent, one can again repeat the process of identification and vicariously relive the youthful hopes and deeds of still the next generation (55).

hostile element which he attributes to the unavoidable "social disjunction" inherent in the relationship. While grandchildren are newly entering into social transactions, their grandparents are simultaneously retiring from them. Thus, the grandchildren, in essence, displace their elders.

Creativity, another achievement which Kohut maintains is related to the mature expression of narcissistic drives, has not been directly discussed in relationship to grandparenthood. However, this capacity is included in Erikson's discussion of generativity (18), a quality which potentially emerges in middle adulthood. Mature man, according to Erikson, needs encouragement from that which he has produced and nurtured, and must be able to identify with his products. While the concept of generativity stresses the concern with establishing and guiding succeeding generations, it also involves the more general relationship to one's creative products. Erikson regards generativity as an essential life stage which enables man to expand his ego interest and "libidinal investment to that which is being generated." Stagnation and personal impoverishment result from a failure of the development of this capacity. Erikson attributes the inability to develop this stage to early deficiencies in "basic trust," or to "excessive self-love," implicitly suggesting a deficiency in the narcissistic sector of the personality. This complements Kohut's claim that creativity, as one aspect of generativity, involves a transformation of narcissism in the sense that it manifests the ego's ability to harness relatively primitive structures into complex and new configurations (38).

The mechanisms through which generativity prevents emotional impoverishment need to be further clarified through an examination of the symbolic meaning of the grandchild to the grandparent. While early psychoanalytic writing elegantly discussed the symbolic meaning of grandparents to grandchildren, emphasizing fantasy (1, 19, 32, 33, 56), there has been no equivalent work from the point of view of the grandparent.

Perhaps grandparenthood, in highlighting one's own generative abilities, serves a reparative function which helps to counterbalance some of aging's natural blows to one's self-esteem. Huyck implicitly supports this idea in the following statement: "Grandparenthood . . . can give life a renewed sense of generativity, and provides intimations of immortality" (29). Huyck's suggestion that grandparenthood provides "intimations of immortality" bears exploration, since the ability to come to terms with one's finitude is frequently cited as a significant task of middle adulthood. One characteristic of individuals manifesting severe narcissistic vulnerability would be their inability to conceive of their own death, while the transformation of such energies would be evident in an individual who emotionally accepts his own transience. Entry into grandparenthood may specifically highlight this issue of one's finitude.

Narcissism and Finitude

An important shift in one's outlook on time and life has been observed during middle adulthood, when, rather than thinking of one's age in terms of number of years since birth, an individual begins to consider the amount of time left in the life span before death (17, 21, 30, 45). This time reversal and budding awareness of one's own mortality are frequently observed in connection with grandparenthood (8), as is Huyck's idea that through one's family one gains a sense of immortality and more easily accepts one's own physical transience. Benedek emphasizes the parents' longing for: "something beyond their ken . . . and the wish to survive in the grandchildren" (8). Fried and Stern (20) mention the pleasure their sample of grandparents derived from the sense that their physical lives continued, as it were, "through" their grandchildren.* This ability to feel that some aspect of one's life continues with succeeding generations requires that one is relatively at peace with one's finitude and physical limitations and, in some measure, albeit perhaps unconsciously, able to tolerate the idea that one must die. What is the process by which one accomplishes this attitude in middle adulthood? Freud, in 1915, depicted the enormity of the task of accepting one's own death:

> We were prepared to maintain that death was the necessary outcome of life. . . . In reality, however, we were accustomed to behave as if it were otherwise. We displayed an unmistakable tendency to "shelve" death, to eliminate it from life. We tried to hush it up. . . . That is our own death, of course. . . . No one believes in his own death. . . . In the unconscious everyone is convinced of his own immortality (quoted in Jaques, 31).

Levinson (40) describes the massive, tumultuous reappraisal of one's life and the considerable task of "de-illusionment" which confronts men during the mid-life transition. One result of this loss or reduction of illusions, fre-

---

*A cross-cultural example in which this relationship was consciously acknowledged was found by Gorlitz among the Kamano in the Eastern Highlands of Papua New Guinea. There is a reciprocal term used for both grandparent and grandchild (*tata*), and the birth of the first grandchild is said to enable the paternal grandparents to die fulfilled, knowing that they have been replaced. This also exemplifies the importance of lines of filiation in certain cultures. In this patrilineal society, the maternal grandparents are not said to be replaced.

quently a painful process, is the freedom "to admire others in a more genuine, less idealizing way." In the move from early to middle adulthood, one gives up the "youthful dream" which is derived in part from the normal fantasies of omnipotence in early childhood. Levinson stresses that "some degree of normal omnipotence," however, is also necessary in young adulthood, when the self is frail and vulnerable. The idealization of external entities, he maintains, serves to protect one's illusions about the self.

Elliot Jaques (31) discusses the mid-life crisis in terms similar to Levinson's (although his theories extend to women) as the time in which one must confront one's own imperfections and the inevitability of one's own death, as well as the inherently destructive impulses within each of us. He, like Levinson, stresses the idealism and optimism in the unconscious fantasies of early adulthood.

While Jaques and Levinson adopt disparate conceptual frameworks* through which to explain similar phenomena, the changes noted by both as integral parts of accepting one's own mortality can be usefully examined within Kohut's framework of the psychology of the self. Kohut (38) delineates two normal developmental phases of the self during infancy—one in which the infant experiences himself as flawless, and the other in which security is attained by basking in the reflection of the idealized perfect object's love. Levinson and Jaques describe the adaptive use of the derivatives of both this grandiose stage and what Kohut calls the stage of the idealized parental imago in moving from early to mature adulthood and in beginning to accept one's mortality. It seems feasible that many of the capacities which emerge or reemerge during middle adulthood might involve the transformation of archaic narcissistic energies, and that this paradigm may be productive.

Jaques contends that if an individual does not adjust to the conscious contemplation of his own death in mid-life, death becomes equated with depressive chaos and confusion. Such middle-aged individuals who compulsively deny death to mitigate a chaotic and helpless internal environment may manifest symptoms including: "hypochondriachal concern over health and appearance, emergence of sexual promiscuity to prove youth and potency, . . . lack of genuine enjoyment of life, (and) frequency of religious concern" (31). Each of these symptoms noted by Jaques is, in fact, charac-

---

*Levinson discusses mid-life "individuation" within an ego-analytic framework, while Jaques' analysis is derived from a Kleinian perspective. Jaques contends that the task of moving from young adulthood to mature adulthood involves reworking the "depressive position" of infancy, a normal developmental phase described by Melanie Klein (35), during which the infant begins the task of tolerating ambivalence and of accepting extreme instinctual urges of both love and hatred toward the primary object.

teristic of a regression to an early narcissistic phase of development.

Thus, the work of Jaques and others, when viewed from the perspective of the psychology of the self, suggests that the mid-life task of accepting one's own imperfections and finitude requires a transformation of narcissistic energies. Breakdown during this period, according to Jaques, involves a depression or an attempt to defend against depressive anxieties. But the symptoms he presents may also be viewed as restitutive attempts to protect a defective or depleted self.

Grandparenthood is one of the few life roles which an individual does not elect. In fact, it is an unwelcome reminder of aging for many middle-aged individuals, and may evoke painful memories of the past (29). The lack of control inherent in this transition may be experienced as a narcissistic injury, especially in individuals already sensitive to some of the losses inherent in aging. Mead poignantly describes her own personal struggle with this element of the transition into grandparenthood:

> I suddenly realized that through no act of my own I had become biologically related to a new human being. This was one thing that had never come up in discussions of grandparenthood and had never before occurred to me. . . . I had never thought how strange it was to be involved at a distance in the birth of a biological descendent . . . the idea that as a grandparent one was dealing with action at a distance—that somewhere, miles away, a series of events occurred that changed one's own status forever—I had not thought of that and I found it very odd (43).

This convergence of narcissistic issues with increasing age is noted by Parens and Saul (51), who emphasize the significance of inner sustainment and self-reliance in determining an individual's resilience during late adulthood. But aging deals a harsh blow to both; self-reliance is attacked by the reduction of individual capacities and the loss of objects, while inner sustainment is undermined by the inevitable losses in ego achievements which provide a crucial source of self-esteem (such as the loss of a job). "Where self-esteem is still largely based on infantile narcissistic residuals, the subject will suffer from self-devaluations accompanying aging" (51).

Gutmann (26) too, describes the resurgence of narcissism during the post-parental years, which can take the form of hypochondriasis or a repetitive need for reminiscence, in which "the older person, unable to dramatize his present depleted self, seeks confirmation in an idealized past." In his view, this "post-parental crisis of narcissism" results from the reinvestment of narcissistic claims in the self, once the grown children have become autonomous, and are consequently less available to the parents as self-extensions.

Those individuals who have reached satisfactory levels of emotional maturity, however, in both the narcissistic and object-related sphere of the personality, should be able to suffer "less narcissistic devaluation by the aging process and to maintain 'integrity' of ego functioning and ego identity in Erikson's sense" (51).

In sum, if the post-parental years represent a time of narcissistic vulnerability, one must be especially attuned to the ways in which grandparenthood meshes with these issues. The literature raises issues which suggest that, depending upon an individual's maturational achievements within this sector of the personality, grandparenthood may exacerbate the narcissistic injuries of aging or may help to soothe them.

Thus, for persons with narcissistic fixations or deficiencies in the self, one might expect to see the emergence of any of the following symptoms with entry into grandparenthood:

1. Hypochondriasis.
2. Renewed fears about aging and death, manifest in a preoccupation with these issues or in a rigid system of denial.
3. A rekindling of painful memories of one's own (or one's wife's) pregnancy and early years of parenting, manifest in an over-identification with one's daughter.

By the same token, entry into grandparenthood may serve the specific function of channelling and transforming revitalized narcissistic energies for an individual relatively free of narcissitic fixations. In this case, one might expect to see:

1. Heightened awareness of one's own transience and limitations.
2. The reparative effects of generativity manifest in:
   a. The rekindled memories of one's past gratifications, in an identification with one's daughter (especially for the grandmother).
   b. The symbolic identification with one's grandchild, providing a sense of continuity with the future, and thus making more acceptable the concept of one's own finitude.
3. The use of humor as a buffer against the narcissistic injuries inherent in the impending stages of aging and death, and as an adaptive means of expressing ambivalence toward the younger generation.
4. Shifts in the capacity for empathy.

GRANDPARENTHOOD AND THE SECOND HALF OF LIFE

The transition into grandparenthood is an event which must be viewed within the larger life-cycle context in which it occurs. As grandparenthood today usually comes within middle, rather than old age (29), the independent and yet converging issues of middle life must be considered. In addition to the mid-life awareness of one's mortality, Margaret Huyck (30) identifies two broad themes of middle-age in the literature: aging as loss, and middle-age as emergence.

Aging as Loss

One of the tasks appropriate to middle life, in preparation for aging and for one's eventual death, is a coming to terms with losses (30, 31, 47). Losses are significant during the later half of life, be they tangible personal losses, as in the death of someone close; social losses, such as the loss of an important life-role or an accustomed means of livelihood (5); or losses of capacities, such as beauty or strength. The disengagement point of view (14) envisions aging primarily in terms of these inevitable losses, and stresses the necessity of emotionally withdrawing from the attitudes and activities of early and middle adulthood.

Paradoxical findings in the grandparenthood literature are frequently rendered intelligible when viewed within the broader context of the author's view of aging. Much of the research, for instance, which stresses the negative influence of the grandparent upon children, or grandparent's domineering behavior, seems derived from the above-mentioned narrow focus on aging as decline. Fried and Stern (20), for example, seem to regard the preference of parents to remain relatively independent from their adult children as a defensive attempt to cope with the loss of function and prestige in the family. And Vollmer's theory (65) about the grandmother's inability to maintain appropriate distance from her grandchildren typifies the disengagement perspective at its extreme. Based on a small number of clinical cases, Vollmer portrays the grandmother's tendency to use the grandchild as a means of relieving her from her life of futility and boredom, and of compulsively denying her incipient death. Because she is old, she is rigid and insensitive; she infantilizes the child while disparaging her daughter out of jealousy. These attitudes result from the attempt to:

> relive the central experience of a former period of life during which she stood at the zenith of her career as a woman. . . . Unfortunately

the grandmother's situation is entirely different from that in which she first experienced motherhood: . . . then her life was crammed with duties, tasks, and interests; now the scope of her practical activities has dwindled to boredom. . . . The grandmother is not a suitable custodian of the care and rearing of her grandchild; . . . She is a disturbing factor against which we are obligated to protect the child, according to the best of our ability (65).

Rheingold, too, describes a "poignant sense of loss" disturbing women at the menopause, and their "desperate attempt to turn time backward" (57).

These pessimistic views of aging which stress massive social losses converge with the common stereotypes of our youth-oriented culture which equate age with decay. In this view, all of the changes which occur during the later stages of adulthood are regarded as losses; the potential gains of this period of life are ignored, as is individual variability.

In fact, the University of Chicago group who developed the disengagement theory later reexamined the process of adjustment to loss in aging within a large multidimensional approach. Contrary to the earlier finding, suggesting that high morale was maintained for people over 65 years old by disengaging, this study found high life satisfaction to be positively correlated with an active and involved social life. Bernice Neugarten summarized the revised theory as one which postulated that personality organization was the mediating factor in influencing adaptation among the elderly (45). From a social psychological perspective, these investigators have found the critical element in aging to be neither engagement nor disengagement, but the personality's ability for adaptation and change.

Middle Age as Emergence

One approach to measuring an individual's perception of his life span is to focus specifically on meaningful transitions, as opposed to viewing lifetime as a continuum (45). Exemplars of this tradition are Erikson (18), Lowenthal, Thurnher, and Chiriboga (41), Sheehy (59), and Levinson (40), who have attempted to adapt a stage theory approach to middle and later adulthood. Within their various schemas, an individual is thought to progress from one specific, invariate structural phase to the next, each phase posing its own challenges for growth and conflict.

An important implication of this approach is its view that the significance of a major life-cycle event, such as entry into grandparenthood, will be largely dependent upon the developmental frame and life structure in which it occurs, and therefore must be seen within the context of the whole person. This viewpoint points to a methodological flaw in much of the literature, which treats grandparenthood as an isolated variable in a person's life.

The second major approach to conceptualizing middle adulthood as a period of emergence involves the view that nascent capacities with the self, hitherto latent within the psyche, are allowed to emerge and find expression.

Gutmann posits a later life intrapsychic shift in sex-role characteristics (22, 24, 25, 26). Such age-graded changes in sex role occur with regularity across a wide range of cultures and according to Gutmann are intrinsic and developmental in nature. Utilizing naturalistic interviews and TAT data, Gutmann found a later life reversal in personality characteristics between the sexes (22, 23). Thus, men in early adulthood were characterized by active mastery of the environment, aggressivity, and a "phallic stance" concerned with power, while those in middle and later adulthood were more affiliative and accepting of their diffuse pregenital longings and sensuality. Women, on the other hand, were found with increasing age to shift to active mastery and a more assertive stance in which the urge for instrumentality, long denied in the service of tending children and the home, could finally emerge. There was a concurrent reorientation among women away from the family-dominated concerns of the maternal caretaker and toward the self and personal needs. This turnover in sex role characteristics during the post-parental years moves toward what Gutmann dubs "the normal unisex of later life" (24).

The transcultural regularities in sex-role distinctions during the phase of early parenthood, and in response to the decline of this "chronic emergency," suggest to Gutmann that sex-role distinctions have been shaped and have evolved in response to the requirements of infant care. During the early years of parenthood the woman must suppress her own outer-directed strivings in the service of nurturing her young within the home. By the same token, the man's passive and dependent longings are denied in order to protect the home and procure a livelihood for his family. During early adulthood, therefore, the male vicariously satisfies his own dependency longings via caring for his wife and children, while she lives out her desire for active mastery and instrumentality through her husband. Later life, however, provides the opportunity for those previously suppressed capacities to emerge. Men may reclaim aspects of themselves often regarded as "feminine," such as a concern for the family and nurturance, while women may realize their strivings for power. In sum, then, the trend in later life is toward a bisexual modality and what Gutmann calls the desire for omni-potentiality (26).

Neugarten and Associates (47) utilized a multidimensional approach to study intrapsychic continuity and change in middle adulthood. Age-related changes in the preferred modes of handling impulses and affects were noted; in both sexes there was a shift from an outer world orientation to a preoccupation with inner life, called "interiority." There seemed to be a decreased "emotional cathexis toward persons and objects in the outer world" (47), in which individuals attended increasingly to the satisfaction of their personal needs. These views are complementary to the research reviewed earlier, indicating a resurgence of narcissistic issues and egocentricity with increased age.

Fried and Stern (20) found evidence in a few of their subjects of a grandfather's excessive warmth toward his grandchild, attitudes which the subjects' wives ascribed to guilt over the relative neglect and lack of nurturance expressed toward their own children when they were young. While this interpretation of compensatory warmth may accurately assess their husbands' motivation, the theory of a male late-life shift toward increased receptivity of affiliative needs enriches such data and may explain why such a change in attitude occurs at this time. Perhaps grandfatherhood provides a timely opportunity for men to give expression to their newly emergent "maternal" instincts in a manner which was unavailable to them or prohibited when their own offspring were infants.

Fried and Stern (20) also noted that women were more absorbed by their relationship to their children than were their husbands, and experienced more friction with their offspring as well. The woman's continued greater involvement in the family probably represents a carryover from earlier years, but the friction may involve the older woman's shift away from such concerns with the family toward a greater concern with herself and her own needs. Lowenthal et al. (41) found that, while the women in their study experienced the late-life developmental shifts discussed earlier, often the only culturally available outlet for the emergent self-assertiveness was through the family. In this case, women became more dominant toward their husbands and sometimes toward their grown children.

Albrecht (3) found men to have a greater tolerance for accepting the independence of their offspring, a finding which, if borne out, might also reflect some women's need for dominance within the family. In some families one might see the husband's reluctance to relinquish or even share his wife, the object toward whom his long-repressed dependency strivings have finally emerged. Hence, the male's greater "tolerance" for accepting the emptying of the nest might actually mask his *preference* for being alone, once again, with his wife. In this regard, one should be sensitive to the prospective and new grandfather's potentially rivalrous feelings toward his daughter and grandchild, both of whom encroach upon his newly claimed territory.

Thus, grandparenthood can be understood only within the wider context of the life-cycle. Salient changes occurring within middle life impact upon grandparenthood and help to shape the individual experience, just as the experience of grandparenthood may give a focus to middle-life changes within the self, or perhaps provide an arena for their expression.

REFERENCES

1. ABRAHAM, K. (1913). Some remarks on the role of the grandparent in the psychology of neurosis. *Clinical Papers and Essays on Psycho-analysis* (Vol. I), London: Hogarth, 1955. (Reissued, 1979, New York: Brunner/Mazel)
2. ALBRECHT, R. (1954). The parental responsibilities of grandparents. *Marriage and Family Living, 16*, 201-204.
3. ALBRECHT, R. (1954). Relationships of older parents with their children. *Marriage and Family Living, 16*, 32-35.
4. APPLE, O. (1956). Social structure of grandparenthood. *American Anthropologist, 58*, 656-663.
5. BART, P. (1974). Depression in middle-aged women. In: M. Huyck (ed.), *Growing Older*. Englewood Cliffs, N.J.: Prentice-Hall.
6. BELL, N. (1962). Extended family relations of disturbed and well families. *Family Process, 1*, 175-193.
7. BENEDEK, T. (1959). Parenthood as a developmental phase: A contribution to the libido theory. *Journal of the American Psychoanalytic Association, 7*, 389-417.
8. BENEDEK, T. (1970). Parenthood during the life cycle. In: Anthony, E. and Benedek, T. (eds.) *Parenthood: Its Psychology and Psychopathology*. Boston: Little, Brown.
9. BENEDEK, T. (1970). The psychobiology of pregnancy. In: Anthony, E. and Benedek, T. (eds.), *Parenthood: Its Psychology and Psychopathology*. Boston: Little, Brown.
10. BOSZORMENYI-NAGY, I., and SPARK, G. (1973). *Invisible Loyalties: Reciprocity in Intergenerational Family Therapy*. New York: Harper and Row.
11. BOYD, R. (1969). The valued grandparent: A changing social role. In: Donahue, W. (ed.), *Living in a Multigenerational Family*. Ann Arbor, MI: Institute of Gerontology, 1969.
12. COHLER, B., and GRUNEBAUM, H. (in press). *Mothers and Grandmothers: Personality and Childcare across Three Generations*. New York: Wiley.
13. COHLER, B., GRUNEBAUM, H., WEISS, J., and MORAN, D. (1969). *The Childcare Attitudes of Two Generations of Mothers*. Revision of paper presented at the Annual Meeting of the American Orthopsychiatric Association, New York, 1969.
14. CUMMING, E., and HENRY, W. (1961). *Growing Old*. New York: Basic, Books.
15. DEUTSCH, H. (1945). *The Psychology of Women (Vol. II, Motherhood)*. New York: Grune & Stratton.
16. DEUTSCHER, I. (1968). The quality of postparental life. In: Neugarten, B. (ed.), *Middle Age and Aging*. Chicago: University of Chicago Press. (Originally published, 1964).
17. EISSLER, K. (1955). *The Psychiatrist and the Dying Patient*. New York: International Universities Press.
18. ERIKSON, E. (1963). *Childhood and Society* (Rev. ed.). New York: Norton.
19. FERENCZI, S. (1950). The grandfather complex. In: *Further Contributions to the Theory and Technique of Psychoanalysis*. London: Hogarth Press, 1950. (Originally published, 1913.) (Reissued, 1980, New York: Brunner/Mazel)

20. FRIED, E. G., and STERN, K. (1948). The situation of the aged within the family. *American Journal of Orthopsychiatry, 18,* 31-54.
21. GAP Report. (1973). *The Joys and Sorrows of Parenthood.*
22. GUTMANN, D. (1964). An exploration of ego configurations in middle and later life. In: Neugarten, B. and Associates (eds.), *Personality in Middle and Later Life.* New York: Atherton Press.
23. GUTMANN, D. (1974). Alternatives to disengagement: The old men of the Highland Druze. In: LeVine, R. (ed.), *Culture and Personality: Contemporary Readings.* Chicago: Aldine.
24. GUTMANN, D. (1975). Parenthood: A key to the comparative study of the life cycle. In: Datan, N. and Ginsberg, L. (eds.), *Life-Span Developmental Psychology: Normative Life Crises.* New York: Academic Press.
25. GUTMANN, D. (1977). The cross-cultural perspective: Notes toward a comparative psychology of aging. In: Birren, J. E., and Schaie, K. W. (eds.), *Handbook of Psychology and Aging.* New York: Van Nostrand Reinhold.
26. GUTMANN, D. (1978). *Personal Transformations in the Post-Parental Period: A Cross-Cultural View.* Paper presented at the meetings of the American Association of the Advancement of Science, Washington, D.C.
27. HADER, M. (1965). The importance of grandparents in family life. *Family Process, 4,* 228-240.
28. HILL, R., and ALDOUS, J. (1969). Socialization for marriage and parenthood. In: Goslin, D. (ed.), *Handbook for Socialization Theory and Research.* Chicago: Rand McNally.
29. HUYCK, M. (1974). *Growing Older.* New Jersey: Prentice-Hall.
30. HUYCK, M. (1977). Aging: The ultimate experience. *The Vassar Quarterly,* 16.
31. JAQUES, E. (1965). Death and the mid-life crisis. *The International Journal of Psychoanalysis, 46,* 502-513.
32. JONES, E. (1956). The phantasy of the reversal of generations. In: Wood, W. (Ed.), *Papers on Psychoanalysis* (5th ed.). Baltimore: William Wood & Company. (Originally published, 1913.)
33. JONES, E. (1938). The significance of the grandfather for the fate of the individual. In: Wood, W. (ed.), *Papers on Psychoanalysis* (4th ed.). Baltimore: William Wood & Company. (Originally published, 1913.)
34. KAHANA, E., and KAHANA, B. (1971). Theoretical and research perspectives on grandparenthood. *Aging and Human Development, 2,* 261-268.
35. KLEIN, M. (1948). A contribution to the psychogenesis of manic-depressive states. In: *Contributions to Psycho-Analysis.* London: Hogarth. (Originally published, 1935.)
36. KOHUT, H. (1966). Forms and transformations of narcissism. *Journal of the American Psychoanalytic Association, 14,* 233-272.
37. KOHUT, H. (1968). The psychoanalytic treatment of narcissistic personality disorders. *The Psychoanalytic Study of the Child, 23,* 86-113.
38. KOHUT, H. (1971). *The Analysis of the Self.* New York: International Universities Press.
39. KOHUT, H., and WOLF, E. (1978). The disorders of the self and their treatment: An outline. *International Journal of Psychoanalysis, 59,* 413-425.
40. LEVINSON, D. (1977). The mid-life transition: A period of psychosocial development. *Psychiatry, 40* (2), 99-112.
41. LOWENTHAL, M., THURNHER, M., and CHIRIBOGA, D. (1975). *Four Stages of Life: A Psychosocial Study of Women and Men Facing Transition.* San Francisco: Jossey-Bass.
42. MAHLER, M. (1972). On the first three phases of the separation-individuation process. *International Journal of Psychoanalysis, 53,* 333-338.
43. MEAD, M. (1972). *Blackberry Winter.* New York: Simon & Schuster.
44. NADEL, S. (1953). *The Foundations of Social Anthropology.* Glencoe, Ill.: Free Press.
45. NEUGARTEN, B. L. (1977). Personality and aging. In: Birren, J. E. and Schaie, K. W. (eds.), *Handbook of the Psychology of Aging.* New York: Van Nostrand Reinhold.

46. NEUGARTEN, B. L., WOOD, V., KRAINES, R. J., and LOOMIS, B. (1963). Women's attitudes toward the menopause. *Vitae Humana, 6,* 140-151.
47. NEUGARTEN, B. L., and Associates. (1964). *Personality in Middle and Late Life.* New York: Atherton.
48. NEUGARTEN, B. L., and WEINSTEIN, K. (1968). The changing American grandparent. In: Neugarten, B. (ed.), *Middle Age and Aging.* Chicago: University of Chicago Press. (Originally published, 1964).
49. NOON, K. (1977). Maybe by next week I'll be a grandmother. *Voices, 12* (4), 60-62.
50. OLDEN, C. (1953). On adult empathy with children. *The Psychoanalytic Study of the Child, 8.,* 111-126.
51. PARENS, H., and SAUL, L. (1971). *Dependence in Man: A Psychoanalytic Study.* New York: International Universities Press.
52. PAUL, N. (1970). Parental empathy. In: Anthony, E. and Benedek, T. (eds.), *Parenthood: Its Psychology and Psychopathology.* Boston: Little, Brown.
53. RADCLIFFE-BROWN, A. (1951). A study of kinship systems. In: Parsons, T. et al. (eds.), *Theories of Society.* Glencoe, Il: Free Press. (Originally published, 1950.)
54. RADCLIFFE-BROWN, A. (1952). *On Joking Relationships: Structure and Function in Primitive Society.* New York: Free Press.
55. RANGELL, L. (1970). The return of the repressed "Oedipus." In: Anthony, E. and Benedek, T. (eds.), *Parenthood: Its Psychology and Psychopathology.* Boston: Little, Brown. (Originally published, 1955.)
56. RAPPAPORT, E. (1958). The grandparent syndrome. *The Psychoanalytic Quarterly, 27,* 518-537.
57. RHEINGOLD, J. (1964). *The Fear of Being a Woman: A Theory of Maternal Destruction.* New York: Grune & Stratton.
58. ROBERTSON, J. (1976). Significance of grandparents' perceptions of young adult grandchildren. *The Gerontologist, 16.*
59. SHEEHY, G. (1976). *Passages.* New York: Bantam.
60. SPARK, G. (1974). Grandparents and intergenerational family therapy. *Family Process, 13,* 225-237.
61. STAPLES, R., and SMITH, J. (1954). Attitudes of grandmothers and mothers toward child-rearing practices. *Child Development, 25,* 91-97.
62. STIERLIN, H. (1977). *Psychoanalysis and Family Therapy.* New York: Jason Aronson.
63. SUSSMAN, M. (1965). Relationships of adult children with their parents in the United States. In: Shanas, E. and Streib, G. (eds.), *Social Structure and the Family: Generational Relations.* Englewood Cliffs, NJ: Prentice-Hall.
64. TROLL, L. (1975). *Early and Middle Adulthood.* Monterey, Ca: Brooks/Cole.
65. VOLLMER, H. (1937). The grandmother: A problem in childrearing. *American Journal of Orthopsychiatry, 7,* 378-382.
66. WINNICOTT, D. (1970). The mother-infant experience of mutuality. In: Anthony, E. and Benedek, T. (eds.), *Parenthood: Its Psychology and Psychopathology.* Boston: Little, Brown, 1970.
67. ZINKER, J. (1977). On grandparently love. *Voices, 12* (4), 63-75.

12

ON PARENTING
ONE'S ELDERLY PARENT

RITA R. ROGERS, M.D.

Clinical Professor of Psychiatry,
Chief, Division of Child Psychiatry,
Harbor-UCLA Medical Center,
Torrance, California

INTRODUCTION

The transition to becoming a parent to one's elderly parent is not heralded by any rite of passage. There is no ceremony, no acknowledgment, no visible or tangible external change. There is only a subtle, almost imperceptible inner transformation for which external reality offers no cushions, while one's emotional resources are drawn off in a new direction.

Although a visible status change and awareness of what is occurring may be lacking, this experience of becoming a parent to one's elderly parent is a truly important event in the emotional calendar of a person. Because of the profound intergenerational impact which takes place, it has clinical significance for the understanding of the adult phase of parenting.

THE ONSET

Men and women usually find themselves faced with the dependency of their parents at a time in their own lives when they have to face themselves in a new light and from a new perspective. They have reached a stage when, looking squarely at their accomplishments and aspirations, they are forced to evaluate the balance between what they dreamed of becoming and what they actually became.

No longer can one with any pretense of emotional health anticipate the

187

possibility of becoming a piano virtuoso acclaimed by the world, while re- alizing the actuality of being an ineffectual housewife. No longer can one's cravings for glory be gratified by firm expectations that the children will achieve what was not quite accomplished by the parent. It is clear by this stage in an individual's life that one's children will or will not achieve their potential and are not hesitating to give strident messages to their parents of what they can, will, or want to do with their own lives. If they are emotionally healthy, they make it clear that what they do and are is for themselves and not for their parents. Integrating this message into one's selfhood necessitates fierce confrontation with oneself.

Invariably, when one has to look so starkly at oneself, one is inclined to look at one's parents. First, one turns to them and attempts to reach out for protection, for nurturing, for comfort, as in the days of faraway childhood. It is then that one notices, with a new painful awareness, what one's parents have attempted to convey for quite a while. It is they who now crave nur- turing, care, and support! Initially, their external reality frequently demands attention. Their health is deteriorating, their finances are strained, their locomotion hindered, their access to places and people limited, their op- portunities decreased. While their needs and wants have increased, for these very reasons fewer people and places want them. Thus, their emotional hurts and needs are augmented. For quite a while they have been signaling towards their children, usually unsuccessfully, that a shift has occurred, that they are the ones who now need to be looked after, cared for, and thought about. The more the external world decreases its contact with the elderly, the more they reach out for their grown-up children.

PARENTING UNDER THE IMPACT OF HOW ONE HAS BEEN PARENTED

There is a strong emotional reaction whenever our inner demand for being given to is not acknowledged. This upheaval is markedly intensified when, instead of being given to, more is demanded of us at a time when we ourselves feel depleted. The elderly parent and his/her demands are spe- cifically difficult to respond to. Whenever we face disappointments, rightfully or in a skewed form, we focus on our early childhood relationships, on our parents, on our old grievances, which proceed to become accentuated and caricatured. As we look at ourselves, we experience the constant impact of whom we begot and by whom we were begotten. As we crave for increased nurturing, we reevaluate how we nurtured our children through the prism of how we ourselves have been nurtured. The past becomes exacerbated.

Old hurts, old views, old distortions blend into the present needs, enmeshed and entangled.

Case Illustration

Mrs. R. is a 55-year-old married woman, tense, controlling, conscientious, mastering her life through painstaking attention to doing what is right. She has raised four daughters while beset by an overwhelming fear of possibly not being the kind of mother her mother was. The pain and hurt of ungratified mothering have permeated all aspects and yearnings of her life. Whenever somebody deals with her, be it in a grocery store, restaurant, office, or elsewhere, she always feels slighted and uncared for. Since her earliest childhood she has walked around with a hungry heart. Her mother's low esteem of her still resounds in her ears and feelings. Because of what she perceived as her mother's disapproval, she has always felt belittled by everybody. Her mother's low opinion of her academic potential made her attempt an academic career but her mother's disparagement led her to curtail it. Because of her mother's low regard of her as a woman, she has engaged in heterosexual relationships only with disdain and discomfort. Because of her mother's limited respect for her, she has held herself in very low esteem. Not to be a mother like her mother has been the anthem of her selfhood.

One by one the four daughters left the home, which was never a pleasant, happy one. Their leaving diminished her *raison d'être,* for now she could not use her daughters to prove that she was not a mother like her own. Their departure from home with seeming enjoyment at leaving her behind and out of their lives rekindled the feelings of relief she had felt when she escaped her mother, and simultaneously reawakened the guilt she had experienced at that time. When her daughters called, rather than enjoy their contacts, she found herself wondering whether they, too, called out of guilt and remorse rather than because of genuine wishes to be with her.

When her mother became ill and notified Mrs. R. of her impending surgery, Mrs. R. became intensely anxious and agitated and meekly attempted to cancel her therapeutic sessions for an indefinite period of time. Because of the conflict within herself over her mother's need of her as a nurturer, and because of her unwillingness and inability to give to her mother, she felt guilty for enjoying the caring she enjoyed in psychotherapy. She was immensely relieved when this was interpreted to her, and she was assured that it is understandable for her to find it hard to care for somebody from whom she has not experienced a sense of caring, and that in order to be able to give this nurturing she will find herself craving for more psychotherapeutic attention rather than less.

To herself, the therapist has wondered about the number of patients who might discontinue psychotherapy at such times without either the patients or therapists being aware of the actual reasons for their doing so.

Case Illustration

Mrs. B. was a married housewife of 45, who has been separated from her mother since age five because of the mother's chronic illness. She had gone through her entire life with a voracious hunger for mothering. She felt that she had failed her daughters, as a mother, was fixated on her sons, and vacillated irresolutely towards many people because of her special cravings for attention. Although she made various demands on physicians for care, medication and drugs, these experiences were shallow and unsatisfactory. Indeed, her demands were always arranged in such a fashion that they would annul each other. One physician was asked for "uppers" and one for "downers," one for the treatment of one disease while the other for a disease complete opposite to the previous. The patient frequently escaped her wifely and motherly duties by visits to her elderly aunts, whom she frequently referred to as "my mothers." When one of the aunts became terminally ill with cancer, she suddenly informed her therapist that she was going to take a trip to another country with "my family." To the therapist's surprise, it was the aunts whom she referred to as "her family," not her husband and children. An attempt to disentangle her emotionally from this most irrational plan of taking a terminally ill woman to a foreign country made it clear that the burden of caring for somebody who had been a substitute mother to her was being evaded by making-believe that she was a little girl going on a fun trip with "her mothers." Illness, which had robbed her of her own mother, had to be denied.

Case Illustration

Another patient, Mrs. C., had felt burdened throughout her married life with the presence of her mother in her home. She had asked her mother to come and live with her, but then throughout all these years she had never spoken to her mother, bitterly resenting having her there although never acknowledging it. Throughout her mother's years of invalidism she did all she had to do, even spending nights in the emergency room with her mother, but never conversed with her. After her mother's death, when she herself developed a chronic illness, she withdrew to what used to be her mother's room, spending her days as her mother used to, even though she suffered from a completely different condition. Toward her three children she exhibited inappropriate exaggerated mothering. She was always deeply embroiled in their affairs and precipitated all kinds of situations in the children's lives which made it necessary for them to move in and out of her house. When they lived in her home, her condition worsened and so did her psychosomatic disease. As soon as the children left the mother's home, however, another crisis occurred and one of them had to move in with children, dogs, and personal belonging.

Mrs. C. was plagued by these visits, but at the same time feared that her children might feel about her as she had felt about her own mother. She constantly tried to prove to herself that she was close to her children. She precipitated their moving in with her, but also resented having them in her house. Although acutely afraid that they might avoid conversing with her, as she had with her mother, she also could not give genuinely to them what had not been given to her.

PARENTING ONE'S PARENT UNDER THE PRISM OF SIBLING RIVALARY

Case Illustration

Mrs. D. was a quaint, 56-year-old lady who had felt slighted by other women throughout her entire married and professional life. She always thought that "they," the other women, were putting her down and attempting to boss her. By now she recognized that she had never overcome her intense rivalry toward her older sister. This older sister lived with their aged mother. When the mother broke her leg, the sister called Mrs. D.; who was surprised at the sister's "vitriolic outpour at her." She was unable to understand why her sister was so bitter about having to look after their mother. Indeed, she quoted the sister's fierce complaints about all doctors and their care for the elderly and her mistrust of their basic intentions. When asked whether the sister might feel that Mrs. D. should help care for the mother and was angry because she was not doing so, Mrs. D. denied this vehemently. This possibility was completely unacceptable to her emotional realities.

Presenting Dilemmas

The parenting of one's elderly parent exacerbates and revitalizes old sibling rivalries. The realization that one feels burdened by one's elderly parent brings about a revitalization of old unhealed wounds. The unsettled issues with one's siblings are the ones most likely to reopen. This is the time when one sensitively recalls how the mother and older sister shared secrets, how it hurt when the older sister was given coveted special clothing—the first fur coat, the first trip, a special birthday party. The younger sister remembers the alliance that seemed to exist between the mother and the older sister, which had provoked a sense of being small, insignificant, below the status of adult women. Now, years later, when the elderly parent is in need of parenting, the younger sister often yields responsibility to the older sister, as though to say, "You are the older one, therefore you take care of mother or father." At such a stage, a 55-year-old woman can and often does demand suddenly to be "the little sister." The resentment experienced throughout her life as the little sister is converted into a refuge role through which she can retaliate to the "big sister." The little sister role "protects" her from the realization that one has a responsibility to protect, nurture, give to, and care for one's elderly parent. It is an attempt to cushion the hurt that now there is nobody out there strong enough to provide a sense of protection for oneself. However, the attempt to challenge the big sister into this role usually fails because she also craves attention, care, and protection at this time when her parent is the one who needs parenting. Thus, anger and bitterness emerge and the sick, elderly, or dying parent frequently remains unparented in this hour of great need.

CAUGHT BETWEEN ONE'S ELDERLY PARENT AND SPOUSE

Parenting of one's elderly parent frequently adds strain to marital relationships. The demanding elderly parent is frequently resented by the son- or daughter-in-law. There is competition for attention, time, and care; there is resentment for this intrusion in their lives. Frequently, the son- or daughter-in-law starts to recognize existing or imagined similarities between their husband/wife and mother/father. Such recognition brings forth intolerance, which may be tossed at the marital partner at a time when the partner is in a position of particular vulnerability. The spouse is likely to react vehemently if deep down there is a fear of possibly becoming burdensome, unwanted, and difficult like their parents. If, and when, there is vague recognition within themselves of the characteristics despised in the parents, and these are thrown at them by their spouses, then anger, severe marital strain, and even marital dissolution may result.

The illness of elderly parents creates a strain for a marriage not only because of the burdens of time, money, and witnessing and sharing suffering, but also because the fear of inheriting the parents' disease becomes intertwined with the fear of passing this disease on to the children.

Case Illustration

Mrs. E., the mother of three girls, insisted that I see one of her daughters, while remaining vague about the reasons for desiring the consultation. When I saw the daughter, she told me about her paranoid grandfather, who sends threatening letters to his son, her father. I pointed out that grandpa lived far away, but the daughter said, "Yes, but my dad becomes more like him everyday, and the fact that my sister has my dad's personality characteristics worries my mother to death." Later, when I talked to the mother, it became clear that she was so frightened by this realization that she had not even been able to ask me to see the daughter she was most concerned about. She had had to camouflage it to herself!

Beyond the fear of inheriting disease, the advanced age of a parent or parent-in-law brings into focus the son's or daughter's (son- or daughter-in-law's) personality characteristics toward which one's tolerance has decreased. Because of this lessened tolerance, one sees in augmented form the unacceptable character traits of one's parent, in-law, or mate. As one becomes dimly aware of the decreasing tolerance level toward oneself and of the lowered tolerance threshold toward others, one gradually and reluctantly has to recognize other shortcomings and deteriorations within oneself, such as changes in one's appearance, physical strength, stamina, reaction time, sight, hearing, and body configuration. Avoiding confrontation with one's lowered emotional tolerance, one tends to focus more on one's lowered physical abilities. This, then, increases the turmoil of having to face the loss of bowel control in one's parents and reactivates old unsettled loss of control issues in oneself, reviving memories of shame and helplessness. It is an experience which increases the yearning, but also the ambivalence, towards parents and their surrogates.

The needs of the aging dependent parent often present additional strains on an already strained marriage. The son or daughter can react towards the demands of the parent with an increased tone of authority or with presenting his or her own helplessness. (Both are reactions geared to overcome the experienced helplessness in facing the parents' helplessness.) Both the authoritarian approach and the helpless approach create problems for the marriage, with accompanying actions and reactions. Only the mature partner in a mature marriage can accept and, indeed, give to his/her partner what is needed at this time: comfort, understanding, and special kinds of nurturing for the specific situation. The loving mate, acting as a pseudoparent geared to the particular needs of the mate, can give the partner an increased feeling of worthwhileness, protection from other hurts, and a degree of surrogate parenting.

Case Illustration

A middle-aged woman, upon learning of her old father's sudden homelessness, was thrown into an emotional turmoil, vacillating between a feeling that she ought to offer her father her home and her worry about the burden of having her father there. Her husband, out of concern for her guilt in case she did not offer her home to her aging father, decisively advised her to invite her father into their home.

Frequently, however, the children or children-in-law cannot supply definite emotional help because of their own childhood memories of grandparents in their homes as they were growing up.

Case Illustration

A 50-year-old man was bombarded by his mother with problems of her widowed loneliness. She felt threatened by the weather, was suspicious of authorities, deadly frightened of being burglarized, and did not venture out of her house for fear that it might be taken from her while she was gone. Her personality characteristics of mistrust, anger, and stinginess, as well as a persecutory trend, were markedly aggravated by her bitter loneliness since becoming a widow. She had always been angry at her husband and now perceived the loneliness of her existence as another inconsiderate thing her husband had done to her. He went off to die! This feeling, laced into her communications to her son, antagonized him and made him less empathic to her plight. What further hindered his helping her was a childhood memory of what it had been like when his maternal grandmother had lived with them. He remembered her frightening tales about the devil, witches, and terrible things which could happen to a little boy when he is naughty. These memories now permeated his present dealings with his elderly widowed mother as her aged helplessness rekindled his childhood helplessness and fear of his grandmother.

THE MEMORY OF HOW ONE'S PARENTS PARENTED THEIR ELDERLY PARENTS

Many a middle-aged woman remembers the intolerance of her father or mother towards an elderly parent. Although they were children then, they can still feel the sting of how it felt when their parents rejected a helpless grandparent.

Case Illustration

A 55-year-old woman remembered vividly a scene from 48 years ago when her cousin brought a widowed, weak grandfather to their humble dwelling. The cousin, a young boy, tossed down a sack of the grandfather's belongings and yelled out to her parents, "You keep him, we don't have room for him. He cannot stay with us." Even now, 48 years later, she could feel the insult of this scene as she summoned earlier memories of her grandfather as a respected, loved, and appreciated person. It hurt to see him discarded. It hurt even more to see her parents and aunts and uncles rejecting him. It crumbled a whole perception of childhood images. Throughout her child, teen, young adult, and maturing years, this woman had not been able to integrate this picture with her other childhood memories. She had always told herself and others that her childhood had been particularly serene, secure, and comfortable, and that her parents had been kind, concerned people. The memory of this grandfather scene, however, intersected and skewed the other childhood memories. It was dissonant and she could not fit it into her image of her family and herself. The thoughts illustrated by this memory reemerged whenever issues around aging and fulfilling the needs of the aged arose. Her perceptions of her own aging and the aging of her parents were slanted through the prism of this memory.

A child reared by grandparents rather than by parents will have particular dilemmas when he or she has to parent his or her parents or grandparents.

Case Illustration

Mrs. Q. had been reared by her grandparents because her own mother divorced and, according to Mrs. Q.'s memory, did not want to raise her. "She did not want to be tied down with me," she explained. She was determined not to be a mother like her mother, but was always insecure in her maternal role and panicked when her children accused her of selfishness. The children, of course, recognized this vulnerability and frequently accused her of selfishness as a way of achieving their goals. They also did this in order to master their discomfort with their mother's vulnerability. When Mrs. Q.'s old grandfather needed a home, her first impulse was to take him into her home and look after him as he had done for her when she needed him. However, she also felt that she was "only the granddaughter," while her mother was the daughter who really "ought" to look after her own father. She wanted the mother to do for grandpa what she felt her mother owed her from her own childhood. The mother, on the other hand, had felt jealous of her father's relationship with her only child. She also could not tolerate the thought that she had abandoned her child to her father and had had to distort this into the perception that her father had alienated her child from her. Anger at the memory of her behavior as a mother became intermixed with her memories of how she had been parented. The result was a feeling of increased discomfort and anger at having now to assume responsibility for parenting the elderly, shriveled father. This very old man became an unwanted ball tossed between the frustrated memories of the two bitter women, mother and daughter.

The children of Mrs. Q. in all likelihood will remember, if only vaguely, that their great-grandfather was not wanted by their mother and grandmother and this memory is likely to influence their parenting of Mrs. Q. later on in life when she will need their parenting.

SUMMARY AND CONCLUSION

The loss of independence and security, failing health, decreasing financial resources, limitation of social contacts, and decreasing mobility all are difficult burdens for the elderly. The fear of dying and the realization that he/she is progressively declining in vigor increase dependency needs in the aging parent. The son or daughter, now in middle or advanced age, frequently has difficulty in parenting the elderly parent. The reasons are manifold. External factors are not geared towards acknowledging this relationship. Indeed, the term "parenting one's parent" usually demands explanation and interpretation. In our society there are no explicit roles, rituals, acknowledgments or rewards to cushion this transition and render it respectable and worthy of esteem. The gradual helplessness of one's parents exacerbates in aging adults their fears of dying and their childhood helplessness. Old unresolved conflicts over helplessness, ungratified dependency needs, and simmering memories of hurts and vulnerabilities are reinforced. The perception of the helplessness of one's parents has a direct impact on one's cravings for having and being a perfect parent. The relationship to one's children becomes heavily overshadowed by one's childhood. Nurturance cravings in marriages become accentuated and augmented. Weak relationships become brittle, and mature relationships can, indeed, become strengthened and more meaningful.

Sibling rivalries often are reactivated. The anger one experiences about not being able to give to one's elderly parent ignites old angers. The younger sibling suddenly demands that the older one assume the responsibility of parenting the parent. The older one might, at such an occasion, face the younger one with what he had been most jealous of. This is the time when the older sibling may remark, "After all, you are a physician, you know what needs to be done for mother or father." Or, "You are worried, so you can take him/her. You are wealthy so you can care for him/her. You have a college education. You live in the city (or country)." Or, directly, "You always got along so much better with mother or dad, she/he would be much better off with you."

Witnessing in one's parent the loss of health, loss of control (body, bowel, urine, sight, or emotions) reawakens one's worst fears of body hurt, abandonment, desertion, and loss of love. The childhood fears are suddenly there, overwhelming, overpowering, and bewildering. One wants to stretch out a hand asking for protection and care, like one used to do when one was a small child. However, the person one wants to reach out to, one's parent, is the one who at that moment is reaching out for protection, and one can give that protective parenting only when there are emotional cushions in one's own internal and external realities.

CLINICAL ISSUES

13

THE EPIDEMIOLOGY OF PSYCHIATRIC DISORDERS OF MIDDLE AGE: DEPRESSION, ALCOHOLISM, AND SUICIDE

JEFFREY H. BOYD, M.D.

Department of Psychiatry,
Yale University School of Medicine,
New Haven, Connecticut

and

MYRNA M. WEISSMAN, PH.D.

Associate Professor of Psychiatry and Epidemiology,
Departments of Psychiatry and Epidemiology,
Yale University School of Medicine;
Director, Depression Research Unit,
Connecticut Mental Health Center, New Haven, Connecticut

INTRODUCTION

This chapter will present current epidemiologic information on the rates and risk factors for depression, alcoholism and suicide, since these are the most prevalent psychiatric disorders of middle-aged people. Until quite

This work was supported in part by US PHS research grant #1 R01 #R01 MH25712 from the Center for Epidemiologic Studies, National Institute of Mental Health; Alcohol, Drug Abuse, and Mental Health Administration (ADAMHA), Rockville, Maryland.

recently, accurate information about the prevalence of psychiatric disorders based on community surveys of treated and untreated persons, using precise diagnostic criteria, was not available. One major obstacle to obtaining this information was the problem of diagnosing psychiatric disorders in a reliable way in the community. Past epidemiologic studies avoided the unreliability of diagnosis by assessing "symptomatology" or "impairment" without differentiating distinct psychiatric diagnoses (27, 39). However, such global information could not readily be translated into clinical terms. Consequently, there was a gap between psychiatric epidemiology and clinical psychiatry.

PSYCHIATRIC DIAGNOSES

The unreliability of psychiatric diagnoses impinged on clinical as well as epidemiologic research in psychiatry. This was highlighted by the United States-United Kingdom collaborative study in the late 1960s. This study set about to discover why the prevalence of schizophrenia in the United States was greater than in England, while the reverse was true for manic-depressive disorders diagnosed in the United States (16, 17, 52). The U.S.-U.K. study found that patients with similar symptoms were given different diagnoses in the two countries. Furthermore, even within each country there was considerable variation in diagnostic practices between clinicians. This unreliability of diagnosis was primarily, but not exclusively, due to variation from one physician to another in the criteria used to make a diagnosis (34, 35). Each physician carries in his mind a set of "typical clinical pictures" against which he matches the symptoms of a patient, but such an approach provides little agreement between different clinicians about the diagnosis of a given patient (48).

There have been two recent parallel lines of development of diagnostic criteria in England and in the United States. Both have dealt with the problem of diagnostic unreliability and have developed diagnostic methods which have been applied to epidemiologic studies of psychiatric disorders.

England

Wing and his collaborators (47-49) in England "have shown that it is possible to apply a standard system of defining, eliciting, and recording symptoms (known as the Present State Examination (PSE) with reasonable reliability. When classificatory rules are specified precisely enough to be incorporated in a computer program (CATEGO) and applied to the symptom ratings, the resulting broad categories agree very well with the diagnoses made by clinicians" (23).

United States

Feighner and his collaborators (12) in the United States developed inclusion and exclusion criteria for making specific psychiatric diagnoses. Spitzer, Endicott, and Robins (32-34) expanded this idea by developing a structured interview called the "Schedule for Affective Disorders and Schizophrenia" (SADS), which elicits information needed to make 25 major psychiatric diagnoses. The Research Diagnostic Criteria (RDC) provide criteria for making the diagnoses.

The SADS-RDC technique has been so successful in providing reliable diagnoses that it was the model for the development of an official clinical diagnostic system used by all psychiatrists and clinicians, namely, the *Diagnostic and Statistical Manual, Third Edition (DSM-III)*.

The Application of Precise Diagnostic Techniques to Epidemiologic Surveys

These new diagnostic techniques are now being applied to community samples to obtain rates of psychiatric disorders which include both treated and untreated cases. Wing et al. have used the PSE-CATEGO system to make diagnoses in two separate community surveys: one of a London suburb and the other of two African villages (23, 47). Similarly, the SADS-RDC has been used in a community survey of New Haven, Connecticut (43). These surveys represent the first application of precise research diagnostic techniques to community samples.

In the 1975-76 New Haven survey (41-43), a follow-up of a probability sample of the general population was interviewed, using the SADS. Then, using RDC criteria, a diagnosis was made for each person interviewed. Figure 1 shows the current point prevalence rates (the percentage of persons having the disorder at the time of the interview) for middle-aged persons.

It can be seen from Figure 1 that the most common psychiatric disorders of middle age were depression and alcoholism. Both depression and alcoholism predispose to suicide, and the risk of suicide is relatively great in the middle-aged population. Therefore, this chapter will focus on depression, alcoholism, and suicide.

While these three disorders are quite common among middle-aged persons, clinicians see only a fraction of the people with these disorders. Many depressed, alcoholic, and suicidal people do not see any clinician for emotional problems (24).

FIGURE I

CURRENT POINT PREVALENCE PER 100 OF
PSYCHIATRIC DISORDERS AMONG PERSONS AGED 40-65
FROM THE 1975-76 NEW HAVEN COMMUNITY SURVEY

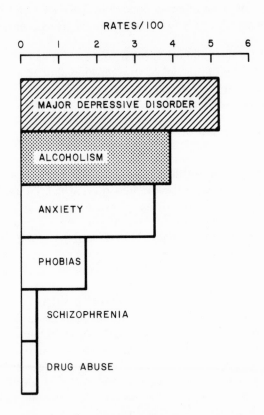

DEPRESSION

The term "depression" has multiple meanings, which tends to confuse discussions of the topic. One can delineate at least three different meanings of "depression":

1. as a mood or affect of sadness;
2. as a decrease in activity of an organ system, such as is produced by anesthesia, sedatives and "central nervous system depressants" (16);

3. as a syndrome, consisting of the following clusters of symptoms and signs: sad mood, loss of energy, sleep and appetite disturbance, loss of interest, distraction, low self-esteem, guilt, suicidal thoughts, agitation or retardation.

In the discussion that follows we will be referring to depression only in the third sense, as a syndrome.

The SADS-RDC makes a diagnosis of "major depressive disorder" based on the type of questions set forth in Table 1. Most of the patients diagnosed as having a major depression would likely be diagnosed as having "neurotic depression" in PSE-CATEGO and in the International Classification of Disease.

Rates of Depression

The recent New Haven survey found a current point prevalence (i.e., the number of persons depressed at the time of the interview) of 5.2% for "major depression" in the population aged 40-65. The London study and the other recent studies thus far have not reported rates of depression by age. However, if we look at the rates of depression in the entire population (without restriction to middle age), then we can compare the rates found by other studies with similar rates found in New Haven. Use of the PSE-CATEGO

TABLE 1

SADS Interview for Depressive Syndrome (32)

1. Did you ever have a period that lasted at least one week when you were bothered by feeling depressed, sad, blue, hopeless, down in the dumps, that you just didn't care anymore, or worried about a lot of things that could happen? What about feeling irritable or easily annoyed?
2. During the most severe period were you bothered by any of the following:
   Poor appetite or weight loss, or increased appetite or weight gain?
   Trouble sleeping or sleeping too much?
   Loss of energy, being easily fatigued, or feeling tired?
   Loss of interest or pleasure in your usual activities or in sex?
   Feeling guilty, worthless, or down on yourself?
   Trouble concentrating, thinking, or making decisions?
   Thinking about death or suicide?
   Unable to sit still and have to keep moving or the opposite—feeling slowed down and having trouble moving?
3. Did you seek help from anyone, like a doctor or minister or even a friend?
   Did it affect your functioning in any way—socially, your family, your work?

system has yielded rates of depression in London and in Canberra, Australia, which are similar to the rates of depression for persons of any age in New Haven. Other surveys in various countries, using less precise methods, have produced figures varying between 1% and 7.2% of persons of all ages who have neurotic depression (31).

About 10-15% of depressed patients have a manic attack some time in their life (18). A manic attack is characterized by euphoria or irritability, increased activity and talkativeness, flight of ideas, inflated self-esteem, decreased sleep, distractibility, and poor judgment (RDC-SADS). Although the Kraepelinean diagnostic system uses the term "manic depressive" for all patients with depression or mania, in the forthcoming diagnostic system in the United States the term "manic depression" is not used, and "bipolar" is used for those depressives with one or more manic attacks. This group of bipolar patients is in many respects different from depressives without mania—they have an earlier age of onset of the disorder, a greater genetic contribution, and they are much less common than are depressed persons (18).

Risk Factors for Depression

A "risk factor" is an epidemiologic concept for a characteristic which increases the likelihood of a person developing the disorder under study.

Sex

The higher rate of depression among women as compared to men has been documented by innumerable studies (38). The current point prevalence is 7.0% of middle-aged women versus 2.9% of middle-aged men, in the New Haven survey. However, from the point of view of a clinician, the proportion of depressed women coming for treatment is even greater than it is in the community because of the different help-seeking behaviors of the two sexes. Women seek professional help more frequently than men, for all medical and psychiatric disorders, including depression. Men may treat their depression with alcohol, and do not seek help until their depression is so severe that they may require hospitalization. When a depressed man presents himself to a physician, he is likely to describe his problem as sexual impotence, work difficulties, or problems with alcohol, rather than sad mood, thus obscuring the underlying depression.

The sex difference in the rate of depression exists at all ages, including middle age, although the reasons for this sex difference are unclear. It is no longer thought that menopause (climacteric) precipitates depression in women: The risk of depression is no greater for a woman at the time of menopause that at other periods, nor are depressions which occur during menopause different in quality (14, 37).

Age

For women, the risk of depression increases up until their early 50s and then declines. For men, the rate of depression continues to increase with age, so that a man's risk of depression is slight when he is young, but by the time he reaches his late 50s he is likely to become depressed. Not only is the older middle-aged man prone to depression, but he is also at very high risk of suicide when he is depressed, as we will discuss later.

Social isolation

The absence of an intimate, confiding relationship increases the likelihood of depression, especially for women. Social isolation becomes increasingly common as a person passes through the middle years, facing departure of one's children and the possible loss of the spouse. For those who are married, conflict in the marriage, lack of intimacy, and emotional isolation are chronic stresses predisposing to depression. Arguments with the spouse and marital disputes are the problems most often discussed by middle-aged, depressed women coming for therapy.

Losses

Losses predispose to depression. For women, a depression is often precipitated by grief over the death of a family member, or the departure of one's children from the home. For men, the losses can be related to mid-life career difficulties, loss of one's job, or breakup of the marriage.

Emotional deprivation as a child

Persons who had been deprived of the love and warmth of a parent as children are at higher risk for developing a depression as adults. Parental deprivation can occur if a parent had left through death or geographic separation, or if the parent had been abusive, rejecting, or disinterested in the child, or if the childhood home had been a hotbed of parental discord.

Family history

A family history of depression in first degree relatives increases the risk of depression (51).

Morbidity of Depressions

Depression leads to considerable impairment of a person's daily life, affecting one's function as a spouse, parent, worker, and member of the community. The marriage of depressed people is often characterized by open warfare. There is frequently a lack of affection, diminished communication, diminished or absent sexual relations. The depressed person can be quite angry and hostile at home. Contrary to earlier psychoanalytic theories about depression being due to a diminished capacity to express anger, systematic study has demonstrated that depressed persons express *increased* levels of anger, irritability, and hostility. However, this anger is often expressed at home with close family members and not in the doctor's office. Consequently, conflict within the home escalates.

Depression seriously impairs one's ability to care for children. There is diminished involvement, interest, and affection for the children. Irritability, distraction, and anergia prevent the middle-aged parent from meeting a teenage child's normal demand for affection, limit-setting and rules. Communication decreases and the teenager finds someone else to talk to, withdrawing from the depressed parent.

Depressed people perform poorly at work, are often absent from work, and are subject to making decisions that reflect poor judgment, such as the decision to quit one's job because of low self-esteem (51).

Mortality of Depression

The lifetime risk of suicide for a person with unipolar or bipolar depressions is about 15% (13). An increased risk of suicide is associated with being a middle-aged man. This and other risk factors for suicide will be discussed below.

Treatment of Depression

The efficacy of several forms of treatment for depression, including pharmacotherapy and psychotherapy, have been demonstrated by randomized clinical trials (9, 40, 44). These studies have shown that antidepressants and psychotherapy in combination are significantly more effective in the treatment of depression than is either treatment alone, and that either treatment alone is significantly better than placebo (45). There is a suggestion that pharmacotherapy and psychotherapy have different modes of action. The tricyclic medication mainly improves sleep disturbance, agitation, anxiety, and appetite disturbance (i.e., the "vegetative symptoms" of depression).

The main effects of psychotherapy are in the areas of mood, interest, activity, suicidal feeling, and generally in improving the person's functioning in intimate interpersonal relationships (9). Several types of psychotherapy have been developed for use with depressed patients; these are marital, cognitive, group and interpersonal therapies.

Prevention of Depression

Prevention can be one of three types: primary, secondary, and tertiary. Primary prevention means the preventing of the disorder altogether by altering susceptibility or reducing exposure for susceptible individuals. Since the "causes" of the depression are poorly understood, in this sense there is no primary prevention beyond trying to alter or prevent the risk factors previously described. Secondary prevention is early detection and treatment of the disorder. Secondary prevention is possible because good methods for diagnosing and treating depression are available. However, less than 20% of depressed people ever receive treatment for their depression. For those who do seek treatment the great majority go to their primary physician complaining of various depressive and somatic symptoms. Frequently depression is undetected and untreated. The result is that the opportunities for secondary prevention are often lost. Much work is needed in training primary care physicians to effectively diagnose and treat depression (24).

Tertiary prevention means preventing disability from the disorder and restoring effective functioning. It has been shown that maintenance on tricyclic antidepressants prevents a recurrence of the depression in many patients and that maintenance psychotherapy can enhance social functioning (40).

ALCOHOLISM

There is still scientific disagreement about how to define alcoholism. While everyone would agree about the diagnosis in a skid row alcoholic, 95% of alcoholics are not skid row types (7). All definitions of alcoholism include some combination of five sorts of criteria (8):

1. Length, amount, and pattern of drinking (steady versus episodic drinking, binge drinking).
2. Social problems as a result of drinking (loss of job, divorce, traffic violations, arrests, etc.).
3. Psychological dependence (loss of control, preoccupation with alcohol).

4. Physiological dependence (tolerance to high blood alcohol levels, various withdrawal syndromes: tremors, hallucinations, delirium tremens, seizures).
5. Medical diseases caused by alcohol (liver damage, upper gastrointestinal bleeding, neuropathy, Wernicke-Korsakoff's syndrome, etc.).

The SADS-RDC makes a diagnosis of "alcoholism" based on the type of questions set forth in Table 2.

TABLE 2

SADS Interview for Alcoholism (32)

1. What have your drinking habits been like?
   Was there ever a period in your life when you drank too much?
   Has anyone in your family—or anyone else—ever objected to your drinking?
   Was there ever a time when you often couldn't stop drinking when you wanted to?
   When you were drinking, how much did you drink?
2. Was there ever a time when you frequently had a drink before breakfast?
   Was there ever a time when, because of your drinking, you often missed work, had trouble on the job, or were unable to take care of household responsibilities (e.g., getting meals prepared, doing shopping)?
   Did you ever lose a job because of your drinking?
   Did you often have difficulties with your family, friends, or acquaintances because of your drinking?
   Were you ever divorced or separated primarily because of your drinking?
   Have you ever gone on a bender? (Definition: drinking steadily for three or more days, consuming each day more than a fifth of whiskey [3/4th of a liter of whiskey] or the equivalent in wine or beer).
   Have you ever been physically violent while drinking?
   Have you ever had traffic difficulties because of your drinking—like reckless driving, accidents, or speeding?
   Have you ever been picked up by the police because of how you were acting while you were drinking?
   Have you ever had blackouts?
   Have you ever had tremors (that were most likely due to drinking)?
   Have you ever had the Delirium Tremens?
   Did you ever hear voices or see things that weren't really there, soon after you stopped drinking?
   Have you ever had a seizure or fit after you stopped drinking?
   Did a doctor ever tell you that you had developed a physical complication of alcoholism, like gastritis, pancreatitis, cirrhosis, or neuritis?

Rates of Alcoholism

Different definitions of alcoholism affect the prevalence rates of alcoholism. Despite this problem, there is a convergence of agreement among studies that about 10% of men and 4% of women are alcoholic at some time in their life (42, 51).

The New Haven survey found the *lifetime* rates of alcoholism (ever having been an alcoholic) were 9.6% for men and 3.8% for women. However, half of these people were no longer alcoholic at the time of the interview but had recovered. There is a popular belief that if one is ever an alcoholic, then one remains an alcoholic for life. Contrary to this belief, several studies have found a substantial remission rate (1). Although the lifetime rates were considerably higher, only 4.9% of middle-aged men and 3.1% of middle-aged women were alcoholic at the time of the interview in the New Haven survey. Therefore, many persons who had a previous history of alcoholism had recovered (42).

Risk Factors for Alcoholism

Sex

Alcoholism is more prevalent among men than it is among women. Furthermore, alcoholism is harder to detect among women. Because women tend to drink unobtrusively at home, and do not have so much difficulty from the police or employers, a clinician must maintain a high index of suspicion in order to detect those women who are alcoholic (29, 30, 46).

Age

Men tend to begin heavy drinking as teenagers or in their early 20s, whereas women begin heavy drinking later—in their 30s (50). But for both sexes the medical complications of alcohol use and the beginning of hospitalization for these complications occur during the middle-aged years. A level of alcohol consumption which the person had previously accepted as "normal" may cause cirrhosis of the liver, gratrointestinal bleeding, or various neurological problems in middle age (5, 6, 51).

Race

The New Haven survey found alcoholism to be five times as prevalent among nonwhites (blacks and Puerto Ricans) as among whites. However, this difference partly reflects the fact that most nonwhites in New Haven fall into the lowest social classes, and lower social class people of any race have much higher rates of alcoholism.

Class

The rates of alcoholism are three to five times as high among the lower socioeconomic classes as among middle or upper classes. The lower-class drinker gets into trouble from his drinking out of all proportion with the difficulties suffered by an upper-middle-class person who drinks as heavily (5). For example, a lower-class heavy drinker is apt to be repeatedly fired from jobs and end up unemployed by the time he is middle-aged; however, his upper-middle-class counterpart might be tolerated in a managerial position despite his drinking.

Ethnic group

Different cultures develop different patterns of drinking and have very different rates of alcoholism. In the United States, for example, Jews, Italian immigrants and Chinese immigrants have very low rates of alcoholism, presumably because the use of alcohol is culturally moderated. However, as subsequent generations of Italian and Chinese immigrants' children become acculturated to American drinking patterns, the rates of alcoholism rise (7).

Occupation

Certain occupational groups (waiters, bartenders, longshoremen, musicians, authors, and reporters) have higher rates of alcoholism (51).

Family history

The children of alcoholics are at higher risk of alcoholism than are other people. In particular, a father's alcoholism predisposes his son to the disorder. While much of the reason for this transmission is undoubtedly due to children learning the behavior pattern of their parents, recent adoption and twin studies have indicated that there is also a genetic contribution to the transmission of alcoholism to the children (50, 51).

Morbidity of Alcoholism

The morbidity of alcoholism is enormous, especially in the middle-age years, and affects all areas of life. Alcoholics are involved in about half of all traffic accidents. Half of all convicted felons are alcoholic; about half of all police work is involved with alcoholics (7). Alcoholism produces absenteeism from work and loss of jobs, disruption of marriages and divorces (51). Drunken middle-aged parents can't be good role models for their teenage children.

Cirrhosis of the liver and portal hypertension are prominent middle-aged complications of heavy alcohol use, affecting 10% of all alcoholics (51). Other medical complications can be found in any medical or psychiatric textbook.

Mortality of Alcoholism

The mortality rate for an alcoholic is two to three times that of the general population at the same age (51). An episode of delirium tremens carries a 15% mortality rate, which is comparable to the risk of death during an episode of acute myocardial infarction (7). In addition to death from medical illnesses, and death from traffic accidents, alcoholics die of suicide. As we will discuss below, about one-fifth of all suicides are alcoholics.

Treatment of Alcoholism

There have been few controlled clinical trials of treatment programs for alcoholics. One of the few prospective studies was done at the Maudsley Hospital (Institute of Psychiatry, London) (10). One hundred alcoholic men were randomly assigned to either an advice group (in which the man and his family had only one session of counseling) or a treatment group (in which the man and his family were offered intensive outpatient and inpatient treatment for a year). Evaluation at 12 months and 24 months revealed no difference between men who received treatment and those who did not. Both groups did equally well (10, 22).

There is some reason to be optimistic about the prognosis of alcoholics, whether or not they are treated for alcoholism. A major report in the United States found a 50% remission rate among untreated alcoholics, and a 70% remission rate among treated alcoholics (1). The New Haven survey likewise found a high rate of remission among alcoholics. However, the word "remission" here does not mean abstinence from alcohol; it means either abstinence or drinking less than before, in a manner which does not produce problems and which, therefore, does not warrant the diagnosis of "alcoholism." Many treated (and untreated) alcoholics continue to drink in moderation. One study found that most former alcoholics who drink in moderation run no greater risk of relapse into full alcoholism than do former alcoholics who are abstinent (1).

Diagnostic Heterogeneity of Alcoholics

Many alcoholics have had another psychiatric disorder at some time in their life, most commonly depression (29, 30, 42). This raises the question whether a certain number of alcoholics, particularly men, are using alcohol to medicate the feelings arising from a separate psychiatric disorder. It is important for clinicians to recognize the diagnostic heterogeneity of alcoholics because of the implications for treatment: A bipolar manic-depressive may no longer need alcohol if he is maintained on lithium; a depressed alcoholic may warrant treatment with a tricyclic antidepressant (25).

Prevention of Alcoholism

An emerging consensus among many epidemiologists is that "primary prevention" of alcoholism depends on reducing the total amount of alcohol consumed by everyone in the society (6).

"Secondary prevention" consists of early detection of alcoholism and effective intervention. Clinical experience suggests that the decisive step may be detecting the existence of alcoholism and helping the patient to overcome his denial of the problem. Once alcoholism is diagnosed, the patient may be convinced to enter a treatment program, or his family may drag him into treatment.

Alcoholics Anonymous is an important resource in the community for "secondary" or "tertiary" prevention of alcoholism. There are few statistics concerning the efficacy of Alcoholics Anonymous because its members have often resisted scientific study. However, it is clear that Alcoholics Anonymous is capable of offering many alcoholics a degree of availability and support at all hours of the day and night which no physician or mental health professional would be able to offer an alcoholic patient. Alcoholics Anonymous makes strong use of group norms and pressure, and offers a gratification of dependency needs through membership in the group. Alcoholics Anonymous groups have become a standard part of many inpatient treatment programs (1).

SUICIDE

Successful suicide must be distinguished from suicide attempts (unsuccessful suicide) (36), since they affect different populations and have different risk factors. Many persons who commit suicide have never previously made a suicide attempt; likewise, the majority of suicide attempters never go on to commit suicide (see Figure 2). Those who commit suicide are usually men

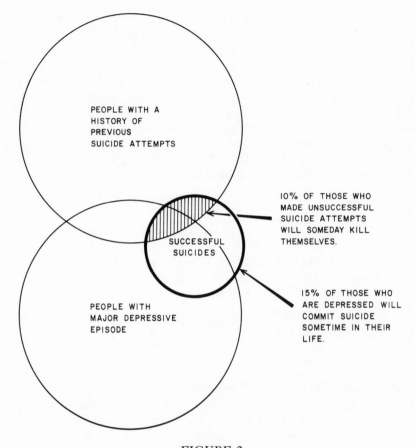

FIGURE 2

The Relationship of Successful Suicide to Suicide Attempts
and to Depression

who are middle-aged or older, whereas those who attempt suicide unsuccessfully are usually younger women (36). We will focus on suicide because
of its relevance for a middle-aged population.

Rates of suicide are affected by coroners' habits and public recording
methods (4) and the tendency to hide suicides due to the stigma and threatened loss of insurance. Moreover, there can be uncertainty about whether
a given death was due to suicide or to accident. Poisoning, for example, is
sometimes called "suicide" and sometimes called "accident." The same death

could be judged either way, depending on what the deceased person intended to do. Frequently, the intent can't be determined.

"Psychological autopsies," i.e., interviewing the deceased person's family and friends looking for hints of suicidal intent, may clarify the diagnosis in cases in which the diagnosis is uncertain (19, 28). Many suicides fall into a grey zone, or spectrum: At one end are those who intend to kill themselves on a conscious level, but have some ambivalence; at the other end of the spectrum are those whose fatal accident may have had some unconscious element of suicidal intent (19). A recent study in Finland used a five-point classification scale: certain suicide, almost certain suicide, undetermined, almost certain accident, and certain accident (19).

Rates of Suicide

The variability in rates of suicide from country to country probably has more to do with different detection and recording methods than with real differences (4). Despite the variability, suicide is one of the major causes of death for middle-aged white men (28). Suicidal risk is quite common among middle-aged people. The data on risk factors, given below, are more reliable than are the data on the rates of suicide.

Risk Factors for Suicide

Sex

Men commit suicide about three times as often as do women. This is different from suicide attempts and suicide threats, in which women predominate over men by three to one. Therefore, a middle-aged man who talks about suicide should be taken seriously. When men set about to commit suicide they choose more violent means with a greater assurance of lethality, such as guns, whereas women more often overdose, a form of suicide attempt that may not always be lethal (28).

Marital status

Widowed and divorced men commit suicide four or five times as often as married men. Single men who have never married commit suicide twice as often as married men (20). Living alone is also a risk factor.

Age

The risk of suicide increases with age (20).

Previous suicide attempts

The Venn diagram in Figure 2 illustrates the relationship between successful suicides, suicide attempters, and depressives (2). The hatched area of the diagram represents those people with a previous suicide attempt who finally kill themselves. A previous suicide attempt is much more serious if a highly lethal method was chosen (such as a gun) or if the likelihood of rescue was low (such as a person who goes off alone without telling anyone where he is) (28).

Psychiatric illness

Suicide by someone who has no psychiatric disorder is uncommon. Some history of psychiatric disorder was found in 85-95% of suicides based on interview of the family and friends (3, 26). Most people who commit suicide are having a major depressive episode at that time. This is illustrated in the lower half of the Venn diagram in Figure 2 (2). Anyone who is seriously depressed and who also begins to make hints about suicidal feelings or thoughts is at high risk of suicide.

Between 15% and 23% of successful suicides have been alcoholics (3, 26). Other men drink heavily in order to work up the courage to commit suicide.

Medical illness

Medical illness and chronic pain increase the risk of suicide (11).

Giving hints of suicidal intent

A majority of those who kill themselves have seen a doctor in the previous month, and have told someone that they intend to kill themselves. The message may be disguised, such as saying that they are preoccupied with death or wished they were dead (3, 26).

Prevention of Suicide

The most effective form of prevention of suicide is an impractical one, i.e., to hospitalize all persons who threaten to commit suicide (3, 26). Since you can't predict for sure who will commit suicide, the choice of who should be hospitalized is not simple. Effective prevention depends on understanding the risk factors (see Table 3). The more risk factors the patient has, the more likely he is to actually kill himself, and the more advisable is hospitalization.

Physicians and mental health professionals are in a position to detect those

TABLE 3

Risk Factors for Suicide

Male
Living Alone: Widowed, Divorced, or Single
Over Age 40
History of a Previous Suicide Attempt (especially use of a lethal method and little likelihood of being rescued)
Depression
Alcoholism
Other Psychiatric Diagnosis
Medical Illness and/or Chronic Pain
Suicidal Thoughts and/or Suicidal Plan

persons who are going to go on to commit suicide. In one sample of suicides, two-thirds of the people had seen a physician, usually their primary care physician, within a month (3). However, as Murphy has pointed out, for the most part primary care physicians are not sensitive to the evidence of suicidal risk factors, and do not ask the patient the relevant questions. The result is that the suicidal risk is never recognized, and the physician may even hand the patient a prescription for medication with which the patient subsequently overdoses (21).

The effectiveness of suicide prevention centers and Samaritan centers in preventing suicide has been equivocal. Four separate controlled studies have been done, and only one found any impact on the suicide rates. The study using the most careful methods demonstrated that Samaritan centers (the British equivalent of American suicide prevention centers) have had little impact on the suicide rate (15). These centers may, however, play an important role in crisis intervention and in allaying distress.

CONCLUSIONS

The most prevalent psychiatric disorders of middle-aged people are depression, alcoholism, and suicide. We have discussed the rates, risk factors, treatment, and prevention of each of these three problems. Certain common themes emerge.

With all three disorders there is a high degree of human misery, a substantial morbidity, and some mortality. Persons afflicted with these disorders often come to their primary care physician seeking help, although they may not be able to articulate clearly what it is that is troubling them. Someone who is depressed, for example, may complain to the physician about impotence, fatigue, insomnia, or various aches and pains, leaving it to the physician to discover that these symptoms are manifestations of an underlying depression. Tables 1, 2, and 3 summarize the questions a physician might ask in order to make a diagnosis of depression, alcoholism, and suicidal risk.

Depression and alcoholism share in common the fact that they predispose middle-aged people to committing suicide. The great majority of suicides are either depressed or alcoholic. The great majority of suicides are also men over the age of 40. Any middle-aged man who is depressed or alcoholic is at substantial risk for suicide, by virtue of having three major risk factors (diagnosis, sex, and age). If he has other risk factors (see Table 3), such as giving hints that he is ruminating about death, then his risk of death from suicide is alarmingly high.

The primary care physician who is sensitive to the psychiatric problems of the middle-aged is in an excellent position to do important preventive work, since patients with such problems are more apt initially to seek out the help of a nonpsychiatric physician. There exists a range of therapies with reasonably well-established efficacy for some of the psychiatric disorders of this population. Moreover, most of these therapies usually can be administered by the nonpsychiatric physician alone or in occasional consultation with a psychiatrist.

The reduction in morbidity, and possibly mortality, which can occur with the detection and treatment of the psychiatric problems of the middle-aged population, makes the physician's efforts most important and rewarding.

REFERENCES

1. ARMOR, D. J., POLICH, J. M. and STAMBUL, H. B. (1976). *Alcoholism and Treatment*. Santa Monica: Rand Corporation.
2. AVER, D. and WINOKUR, G. (1978). Suicide, attempted suicide and relapse rates in depression. *Arch. Gen. Psychiat, 35*, 749.
3. BARRACLOUGH, B., BUNCH, J., NELSON, B. and SAINSBURG, P. (1974). A hundred cases of suicide: Clinical aspects. *Brit. J. Psychiat, 125*, 335.
4. BROOKE, E. M. (ed) (1974). *Suicide and Attempted Suicide*. Geneva: World Health Organization.
5. CAHALAN, D. and ROOM, R. (1972). Problem drinking among American men aged 21-59. *Amer. J. Public Health, 62*, 1473.
6. CARTWRIGHT, A, K. J. and SHAW, S. J. (1978). Trends in the epidemiology of alcoholism. *Psychol. Med, 8*, 1.
7. CHAFETZ, M. D. (1975). Alcoholism and alcoholic psychoses. In: Freedman, A. M., Kaplan, H. I. and Sadock, B. J. (eds.), *Comprehensive Textbook of Psychiatry—II*. Baltimore: Williams & Wilkins.

8. Criteria Committee, National Council on Alcoholism (1972). Criteria for the diagnosis of alcoholism. Am. J. Psychiat, 129, 127.

9. DiMascio, A., Weissman, M. M., Prusoff, B. A., Neu, C., Zwilling, M. and Klerman, G. L. (in press). Differential symptom reduction by drugs and psychotherapy in acute depression. Arch. Gen. Psychiat,

10. Edwards, G., Orford, J., Egert, S., et al. (1977). Alcoholism, a controlled clinical trial of treatment and advice. J. Stud. Alcohol, 38, 1004.

11. Fawcett, J. (1972). Suicidal depression and physical illness. JAMA, 219, 1303.

12. Feighner, J. P., Robins, E., Guze, S. B., et al. (1972). Diagnostic criteria for use in psychiatric research. Arch. Gen. Psychiat. 26, 57.

13. Guze, S. B. and Robbins, E. (1970). Suicide and primary affective disorders. Brit. J. Psychiat: 117, 437.

14. Hallstrom, T. (1973). Mental Disorder and Sexuality in the Climacteric. Goteborg, Sweden: Scandinavian University Books.

15. Jennings, C., Barraclough, B. M. and Moss, J. R. (1978). Have the Samaritans lowered the suicide rate? A controlled study. Psychol. Med., 8, 413.

16. Klerman, G. L. and Barrett, J. E. (1973). The affective disorders: Clinical and epidemiologic aspects. In: Gershon, S. and Shopsin, B. (eds.), Lithium: Its Role in Psychiatric Research and Treatment. New York; Plenum Press.

17. Kramer, M. (1969). Corss national study of diagnosis of the mental disorders: Origin of the problem. Am. J. Psychiat. (supplement), 125, 1.

18. Krauthammer, C. and Klerman, G. L. (1979). The epidemiology of mania. In: Shopsin, B. (ed), Manic Illness. New York: Raven Press.

19. Lonnquist, J. (1977). Suicide in Helsinki. Espoo, Finland: Psychiatria Fennica.

20. Monk, M. (1875). Epidemiology. In: Perlin, S. (ed.), A Handbook for the Study of Suicide. New York: Oxford University Press.

21. Murphy, G. E. (1975). The physician's responsibility for suicide: I. An error of commission. II. Errors of omission. Ann. Internal Med., 82, 301.

22. Orford, J. and Edwards, G. (1977). Alcoholism. Oxford: Oxford University Press.

23. Orley, J., Blitt, D. M. and Wing, J. K. (1979). Psychiatric disorders in two African villages. Arch. Gen. Psychiat. 36, 513.

24. Regier, D. A., Goldberg, I. D. and Taube, C. A. (1978). The de facto US mental health services system. Arch. Gen. Psychiat., 35, 685.

25. Reich, L. H., Davies, R. K. and Himmelhoch, J. M. (1974). Excessive alcohol use in manic depressive illness. Am. J. Psychiat., 131, 83.

26. Robins, E., Murphy, G. E., Wilkinson, R. H., Gassner, S. and Kayes, J. (1959). Some clinical considerations in the prevention of suicides based on a study of 134 successful suicides. Amer. J. Public Health, 49, 888.

27. Robins, L. N. (1978). Psychiatric epidemiology. Arch. Gen. Psychiat., 35, 697.

28. Schneidman, E. S. (1975). Suicide. In: Freedman, A. M., Kaplan, H. I. and Sadock, B. J. (eds.), Comprehensive Textbook of Psychiatry—II. Baltimore: Williams & Wilkins.

29. Schuckit, M., Pitts, F., Reich, T., King, L. V. and Winokur, G. (1969). Alcoholism: Two types of alcoholism in women. Arch. Gen. Psychiat., 20, 301.

30. Schuckit, M. A. and Morrissey, E. R. (1979). Psychiatric problems in women admitted to an alcoholic detoxification center. Am. J. Psychiat., 136, 611.

31. Silverman, C. (1968). The Epidemiology of Depression. Baltimore: Johns Hopkins University Press.

32. Spitzer, R. L. and Endicott, J. (1978). Schedule for Affective Disorders and Schizophrenia. New York: Biometrics Research, Evaluation Section, New York State Psychiatric Institute.

33. Spitzer, R. L., Endicott, J. and Robins, E. (1978). Research Diagnostic Criteria. New York: Biometrics Research, Evaluation Section, New York State Psychiatric Institute.

34. Spitzer, R. L., Endicott, J. and Robins, E. (1978). Research diagnostic criteria: Rationale and reliability. *Arch. Gen. Psychiat.*, 35, 773.
35. Spitzer, R. L., Endicott, J. and Robins, E. (1975). Clinical criteria for psychiatric diagnosis and DSM III. *Am. J. Psychiat.*, 132, 1187.
36. Weissmann, M. M. (1974). The epidemiology of suicide attempts, 1960 to 1971. *Arch. Gen. Psychiat.*, 30, 737.
37. Weissman, M. M. (1979). The myth of involutional melancholia. *JAMA*, 242, 742-744.
38. Weissman, M. M. and Klerman, G. L. (1977). Sex differences in the epidemiology of depression. *Arch. Gen. Psychiat.*, 34, 98.
39. Weissman, M. M. and Klerman, G. L. (1978). Epidemiology of mental disorders: Emerging trends. *Arch. Gen. Psychiat.*, 35, 705.
40. Weissman, M. M., Klerman, G. L., Paykel, E. S., Prusoff, B. A. and Hanson, B. (1974). Treatment effects on the social adjustment of depressed patients. *Arch. Gen. Psychiat.*, 30, 771.
41. Weissman, M. M. and Myers, J. K. (1978). Affective disorders in a US urban community. *Arch. Gen. Psychiat.*, 35, 1304.
42. Weissman, M. M., Myers, J. K. and Harding, P. S. (1980). The prevalence rates and psychiatric heterogeneity of alcoholism in a United States urban community. *J. Stud. Alcohol*, 41, 672.
43. Weissman, M. M., Myers, J. K. and Harding, P. S. (1978). Psychiatric disorders in a US urban community: 1975-1976. *Am. J. Psychiat.*, 135, 459.
44. Weissman, M. M., Neu, C., Rounsaville, B. J., Dimascio, A., Prusoff, B. A., and Klerman, G. L. (May, 1979). Short-term interpersonal psychotherapy (IPT) for depression: Prescription and efficacy. Paper read at the American Psychiatric Association Meeting, Chicago, Il.
45. Weissman, M. M., Prusoff, B. A., Dimascio, A., Neu, C., Goklaney, M. and Klerman, G. L. (1979). The efficacy of drugs and psychotherapy in the treatment of acute depressive episodes. *Am. J. Psychiat.*, 136: 555.
46. Wilsnack, S. C. (June 2, 1977). Women are different: Overlooked differences among women drinkers. Paper read at the Symposium on Alcoholism and Women at the Institute for the Study of Women in Transition, Portland, Maine.
47. Wing, J. K. (1976). A technique for studying psychiatric morbidity in in-patient and out-patient series and in general population samples. *Psychol. Med.*, 6, 665.
48. Wing, J. K., Mann, S. A., Leff, J. P. and Nixon, J. M. (1978). The concept of a "case" in psychiatric population surveys. *Psychol. Med.*, 8, 203.
49. Wing, J. K. and Nixon, J. M. (1975). Discriminating symptoms in schizophrenia. *Arch. Gen. Psychiat.*, 32, 853.
50. Winokur, G., Reich, T., Rimmer, J. and Pitts, F. (1970). Alcoholism: Diagnosis and familial psychiatric illness in 259 alcoholic probands. *Arch. Gen. Psychiat.*, 23, 104.
51. Woodruff, R. A., Jr., Goodwin, D. W. and Guze, S. B. (1974). *Psychiatric Diagnosis*. New York: Oxford University Press.
52. Zubin, J. (1969). Cross-national study of diagnosis of the mental disorders: Methodology and planning. *Am. J. Psychiat.* (supplement), 125, 12.

14

DEPRESSION AND SUICIDE
IN MIDDLE AGE

GRAHAM D. BURROWS, M.D., CH.B., B.SC., D.P.M.,
F.R.C.PSYCH., F.R.A.N.Z.C.P

First Assistant and Reader

and

LORRAINE DENNERSTEIN, M.B., B.S., PH.D., D.P.M.

Clinical Supervisor
Department of Psychiatry, University of Melbourne, Australia

INTRODUCTION

Middle age is an ill-defined phase of life characterized by many psychological, sociological and biological changes. Epidemiological studies suggest a high incidence of depression and suicide between the fourth and sixth decades. This chapter will consider the relative roles of biological, psychological and sociological factors in the aetiology and management of depression and suicide in middle age.

DEPRESSION

Terminology

A major source of confusion in both scientific research and clinical practice relates to the different usage of the term "depression." Depression may refer to a mood, symptom or syndrome and has diverse meanings for workers in various fields (56).

A depressed mood is a normal human emotion that all experience at some

222

time or another. Feelings of sadness and disappointment are part of normal experience. Depression becomes a pathological symptom by virtue of its intensity, pervasiveness, duration and interference with normal social or physiological functioning.

Along with other signs, the symptom of abnormal depressed mood occurs as part of a depressive syndrome. This disorder is characterized by abnormal persistent affective changes associated with feelings of worthlessness, guilt, helplessness and hopelessness; anxiety, crying; suicidal tendencies; loss of interest in work and other activities; impaired capacity to perform everyday social functions; hypochondriasis, anorexia, weight change, constipation, psychomotor retardation or agitation, headache and other bodily complaints. Physical symptoms are caused by changes in bodily functions associated with the depressive illness, mediated through the autonomic nervous system.

Workers in different disciplines also use the term depression in varying ways. For the neurophysiologist, depression refers to a decrease in electro-physiological activity. For the pharmacologist, depression refers to drug actions which decrease the activity of target organs. For the psychiatrist, depression connotes changes in affective state ranging in severity from nor-mal mood swings to a major illness.

Classification

Despite extensive debate and research, the classification of depressive illness remains controversial. "Almost every classificatory format that is log-ically possible has been advocated by someone within the last 20 years, and some more or less plausible evidence offered in support" (50). Classificatory schemata suggested include category, dimensional and hierarchical systems.

Different terms have been used to characterize depressive illnesses. These include "psychotic," "neurotic," "endogenous" and "reactive." Some authors regard "psychotic" and "endogenous" as synonymous, and "neurotic" and "reactive" likewise, using either pair of terms to denote two contrasting syndromes (50). The psychotic or endogenous syndrome is characterized by an acute onset and accompanied by retardation, guilt, diurnal variation of mood and severe insomnia and weight loss. In contrast, the neurotic/reactive depression is said to be prone to vary from day to day, often accompanied by anxiety, with self-pity and histrionic outbursts rather than guilt, and complaints of anorexia rather than weight loss.

Other authors have commented that the terms neurotic or psychotic are incapable of precise definition and mean little more than "mild" or "severe" (15). Still other writers have interpreted the terms more narrowly, confining the term "psychotic" to illnesses characterized by delusions, hallucinations or gross loss of insight, the term "reactive" to illnesses preceded by obviously stressful events and the term "endogenous" to illnesses without precipitating stress. These semantic differences have produced widespread confusion.

A classification gaining widespread acceptance distinguishes first between primary and secondary affective disorders. Primary affective disorders are not preceded chronologically by any other psychiatric disorder, whereas secondary disorders are either preceded by another psychiatric illness (such as anxiety, neurosis, schizophrenia, alcoholism) or accompanied by a life-threatening or incapacitating physical illness(78). Primary affective disorders are then subdivided into unipolar and bipolar types (61), the former consisting of depressive illnesses only, the latter of depression and mania combined.

While a number of different subclassifications of the unipolar depressive disorders have been suggested (for example, depressive spectrum disease versus pure depressive disease), it is clinically useful to divide the unipolar depressive disorder into mild, moderate or severe.

"Involutional Melancholia": Depression of Middle Age

The concept of involutional melancholia arose in 1896 with Kraepelin's classification of the functional psychoses into three major groups. These were dementia praecox (later to be called schizophrenia), manic-depressive psychoses and involutional psychoses, the latter including melancholia. Kraepelin's diagnosis of melancholia included "all states of anxiety in more advanced stage which are not episodes in the course of other forms of insanity" (45). Melancholia was characterized by "uniform despondency with fear, various delusions of self-accusation, of persecution, and of hypochondriacal nature, with moderate clouding of consciousness, leading in the greater number of cases after a prolonged course to moderate mental deterioration" (58). No consideration was given to the premorbid personality or to the psychodynamics of this condition. Brief mention was made of *some relation to the climacterium*. Therapy was supportive, with emphasis on bed rest, nutrition, isolation from the family and prevention of suicide. The prolonged course and poor prognosis with probable deterioration were important factors in the diagnosis.

"Melancholia" was used interchangeably with involutional melancholia over the next 30 years. It was probably patients of this group that Freud described in *Mourning and Melancholia* (38).

There was difficulty in finding a clear definition of the concept of involution. Presumably, by involution was meant the cessation of function which takes place in the ovaries at the menopause. Involutional depression was not diagnosed before the age of 40 years. Attempts have been made to define involutional melancholia on the basis of characteristic symptomatology, but no constant symptomatology has been found.

It is now generally agreed that involutional melancholia is not an independent entity. An important reason for this change is that the classical presentation with severe agitation, nihilistic delusions, and bizarre hypochondriasis has become increasingly uncommon.

Other considerations include the fact that the poor prognosis described by Kraepelin was diminished following the introduction of electroconvulsive therapy. A number of clinical studies (1, 75), have shown that agitated depressions were not restricted to the involutional period. The syndrome was also found to be genetically heterogenous (89). Psychiatrists have become familiar with the depressions of older ages and now realize that classical involutional melancholia is only one component of a spectrum of illnesses found in this age group.

The ninth revision of the International Classification of Diseases has left out involutional melancholia. In its place is a category of "other affective psychosis" intended for all agitated depressions regardless of age.

EPIDEMIOLOGY

Epidemiological studies investigate the distribution of diseases in a population and analyse the factors associated with the prevalence and incidence of changes. In any discussion of epidemiological issues it is necessary to recognize the methodological problems involved in gathering data and the consequent difficulties in comparing findings across studies. The problems involved include those of: case definition and identification which may reflect physician diagnostic bias; the presence of the same symptoms in different disorders; the need to monitor symptoms over time in order to make a satisfactory disgnosis in certain disorders; difficulties in classification; techniques used (such as rating scales versus interviews); the sample studied; and the influence of different cultures on the symptoms presented (92).

Minor Affective Changes

In a prospective community study of New Haven, Connecticut, Weissman and Myers (96) found an increased incidence of minor depression in both middle-aged men and women. The prevalence rate was 3.2% for the middle-aged compared with 1.9% for younger adults or 2.7% for older people. Minor depression was significantly more frequent in the lower socioeconomic group. Two other studies which compared middle-aged women with those of other age groups found no statistically significant peak incidence of minor affective changes or related symptoms in middle age (81, 105). When endocrinological status of women was examined in relation to symptoms, a somewhat different picture emerged than when age cohorts alone were examined (28). The findings were that behavioural changes occur with greater frequency in women whose menstrual cycles have changed recently (5, 47, 66, 67, 93). These changes include those of depression, nervousness, irritability, headaches and decreased social adaptation. An important aetiological role for the menopause is suggested by these findings. Two studies found that insomnia was unrelated to menopause but rather increased with increasing chronological age (47, 67).

Major Depression

Weissman and Myers (96) in a U.S.A. study found an increased prevalence of major depression in persons over the age of 45 years. The prevalence rate was 6.3% in middle age compared with 1.9% in young adulthood. Major depression was most frequent in whites, lower social classes, persons not currently married and females, although only the relationship with age was significant at the 10% level. The majority (86%) of major depressions were primary in this community study. The most frequent preceding disorder of the secondary depressions was alcoholism. Winokur (100) examined the relationship between menopausal status and affective disorder requiring psychiatric admission. He found that menopausal status did not produce an increased risk of hospitalisation for affective disorder over that expected for age.

Sex Differences in the Epidemiology of Depression

A review of studies of depressive disorders from different sources indicated that depression is more frequent in women (95). Studies based on patient populations in Western countries confirmed that most diagnosed depressives were women. Community surveys also found that more women get depressed. Possible explanations for this sex difference were reviewed. Weissman and Klerman (95) concluded that women did not have more stressful life events (perceived or actual) than men. While help-seeking patterns differed between men and women, this did not account for the increase in untreated "cases" of depressed women present in the community. Other explanations, such as those based on endocrine or psychosocial factors, are explored in the following section.

AETIOLOGY OF DEPRESSION

Biological

Genetic

There is considerable evidence for some genetic basis for depressive illnesses(101). When all affective disorders are examined as a group, there is a higher incidence in relatives of depressed patients than in the community (104). Concordance for depression is higher in monozygotic than in dizygotic twins (77, 86).

There are genetic as well as clinical differences between the subgroups of primary depressive disorders. Bipolar patients tend to have an earlier age of onset (102) than unipolar patients, who tend to become depressed for the first time in their mid-forties. The relatives of bipolar patients had a greater risk for all affective disorders than did the relatives of unipolar patients. While unipolar patients rarely had a relative with mania, bipolar patients had relatives with both unipolar and bipolar disorders.

Several workers (65, 103) present evidence for an X-linked transmission in bipolar illness. Father to son transmission of bipolar illness in some families suggests that X-linkage is not the sole means of transmission (64).

Winokur (100) suggested a further classification for unipolar depression based on family studies and age of onset. "Depression Spectrum Disease" had an early onset (before age 40), occurred mainly in females, and was characterised by a family history of depression, alcoholism and sociopathy. "Pure Depressive Illness" was of later onset (after age 40), more common in males, and was characterised by a smaller amount of affective illness in the family than in the depression spectrum type, with little or no family history of alcoholism or sociopathy.

Biochemical

Over the last two decades increased interest has been given to the role of neurotransmitters in psychiatric illnesses. Although over 30 substances have been described as possible neurotransmitters, not all have been proven. At least six substances—acetylcholine, noradrenaline, dopamine, serotonin, glycine and γ-amino-butyrate (GABA)—have been well substantiated as neurotransmitters in mammalian brains (4). Research in the affective disorders has focused almost exclusively on the catecholamines, noradrenaline, dopamine and the indoleamine, serotonin. The catecholamine hypothesis grew out of several clinical and pharmacological observations. Reserpine, a drug which produced depression in man, depleted central amine stores (46).

Euphoric effects were observed in patients treated with iproniazid—a mono-amine oxidase inhibitor. Tricyclic antidepressants are believed to act by inhibition of the reuptake of the biogenic amines at the nerve endings. Lithium, an effective agent used in the prevention of mania, also affects biogenic amine uptake in some systems, having an effect opposite to that of the tricyclics (46).

The catecholamine model failed to explain why cocaine, a potent inhibitor of monoamine reuptake, was without clinical antidepressant action (76) or the antidepressant action of iprindole and mianserin, both of which have minimal effects on reuptake of biogenic amines (24, 33, 39, 73). These failings of the pharmacological models led to further metabolic studies in patients with affective illness. Research studies of catecholamines or their metabolites in plasma urine and CSF in depressed patients fail to clarify the role of catecholamine neurotransmitters in this group of illnesses (21).

Studies of indoleamines have been mainly concerned with levels of ser-otonin or its metabolite 5-hydroxyindoleacetic acid (5-HIAA). Brains of su-icide victims showed decreases of both serotonin and 5-HIAA compared with controls (14, 68, 85). There are conflicting reports of the levels of 5-HIAA in the CSF of depressed and manic patients. Asberg et al. (3) found that patients with low CSF 5-HIAA attempted suicide more often than those with higher concentrations.

Although the role of histamine as a neurotransmitter is still debatable recent data suggest a possible role for histamine in the biochemistry of depression. A number of antidepressant drugs affect histamine sensitive brain adenylate cyclase (49). This includes drugs such as iprindole and mian-serin which have little effect on catecholaminergic and serotonergic systems.

In summary, pharmacological evidence strongly points to a role for neu-rotransmitter substances in the aetiology of affective disorders. Conflicting results reflect the effects of age, assay methodology, circadian rhythms and the complex nature of the disease entity studied. The complex relationship between neurotransmitters makes any simple explanation unlikely.

Hormonal

A hormonal basis for minor changes in affect, headache and decreased sexual response was suggested by epidemiological studies which have dem-onstrated an increase in frequency of these symptoms in women in relation to a phase of declining ovarian hormone production. In order to determine the role of hormones, a double-blind crossover trial of an estrogen and a progestogen, alone and in combination, and a placebo was conducted in oophorectomised women. Affect was measured by verbal reports and psychological rating scales. The findings concur with those of other double-blind studies of menopausal therapy which have demonstrated a beneficial effect of estrogens on the symptomatology of anxiety and depression (29). Affect in women was found to be associated with estrogen-progestogen balance such that increasing estrogen had a beneficial influence on affect while increasing progestogen had an adverse influence.

Klaiber et al. (55) have suggested that monoaminergic changes may underlie these mechanisms. They demonstrated changes in plasma monoamine oxidase activity in association with changing estrogen and progesterone levels. In humans computerised electroencephalograms have demonstrated changes in alpha rhythm in association with changing plasma estrogen and progesterone levels which suggest an antidepressant effect of estrogen. In a later study Klaiber et al. (54) found that high doses of conjugated equine estrogens significantly reduced endogenous depression as measured by the Hamilton Rating for Depression. The influence of hormonal factors on affect may at least in part explain the preponderance of females suffering from depression.

Psychological

In the middle years of life there is the greatest demand for adequate emotional adaptation during a rapidly changing phase, frequently involving two people, both separately and together. The importance of premorbid personality during the climacterium was emphasised by Fessler (36), who claimed that climacteric depression was the continuation into the menopause of the patient's preclimacteric condition. Benedek (10) also emphasised previous adaptation, claiming a better outcome for women whose "adaptive capacity has not been exhausted by previous neurotic processes." Weissman et al. (97) found the N score of the Maudsley Personality Inventory to be a good predictor of the clinical course and long-term outcome in a group of non-bipolar depressed women. Patients with long-standing neurotic maladaptation were at risk for persisting depressive difficulty.

Most psychological theories of depression focus on loss. Of past losses only loss of mother before age 11 is associated with an increased risk of depression in women (17). Among female patients all types of past loss by death were associated with psychotic-like depressive symptoms while other types of loss were associated with neurotic-like depressive symptoms. It was postulated that loss of a mother before 11 may lead to a permanent loss of sense of mastery and self-esteem and hence act as a vulnerability factor by interfering with the method of dealing with grief in adulthood. Other vulnerability factors identified by Brown et al. (17) and Roy (80) in working-class women with depressive neurosis included three or more children at home under 14 years of age, lack of a confiding marital relationship and lack of employment.

Significant "losses" occur for both males and females in middle age. Deutsch (30) referred to the loss of reproductive capacity as "a partial death." The depletion and decline in sexual attractiveness, usefulness and biological function were experienced by some women intrapsychically as an object loss (34). Depression resulted when the object loss was invested with the loser's self-esteem. The affects of giving up are said to be those of helplessness and hopelessness. Oral and narcissistic needs are intensified. Other psychological stresses related to actual or feared losses include those of loss of a loved person, substantial property, sexual potency or even his/her own ideals. Yochelson (106) noted a loss of the "fairy tale idea of happiness" as being a precipitant of some depressive episodes. After achieving goals as measured by community ideals, the individual's own stocktaking may reveal that he is still not happy, resulting in disappointment, bitterness, feelings of failure and depression. Others may become depressed when stocktaking reveals that they have failed to reach goals.

Perris and Espvall (72) present case examples of reactive depression occurring in response to being professionally successful. Explanations offered for depression occurring in response to success include the possibility of an overwhelming guilt if the competition in later life is identified with the rivalries of childhood, and success then experienced as murder of competitors. Alternatively, promotion may result in some isolation. The sudden lack of support from peers may be experienced as an object loss. Lastly, success may limit the forward movement dependent on desire and hope.

The role of specific stressful events in the aetiology of depression has received much attention in the last decade. Retrospective studies of psychiatric patients and general population controls indicate that the great majority of depressive illnesses (70) and suicide attempts (71) are preceded by stressful events of one sort or another. Recent studies confirm that the events may not be such major crises as death or financial ruin, but more common (although serious) domestic disturbances such as interpersonal arguments, marital disruptions, separations and difficulties at work (69). Methodological problems limiting the interpretation of these findings include the possibility of distortion of recall (in an attempt to find a cause for the illness) and the fact that psychiatric illness may itself both produce new events and alter perception of events which have occurred. Paykel (69) noted the importance of "the soil" on which the event falls. Such vulnerability factors as early loss, social support, genetic and personality type may determine response to stress. An almost equal frequency of life stressors was reported by endogenous and neurotic depression patients (63). However, there was a difference in their experience. Endogenous patients have their crucial events in the sphere of physical stress and overdemand in the field of performance, whereas in neurotic depression the stress appears to be in conflictive coping with the environment.

Behavioural theorists such as Liberman and Raskin (62) perceive the major feature of depression to be a reduced frequency of adaptive behaviour. This is said to occur because of a decrease in the rate of positive reinforcement, reflecting aversive stimuli, punishment or a sudden change in the environment such as a death of a close relative. Depressive behaviours once manifest may be maintained or strengthened by their consequences. This viewpoint overlaps with psychodynamic concepts of loss but gives less credence to the intrapsychic consequences and places more emphasis on the observable and functional relations between reinforcing environmental events and behaviour. Secondary gain is redefined as social reinforcement. Secondary gains or reinforcements from a depressive episode in middle age may include being temporarily removed from a frustrating job, receiving attention and sympathy, and manipulation of others (90).

Hammen and Peters (43) found experimentally that "depressed" persons were more strongly rejected than nondepressed persons, especially by members of the opposite sex. They suggested that the sex difference in depression may reflect the fact that males are more reluctant to express their depression to friends. When males do talk of depression, it is more often to a female, who is more rejecting of depression in a male than in another female. Thus men learn to express psychological distress in alternative ways. Alcoholism, a condition occurring more frequently in males, is often suggested to be a "depressive equivalent."

Depression has been suggested to be an emotional expression of a state of helplessness, low self-esteem and powerlessness of the ego (11). Seligman (84) using animal experiments showed that uncontrollable and unpredictable traumas led to a state of passive resignation or learned helplessness.

Sociological

Depressive symptomatology may be culturally defined and engendered. Women in many cultures attain increased status and enjoy greater freedom with the menopause. In these cultures the achievement of the menopause is rewarded. In contrast, in Western cultures the menopause appears to be a sign of decline. This is emphasised by the usage of the term "climacteric," which literally refers to something or somebody being around the top of the ladder and starting on the way down (10). Psychosocial stresses necessitating social readjustments which occur at this phase of life include: adolescent rebellion and children leaving home; the arrival of grandchildren; the loss of youth and attractiveness in a youth-orientated society; the forced re-evaluation of expectations; death of parents and increasing physical ill health for the woman and her partner. An increase in psychological symptoms may reflect an inadequate adjustment to these changes.

Role theorists stress the importance of woman's social role performance. The loss of a role, for example, mothering, may be crucial in women who have few role alternatives, unless this is balanced by important cultural gains after menopause. Any consequent loss of self-esteem may result in depression. Bart (8) investigated middle-aged depressed women and found the highest rate of depression amongst housewives experiencing maternal role loss who had overprotective or overinvolved relationships with their children. Children leaving home resulted in a loss of self-esteem and depression in these women. "Middle age is a time when reality catches up with women's image of the future and some women are confronted with the meaningless-ness of their lives. Women who have embraced the traditionally feminine role are most liable to depression" (8). Feminist behavioural scientists such as Bart and Grossman (9) suggest the answer to these problems is for women to structure alternatives for themselves and other women. Some American women's groups are working towards this end. Two recent studies (60, 83) have failed to confirm the loss of parental role or the "empty nest" syndrome as a precipitant of depression. A major criticism of studies investigating social role functioning in relation to depression is that causality is often imputed from studies able to demonstrate an association only. Bothwell and Weissman (13) found that acutely depressed women were considerably impaired in all social role functioning, especially at work and in marriage and parenthood. Social readjustment took longer than symptom recovery. These findings have implications for the therapy of depressive disorders.

Multifactorial

A number of different aetiological theories have been proposed. Modern viewpoints recognise that many factors are important in the causation of depression. The question is not so much what causes depression but how much is contributed to by each factor relevant for any individual.

THERAPY IN DEPRESSION

Depression as a Mood

A biopsychosocial approach to mild depression in middle age is often helpful. Biological therapy includes the treatment of any concurrent physical illness and the use of hormone therapy for women whose depressive mood is related to the climacterium. While it is perhaps easier to recognize and treat hormone-dependent behavioural changes in women who have had an artificial menopause, there is often a dilemma for the physician treating the climacteric woman, especially if she is still menstruating regularly.

A study by Chakravarti et al.(23) demonstrated that behavioural complaints were more likely to respond to estrogen if vasomotor complaints were also present. The plasma estradiol was significantly lowered and follicle-stimulating hormone (FSH) and luteinising hormone (LH) significantly raised when vasomotor symptoms were present. It was suggested that an FSH> 15 U/1 in the presence of vasomotor symptoms constitutes the best method of selecting patients for estrogen replacement therapy (FSH of women who had no vasomotor symptoms—mean 5.4, range 0.8–16.3 U/1; FSH of women with vasomotor symptoms—mean 37.9 range 14.6–84.6 U/1). For all women with an intact uterus, hormone therapy with an estrogen should be cyclical and should include the addition of a progestogen in the last 10 days of each monthly cycle to induce shedding of the endometrium.

Mild depressions in middle age respond well to psychotherapy, usually of the supportive type. Encouragement is given to the patient to express anxiety about fears of aging, decreased sexual drive, attractiveness, usefulness and so on. Social intervention is often helpful where there are interpersonal difficulties with partners, parents or children. Mild depressions may be significantly helped by hypnotherapy (18). If anxiety is great, short-term use of anti-anxiety agents or, rarely, a low dose of an antipsychotic drug may be a better management.

Depression as a Syndrome

A practical approach to the treatment of depression is based on the severity of the illness. This may be assessed initially and regularly by visual analogue scales in the family practice setting, while psychiatrists often use scales like the Hamilton Depression Rating Scale (42). The majority of depressions are mild and usually do not require pharmacotherapy.

The middle group of moderate depressive illness require antidepressant therapy, and in the smallest group of severe depressive illness electroconvulsive therapy is still the optimum treatment. Concurrent psychotherapy in all types of depression is essential.

Psychotherapy

Any treatment which depends upon the formation and continuation of a therapeutic relationship with another person or persons may be called psychotherapy. All but the most severely depressed patients benefit from a supportive psychotherapy. Tanner et al. (91), in a prospective study of moderately depressed women, found that maintenance antidepressants prevented relapse and symptom return better than placebo or no medication. Maintenance antidepressants had no influence on social functioning. In contrast, maintenance psychotherapy enhanced social functioning but did not prevent symptom return. Tanner and co-workers noted that drugs are prescribed for the relief of symptoms but are not agents for relearning faulty habits or inappropriate patterns in relating to others. Noting the continued social maladaptation of women four years after an acute depressive illness, Bothwell and Weissman (13) also emphasised the need for a prolonged therapy, taking into account the social morbidity of the disorder, which may be responsive to psychological therapies.

It is essential to create a sympathetic, accepting atmosphere in which there is an opportunity for reassurance, ventilation of fears and the reinforcement of positive thinking and behaviour, rather than a frontal attack on morbid beliefs and attitudes. Confrontatory techniques have no place in the supportive psychotherapy of depressed patients.

Initially, the patient should be told that he suffers from a depressive disorder or illness and that treatment is available and will most probably be successful. Major life decisions should be postponed until the patient is well again. The patient should be encouraged to discuss attitudes to herself as a person, the people around her and her life situation.

Antidepressant Pharmacotherapy

Having decided to prescribe an antidepressant drug, what decision does the clinician make in choosing from what may appear a bewildering variety of drugs?

Although a number of drugs are termed "antidepressant," the wise doctor would treat his patient best by not limiting himself to only one of the types of antidepressants available. The ideal antidepressant has not yet been developed.

In broad terms, there are four groups of antidepressant drugs: 1. stimulants; 2. tricyclics, and more recently, tetracyclics and bicyclics; 3. monoamine oxidase inhibitors (MAOI); and 4. lithium carbonate.

Stimulants

Examples of stimulants include amphetamine and amphetamine-like substances. There is no real place for the stimulants in the modern-day treatment of depressive illness because of the dependency problems.

Tricyclic antidepressants

Advances in the treatment of depressive illness in the past 20 years are partly the result of the introduction of the tricyclics. Most of these compounds are effective in about 70% of treated depressed patients. Reasons for discrepancy in the results of tricyclic antidepressant drug trials include lack of homogeneity of the illness studied, problems of measuring changes in symptoms, the very large influence extended by non-pharmacological factors on treatment response and the individual differences in the amount of active substance at the site of action.

Briefly, there are no clear-cut differences clinically between members of the tricyclic antidepressants as regards potency, speed of action, and consistency of effect. Early improvement, particularly diminished anxiety, may occur by the end of the first week, but usually takes three to six weeks. Amitriptyline, trimipramine, nortriptyline, and doxepin have sedative effects which are useful in agitated depression. Imipramine, desipramine and nomifensine have comparatively less sedative component.

Responses to therapy appear, in part, to be genetically determined. Previous response, or a good response in a close relative, may help in the choice between the tricyclic group and a MAOI. Tricyclics have been considered the best first choice until recently. The newer bicyclic and tetracyclic compounds are rapidly gaining favour because of fewer side effects, particularly cardiological.

Dosage regimen of tricyclics

The most useful therapeutic dose is 150 mg of the tricyclic per day. A general practice study showed that 150 mg/day of amitriptyline produced significantly better results than 75 mg/day (12). Tricyclic antidepressants, because of their long plasma half-life, can be conveniently given as a single daily dose at bedtime. If the patient responds, smaller maintenance doses should be continued for four to six months.

In some outpatients, it may be advisable to begin with a low dose, particularly in the elderly, but to increase to a maximum tolerated dose within a week or two at the most. Some patients prefer capsules, while others definitely like tablets. If adequate use of a tricyclic has failed to relieve the depression, it is unlikely that another of the same group will prove effective. Changing to a monoamine oxidase inhibitor might be effective, but more commonly electroconvulsive therapy will need serious consideration with specialist referral.

Side effects and toxicity of tricyclics

The side effects of the tricyclics are extensions of their pharmacological actions. Common symptoms are dryness of mouth, sweating, faintness, and fine tremor. Patients must be warned of the possible side effects; patients expecting them do not become overconcerned and tolerate much higher doses with positive therapeutic effect. More serious effects include severe postural hypotension, urinary hesitancy, delayed ejaculation and impotence. Acute brain syndrome occurs in the occasional patient, especially the elderly, when the dosage is too high, as will cardiac toxicity with conduction problems.

Plasma tricyclic levels and clinical response

Over the past decade a growing number of studies have resulted from the improving techniques for measuring tricyclic plasma levels. Although knowledge of the pharmacokinetics, pharmacodynamics, and pharmacotherapy of the tricyclic antidepressants has greatly increased, there is still much more to be investigated. The bioavailability of the tricyclics differs from person to person, compound to compound, and even within individuals. At present it is impossible to define a therapeutic plasma range for all tricyclics. Some workers have found a definite correlation between a plasma level range and therapeutic response but others have not, and at present plasma level determinations of these drugs remain predominantly of research interest (20).

New antidepressants

Many compounds have been developed over the last few years, and include the tetracyclic mianserin, and bicyclic nomifensine, and specific serotonin reuptake blockers such as zimelidine. As yet none of the newer antidepressants have been shown to be consistently superior to the earlier tricyclics in terms of the proportion of patients responding, average improvement shown, or speed of onset. Unwanted toxic or side effects have limited the usefulness of all the older antidepressants and the newer compounds have been developed in an attempt to find less toxic drugs. The very early studies now available show that nomifensine, mianserin and zimelidine are less cardiotoxic.

Mianserin is a tetracyclic compound. It combines presynaptic alpha-adrenoceptor blocking activity with antihistamine properties, but has no central anticholinergic activity and little effect on central serotonergic mechanisms.

Studies with mianserin in both healthy subjects and a small number of patients have not revealed any adverse cardiovascular effects. Crome and Newman (26) in 19 adults and Crome et al. (25) in 44 patients following an overdose of mianserin suggest much less cardiotoxicity than with tricyclic antidepressants. Green and Kendall-Taylor (40) reported first degree heart-block in a patient following ingestion of 600 mg mianserin.

The cardiovascular effects of mianserin 30 or 60 mg daily and placebo in 50 patients with heart disease showed no significant differences between treatments on heart rate, blood pressure or electrocardiograph records (57).

Ten moderately depressed inpatients studied by His bundle electrocardiography initially and following 60 mg/day for a three-week period showed no effects on cardiac conduction (19).

There have as yet been no published comparisons of the relative effects of overdoses of mianserin and tricyclic antidepressants on intracardiac conduction, but in view of the previous study these should be significantly less.

Monoamine oxidase inhibitors (MAOIs)

There is no agreement on the role of these drugs in the treatment of depression. Some authors state that MAOIs are antidepressants of the second choice to be prescribed only after a failed adequate trial of tricyclics. A drug-free period of a week between these two groups of drugs must occur to avoid the possible risk of interaction (see below). A few researchers believe that MAOIs should initially only be prescribed by the specialist.

MAOIs are thought to be the drug of choice in so-called "atypical depressions," frequently of a reactive type, in the younger patient, where there are a number of anxiety symptoms. There is no doubt that depressed patients who fail to respond to adequate dosage of tricyclics frequently respond to a MAOI. There is some genetic evidence that this is a distinct group of patients.

Autonomic, anticholinergic side effects include orthostatic hypotension, constipation, delayed micturition, dry mouth, delayed ejaculation and impotence. These occur also with the tricyclics but are usually less troublesome with the MAOIs.

Interactions with drugs such as tricyclics, amphetamine-like substances (particularly anorexiants, cough and common cold remedies), narcotics such as pethidine and tyramine-rich foods like matured cheese, yeast and meat extracts such as "Marmite," "Bovril" and packet soups, alcohol (especially dark red wine), and dopamine-rich foods such as broad bean pods, may result in a hypertensive crisis. The patient prescribed MAOIs should be warned of the danger of interaction with certain foods and drugs and should be immediately asked to repeat the instructions. A "MAOI card" should be given also, and the family doctor should also be aware of the contraindications of certain foods and drugs.

The usual dosage, say of tranylcypromine, is one or two 10mg tablets prescribed morning and lunchtime; taken later in the day a MAOI often causes insomnia. The dose is increased by one additional tablet every three days, to an upper level of around 40 to 60 mg daily. When the patient responds, a smaller maintenance dose for at least four to six months is warranted in most patients, as with the tricyclics.

It is now recognised that there is more than one functionally active type of MAOI and newer drugs are being developed. This may result in specific inhibitors of isoenzymes and eliminate some of the potential hazards.

Lithium

Lithium is a specific and effective antimanic drug. It may also be effective against recurring depression. Recent research has shown lithium to be nephrotoxic. The value of lithium in recurrent bipolar illness is so great that it should not be withheld in the severely ill patient, particularly where repeated hospitalisation, suicide attempts, or hypomanic and manic behaviour has been present. For unipolar depression in patients who respond only to ECT after failure of adequate trials of antidepressants, then prophylaxis with lithium would again appear to be indicated. For recurrent unipolar depression which responds to tricyclics, a longer-term prophylaxis with a tricyclic compound may be preferable at this stage of our knowledge.

The exact method of action of lithium is obscure. Ideally, initially, the patients should be investigated in special affective or lithium clinics prior to medication. Lithium causes side effects such as a metallic taste, sedation, tremor, a diabetes insipidus syndrome of thirst, polyuria, nocturia, and skin rashes. Long-term use causes thyroid abnormalities with hypothyroidism in 4% of patients. Baseline renal and thyroid function tests are desirable, with at least yearly reviews. The 250 mg lithium carbonate tablets are prescribed in three to four divided daily doses, aiming for a plasma lithium level measured in the morning 12 hours after the last dose of 0.8 mmol/L (mEq/L) prophylactically. Regular weekly plasma monitoring initially until "steady state" is obtained should be followed by at least two to three monthly reviews. Sodium depletion or renal impairment delay renal lithium excretion and increase the risk of intoxication. In view of the potential renal problems, the criteria for lithium use should be strict, based on the nature, severity and frequency of the acute attacks, and specialist opinion should be sought.

TABLE 1

Antidepressant Drugs

General Classification	Generic Name	Dosage (mg/day)
1. Stimulants	Amphetamine	5-60
	Dextroamphetamine	5-60
	Methamphetamine	5-60
2. Tricyclics	Imipramine	75-300
	Desipramine	75-300
	Trimipramine	75-300
	Amitriptyline	75-300
	Nortriptyline	75-300
	Protriptyline	20-60
	Doxepin	75-300
	Dothiepin	75-300
	Maprotiline	75-300
3. Tetracyclic	Mianserin	30-120
4. Bicyclics	Zimelidine	150-300
	Nomifensine	100-300
5. Monoamine oxidase inhibitors		
Hydrazines	Isocarboxazid	20-60
	Phenelzine	45-75
Non-hydrazine	Tranylcypromine	20-60
6. Lithium carbonate		750-2000

Electroconvulsive Therapy (ECT)

The use of electroconvulsive treatment in depressive illness has been well reviewed(51). Various forms of electrotherapy were used in the 18th and 19th centuries. Cerletti and Bini (22) reintroduced the technique of producing convulsions electrically in 1938. The administration of ECT is described in detail by Kalinowsky and Hippius (48). It is customary to modify the convulsions by administering a muscle relaxant following a short-acting intravenous anaesthetic. Until recently, ECT was generally given using bitemporal electrodes, but now many clinicians believe unilateral electrode placement is more desirable. Advantages include reduction of the period of post-convulsive memory disturbance and improvement of memory for events occuring before treatment. Post-convulsive confusion is reduced (27). Unilateral non-dominant ECT is as efficacious as bitemporal ECT. It is usual to give ECT two or three times weekly. The total number of convulsions required to produce a good therapeutic response in depression varies greatly in different patients. The mean number is about six but some may require up to 16 or more. An empirical working rule is to give a sufficient number of convulsions to significantly relieve the patient's symptoms plus two more. It is widely believed that patients with endogenous depression are more likely to respond to ECT than those with neurotic depressions, but there are only a few comparative trials. Relapse rates in the first six months are around 50% (53). In severe depressive illness with agitation and delusions, ECT would appear to be the best initial choice for therapy.

Psychosurgery

Depression is now the prime indication for prefrontal leucotomy (52). The offer of leucotomy to a patient with a depressive disorder is the result of a complex of interrelated assessments, including clinical features such as "tortured self-concern" (2), personal distress (74), history of the illness, evaluation of the patient's biological status, personality, coping ability, prediction of future environment, and a review of the failed treatments. Prognostic factors are seldom absolute. The presence of anxiety, tension, agitation and obsessionality, and a good premorbid personality favour the operation, while hysterical symptoms, hypochondriasis, inadequacy, aggression, antisocial activity, drug dependence and alcoholism appear unfavourable.

There is some evidence that when relapse occurs following the operation the patient responds to antidepressant therapies which previously had been ineffective. This form of therapy for intractable obscure depression still remains controversial, but despite major criticism still appears to have a role.

The general psychiatric clinician has little experience in this area and patients being considered for psychosurgery should be referred to specialist units. The reader is referred to the excellent review by Kiloh (52).

SUICIDE

There is an enormous number of scientific articles on suicide. A bibliography of suicide published in 1969 listed about 3,400 articles, and a rapid increase has continued, with special journals and publication series dealing solely with suicide and suicide prevention. Emile Durkheim's work, "Le Suicide" (31), was published in 1897 and set an example for studies for the following century. Many studies have commenced from various statistics, hospital case records, and other documents concerning the patients. Recent workers suggest that completed suicide cannot be investigated sufficiently on the basis of statistics alone. Interviews with patients' relatives, friends, fellow workers, primary care doctors, and other people who had been associated with them are necessary (35).

Suicide research has produced divergent results in different countries, partly because there had been no internationally accepted definition of suicide to facilitate the use of identical principles in classification. The earlier estimates of the incidence of psychiatric illness and those committing suicide came from records kept by coroners or other officials. About 30-50% of those taking their lives were considered to be suffering from a mental illness. The more reliable sources are from detailed psychiatric histories. Robins and co-workers (79) reported the histories of 134 suicides. They diagnosed a psychiatric illness in 94%, while another 4% had been physically ill. They reported 68% had suffered from either a manic-depressive psychosis or from chronic alcoholism.

Suicide is the result of a combination of interacting factors which may be biological, psychological, social and cultural. Epidemiological studies have shown that the social and demographic characteristics of a population determine its incidence of suicide. From these studies it is known that men always have a higher suicide rate than women but that suicide in women is increasing throughout the Western world. Suicide rates increase with age, while those of high social and economic status have higher suicide rates and married people have a relatively low risk. Social circumstances that isolate a person from domestic, occupational, religious or neighbourhood groups increase the probability of suicide. It has been found that suicide rates are high in socially disorganised urban areas, among separated and divorced people who do not attend church, in those who live alone, and in immigrants.

Suicide falls in wartime but rises sharply in times of socioeconomic crisis. The stresses of life such as loss, bereavement, moving from one area to another, unemployment, and physical illness are strongly associated with suicide. The important questions for this chapter are how the risk of suicide relates to depressive illness, particularly in middle age, how high-risk patients can be identified, and whether treatment and facilities for the potentially suicidal are realistic prevention objectives.

Depression has been noted as a characteristic symptom in many suicide cases. "Depressive illness or melancholia is the mental disorder with the highest suicide rate . . . invariably depressed patients wish to die and many, though not all of them, commit or attempt suicide" (87).

Some psychiatrists would agree with Whitlock (98) that "the assumption that mental illness, particularly severe depression, is an inevitable forerunner of suicide may well be too simple a view. The age and culture need to be considered and there are also those who as far as can be ascertained are seized by an overwhelming desire to take their lives without showing any of the features of a severe affective disorder. Not all depressed people kill themselves, nevertheless the suicide rate among persons diagnosed as suffering from manic-depressive disorders is very high. In 14 follow-up studies reviewed by Guze and Robins (41), it was revealed that approximately 15% had killed themselves.

Most suicide studies do not distinguish between victims with manic-depressive disorders and those with neurotic-depressive reactions. The frequency of the more severe depressive conditions varies from 7.3% (59) to 30.8% (88) and 45% (79). A WHO committee (1968) reported about 20% of suicides have made previous attempts, which suggests the relationship of depressive illness to attempted suicide.

Whitlock (98) reviewed 16 studies of attempted suicide and showed "clearly that reactive or neurotic depression figures more frequently than endogenous depression, manic-depressive psychosis or melancholia as an antecedent state to suicidal behaviour."

To summarise, in most Western societies suicide is an act of older persons, often male, suffering from a serious physical or mental illness, often widowed, separated or divorced, may be socially isolated, or have moved residence recently, and may have more frequently lost one or more parents during early childhood. Men more often than women die violently. Women more often take poisons or psychotropic drugs in lethal amounts.

In contrast, suicide attempts are from a younger age group, females predominantly, from poor social circumstances, high incidence of personality disorder, alcoholism, drug dependence, and low incidence of major psychiatric illness. The suicide attempt appears to be an impulsive, emotional, frustrated or angry act.

Barraclough and co-workers (6) studied 100 suicides from West Sussex and Portsmouth, based on coroners' records and interviews with close relatives of the deceased. They classified 64 as depressed, 15 as alcoholics, 14 with other diagnoses and seven with no formal psychiatric disorder. Three-quarters of the depressed patients were aged over 45 years. When compared with the general population, there were more single and widowed, fewer married but as many divorced as expected. A past history of psychiatric treatment or consultation was found in 52% and 62% of these had a past history of depression. Of the depressed suicides 33% had made previous suicidal attempts. Forty-two percent of the depressed patients had been in contact with their doctor within seven days of their death and a further 20% had contacted doctors less than 30 days prior to suicide.

Whitlock (98) reported data on 1,052 suicides from 19 coroners in England between 1966-1970. He concluded that about 66% of these suicide victims were seriously depressed. The mean age for males was 55.7, S.D. 16.7, and females 57.8, S.D. 14.9. Whitlock also reported an Australian study of 135 suicides from Brisbane in which approximately 41% were primarily depressed. The mean age was 50.1 for males (S.D. 17.4) and females 53.2 (S.D. 17.3).

Fremming (37) followed a group on Barnholm Island from birth through 50 years and Helgason (44) studied all Icelanders born during 1895-97 until 1957. Both authors found that 50% of the deaths in manic-depressive psychosis were suicides, compared with 11% and 17% respectively of all their psychotic patients, but only 6% and 2% of the schizophrenics died in this manner.

Depressed suicides differed significantly from a comparison group of depressive patients (6) in two ways; They had made more previous suicidal attempts (46% compared with 6%) and the duration of the current illness was larger. This confirms the clinical findings that suicide occurs late in an episode of depressive illness and that the intent to die is high in the suicide attempts of depressives (82).

It would seem from studies of suicide in which psychiatrists attempt a diagnosis that the prevalence of mental disorder exceeds 90%, and that a primary depressive illness of the kind normally treated with antidepressant drugs or ECT is the most frequent condition. Alcoholism is the second most common precipitating factor.

The Causes of Suicide

Since the turn of the century research into suicide has largely resulted from two major hypotheses. The sociologists have described suicides as primarily social phenomena, while many psychologists and psychiatrists have regarded suicides as arising from forces within the individual.

Psychopathological theories emphasise the role of overwhelming guilt and aggression turned against the self as a type of punishment and expiation (38). Freud considered depression and suicide were attributable to hatred originally directed at other people. Later he introduced the assumption that in addition to a self-preservative instinct there was a death instinct in man. Suicide was a consequence of the fact that the death instinct proved stronger than the self-preservative instinct.

Adler considered the following were typical of suicides: a pampered lifestyle in which suicidal tendences develop in persons whose method of living has always been dependent on the achievement and support of others; inferiority feelings and self-centred goals, low self-esteem so that suicide may offer a feeling of mastery over life and death; a high degree of activity; veiled aggression in that the suicider hopes to hurt others by hurting himself and manoeuvres to influence others by creating sympathy.

The Jungian view is that suicide is resorted to when a dead-end situation prevails with the feeling that life has no meaning and that meaning can only be regained through physiological rebirth in which the ego is developed by a conflict; resentment may reach murderous proportions, with rage directed against the person responsible, in which instance suicide may amount to an attempt to prevent such murderous acts; and a lack of vitality makes it impossible to find any "acting-out" substitute to release tension. Horney emphasised hopelessness, suffering, alienation, and search for glory (94).

Durkheim (31) was the prominent sociological theorist of suicide. The states of environment and society he termed egoism, anomy, and altruism. To each of these states of society he described a type of suicide specific for it. An egoistic suicide resulted when an individual was not sufficiently integrated with the community. An anomic suicide resulted when the norm system regulating the individual's behaviour suddenly failed. An altruistic suicide occurred where the individual's ties with the community were too strong. Social mobility, as well as social isolation, is associated with higher suicide rates.

A number of studies have shown that a high incidence of those committing suicide were alcoholics: 25% of male and 8% of female suicides (32).

Personality factors likely to predispose to suicide include impulsiveness, cyclothymia, chronic depressive temperament and unstable personalities.

Prevention of Suicide

It is important to recognise that the majority of people who commit suicide give obvious indication of their actions to their relatives, friends, or fellow workers. These include unequivocal statements or covert threats and such behaviour as making a will or hinting at suicidal thoughts. Warnings are most commonly given to the spouse. In the study of 134 suicides (79), 41% definitely stated intent to kill themselves, 60% told their spouse but only 18% told their doctor, even though 50% had seen him during the 12 months prior to death.

Most people committing suicide had very recently seen their general practitioner or psychiatrist and the majority had easily recognisable and eminently treatable psychiatric illnesses (6).

Sainsbury (82), in discussing prevention and management of suicide, considered the possibilities for preventing suicide initially as depending on the skill with which the medical, psychiatric and welfare personnel are able to identify those most at risk and elicit their suicidal feelings and secondly the development of appropriate services.

An informed general practitioner able to assess suicide intent, 24-hour ambulance service, emergency hospital facilities to deal with self-poisoning, adequate psychiatric follow-up, and crisis intervention are essential. The role and success of voluntary suicide prevention services are controversial. A recent study showed no significant differences in suicide rate whether or not a relationship with a Samaritan has been established (7).

It is important for clinicians to recognise that the risk of suicide varies with the duration of treatment. The onset and terminal stages of depression are danger periods, and the depressed patient is a higher risk on discharge from active treatment.

Early treatment of severe depressive illness, including the judicious use of ECT and prophylactic lithium, will obviously result in decreasing the risk of suicide.

REFERENCES

1. Angst, J. (1966). *Zur Ätiologie und Nosologie Endogener Depressiver Psychosen*. Berlin: Springer.

2. ARNOT, R. E. (1949). Clinical indications for pre-frontal lobotomy. *J. Nerv. Ment. Dis.*, *109*, 267.
3. ASBERG, M., TRASKMAN, L. and THOREN, P. (1976). 5-HIAA in the cerebro spinal fluid. A biochemical suicide predictor. *Arch. Gen. Psychiat.*, *33*, 1197.
4. BACHELARD, H. S. (1974). *Brain Biochemistry*. London: Chapman and Hall.
5. BALLINGER, C. B. (1975). Psychiatric morbidity and the menopause: screening of a general population sample. *Brit. Med. J.*, *3*, 344.
6. BARRACLOUGH, B. M., BUNCH, J., NELSON, B. and SAINSBURY, P. (1974). A hundred cases of suicide: clinical aspects. *Brit. J. Psychiat.*, *125*, 355.
7. BARRACLOUGH, B. M., JENNINGS, C. and MOSS, J. R. (1977). Suicide prevention by the Samaritans. *Lancet*, *ii*, 237.
8. BART, P. (1970). Depression in middle aged women. *Trans-Action*, *8*, 69.
9. BART, P. B. and GROSSMAN, M. (1978). *Menopause in the Woman Patient*, Volume 1, Sexual and Reproductive Aspects of Women's Health Care, pp. 337-354. New York: Plenum Press.
10. BENEDEK, T. (1950). Climacterium: A development phase. *Psychoanal. Quart.*, *19*, 1.
11. BIBRING, E. (1953). The mechanism of depression. In: Greenacre, P. (ed.), *Affective Disorders*. New York: International Universities Press.
12. BLASHKI, T. G., MOWBRAY, R. and DAVIES, B. (1971). Controlled trial of amitriptyline in general practice. *Brit. Med. J.*, *1*, 133.
13. BOTHWELL, S. and WEISSMAN, M. M. (1977). Social impairments four years after an acute depressive episode. *Amer. J. Orthopsychiatry*, *47*, 231.
14. BOURNE, H. R., BUNNEY, W. E. and COLBURN, R. W. (1968). Noradrenaline, 5-hydroxytryptamine and 5-hydroxyindoleacetic acid in hind brains of suicidal patients. *Lancet*, *ii*, 805.
15. BOWMAN, K. and ROSE, M. (1951). A criticism of the terms "psychosis," "psychoneurosis," and "neurosis." *Amer. J. Psychiat.*, *108*, 161.
16. BROWN, G. W., BHROLCHAIN, M. N. and HARRIS, T. (1975). Social class and psychiatric disturbance among women in an urban population. *Sociology*, *9*, 225.
17. BROWN, G. W., HARRIS, T. and COPELAND, J. R. (1977). Depression and loss. *Brit. J. Psychiat.*, *130*, 1.
18. BURROWS, G. D. (1979). Affective illness and hypnosis. In: Burrows, G. D. and Dennerstein, L. (eds.), *Handbook of Hypnosis and Psychosomatic Medicine*. Amsterdam: Elsevier/North Holland Biomedical Press.
19. BURROWS, G. D., DAVIES, B., HAMER, A. and VOHRA, J. (1979). Effect of mianserin on cardiac conduction. *Med. J. Aust.*, *2*, 97.
20. BURROWS, G. D., DAVIES, B., NORMAN, T., MAGUIRE, K. and SCOGGINS, B. A. (1978). Should plasma level monitoring of tricyclic antidepressants be introduced in clinical practice? In: Usdin, E. (ed.), *Communications in Psychopharmacology*, pp. 393-408. New York: Pergamon Press.
21. BURROWS, G. D., NORMAN, T. R., MCINTYRE, I. M. and WURM, J. E. (1979). The role of neurotransmittors in psychiatric illness. In: Kiloh, L. (ed.), *Geigy Symposium 1979*. Sydney: Bloxham Press.
22. CERLETTI, U. and BINI, L. (1938). *Arch, Gen. Neurol. Psychiat.*, *19*, 266.
23. CHAKRAVARTI, S., COLLINGS, W. P., THOM, M. H. and STUDD, J. W. W. (1979). Relation between plasma hormone profiles, symptoms and response to oestrogen treatment in women approaching the menopause. *Brit. Med. J.*, *1*, 983.
24. COPPEN, A., GHOSE, K., SWADE, C. and WOOD, K. (1978). Effect of mianserin hydrochloride on peripheral uptake mechanisms for noradrenaline and 5-hydroxytryptamine in man. *Brit. J. Clin. Pharm.*, *5*, 135.
25. CROME, P., BRAITHWAITE, R., NEWMAN, B. and MONTGOMERY, S. (1978). Choosing an antidepressant (letter to the editor). *Brit. Med. J.*, *1*, 859.

26. CROME, P. and NEWMAN, B. (1977). Poisoning with maprotiline and mianserin (letter to the editor). *Brit. Med. J.*, 2, 260.
27. D'ELIA, G. (1974). In: Fink, M., Kety, S., McGaugh, J. and Williams, T. A. (eds.), *Pyschobiology of Convulsive Therapy*. Washington: Winston.
28. DENNERSTEIN, L. and BURROWS, G. D. (1978). A review of studies of the psychological symptoms found at the menopause. *Maturitas, 1*, 55.
29. DENNERSTEIN, L., BURROWS, G. D., HYMAN, G. and SHARPE, K. (1979). Hormone therapy and affect. *Maturitas, 1*, 247.
30. DEUTSCH, H. (1945). In: *The Psychology of Women, Volume 2, Motherhood*, pp. 456-485. New York: Grune and Stratton.
31. DURKHEIM, E. (1897). *Le Suicide*. Paris: Falcan.
32. EDWARDS, J. E. and WHITLOCK, F. A. (1968). Suicide and attempted suicide in Brisbane: 1 and 2. *Med. J. Aust., 1*, 932 and 989.
33. EL-DEIRY, N. K., FORREST, A. D. and LITTMAN, S. K. (1968). Clinical trial of a new antidepressant (WY 3263). *Brit. J. Psychiat., 113*, 999.
34. ENGEL, G. L. (1962). In: *Psychological Development in Health and Disease*, pp. 208-209 and 294-301. Philadelphia: W. B. Saunders & Co..
35. FARBEROW, N. L. and MC EVOY, T. L. (1966). Suicide among patients with diagnosis of anxiety reaction, or depressive reaction in general medical and surgical hospitals. *J. Abnorm. Psychol., 71*, 287.
36. FESSLER, L. (1950). The psychopathology of climacteric depression. *Psychoanal. Quart., 19*, 28.
37. FREMMING, K. H. (1951). *The Expectation of Mental Infirmity in a Sample of the Danish Population*. London: Cassel.
38. FREUD, S. (1953). Mourning and Melancholia (1917). In: *Collected Papers, 4*, 152-170. London: Hogarth Press.
39. GLUCKMAN, M. I. and BAUM, T. (1969). The pharmacology of iprindole: a new antidepressant. *Psychopharmacologia* (Berl.), *15*, 169.
40. GREEN, S. D. R. and KENDALL-TAYLOR, P. (1977). Heart block in mianserin hydrochloride overdose. *Brit. Med. J.*, 2, 1190.
41. GUZE, S. B. and ROBINS, E. (1970). Suicide and primary affective disorders. *Brit. J. Psychiat., 117*, 437.
42. HAMILTON, M. J. (1960). A rating scale for depression. *J. Neurol., Neurosurg. Psychiat., 23*, 56.
43. HAMMEN, C. L. and PETERS, S. D. (1978). Interpersonal consequences of depression: Responses to men and women enacting a depressed role. *J. Abnorm. Psychol., 87*, 322.
44. HELGASON, T. (1964). Epidemiology of mental disorders in Iceland. A psychiatric and demographic investigation of 5,395 Icelanders. *Acta Psychiat. Scandina., Suppl., 173*, 11.
45. HOCH, A. and MACCURDY, J. T. (1922). The prognosis of involutional melancholia. *Arch. Neurol. Psychiat.* (Chic.), 7, 1.
46. JARVICK, M. E. (1970). Drugs used in the treatment of psychiatric disorders. In: Goodman, L. S. and Gilman, A. (eds.), *The Pharmacological Basis of Therapeutics*, 4th Edition, pp. 151-203. New York: Macmillan.
47. JASZMANN, L. (1973). Epidemiology of climacteric and post-climacteric complaints. In: van Keep, P. A. and Lauritzen, C. (eds.), *Ageing and Estrogens*, pp. 22-34. Basel: Karger.
48. KALINOWSKY, L. B. and HIPPIUS, H. (1969). *Pharmacological, Convulsive and other Somatic Treatments in Psychiatry*. New York: Grune and Stratton.
49. KANOF, P. D. and GREENGARD, P. (1978). Brain histamine receptors as targets for antidepressant drugs. *Nature, 272*, 329.
50. KENDELL, R. E. (1977). The classification of depressions: A review of contemporary con-

fusion. In: Burrows, G. D. (ed.), *Handbook of Studies on Depression*. Amsterdam: Excerpta Medica.

51. KILOH, L. G. (1977). The use of electroconvulsive treatment in depressive illness. In: Burrows, G. D. (ed.), *Handbook of Studies on Depression*. Amsterdam: Excerpta Medica.

52. KILOH, L. G. (1977b). Psychosurgery for depressive illness. In Burrows, G. D. (ed.), *Handbook of Studies on Depression*. Amsterdam: Excerpta Medica.

53. KILOH, L. G., CHILD, J. P. and LATNER, G. (1960). Endogenous depression treated with iproniazid—A follow-up study. *J. Ment. Sci.*, 106, 1425.

54. KLAIBER, E. L., BROVERMAN, D. M., VOGEL, W. and KOBAYASHI, Y. (1976). The use of steroid hormones in depression. In: Itil, T. M., Laudahn, G. and Herrmann, W. (eds.), *Psychotropic Action of Hormones*, pp. 135-154. New York: Spectrum Publications Inc..

55. KLAIBER, E. L., KOBAYASHI, Y., BROVERMAN, D. M. and HALL, F. (1971). Plasma monoamine oxidase activity in regularly menstruating women and in amenorrhoeic women receiving cyclic treatment with estrogens and a progestin. *J. Clin. Endocrinol. Metab.*, 33, 630.

56. KLERMAN, G. L. (1977). Anxiety and depression. In: Burrows, G. D. (ed.), *Handbook of Studies on Depression*, pp. 49-68. Amsterdam: Excerpta Medica.

57. KOPERA, H. and SCHENK, H. (1977). Poisoning with antidepressants (letter to the editor). *Brit. Med. J.*, 2, 773.

58. KRAEPELIN, E. (1907). *Lehrbuch der Psychiatrie* 7th Edition. Translated by Diefendorf, A. F., (1970) as Clinical Psychiatry. New York: Macmillan.

59. KRUPINSKI, J., POLKE, P. and STOLLER, A. (1965). Psychiatric disturbances in attempted and completed suicides in Victoria during 1963. *Med. J. Aust.*, 2, 773.

60. KRYSTAL, S. and CHIRIBOGA, D. A. (1979). The empty nest process in mid-life men and women. *Maturitas*, 1, 215.

61. LEONHARD, K. (1959) *Aufteilung der Endogenen Psychosen*. Berlin: Akademie-Verlag.

62. LIBERMAN, R. P. and RASKIN, D. E. (1971). Depression: a behavioural formulation. *Arch. Gen. Psychiat.*, 24, 515.

63. MATUSSEK, P. The structure of the precipitating events provoking neurotic and endogenous depressions. Unpublished paper.

64. MENDLEWICZ, J. (1979). Juvenile and late onset forms of depressive disorder: genetic and biological characterization of bipolar and unipolar illness—a review. *Maturitas*, 1, 229.

65. MENDLEWICZ, J., FLEISS, J. L. and FIEVE, R. R. (1972). Evidence for X-linkage in the transmission of manic-depressive illness. *J. Amer. Med. Ass.*, 222, 1624.

66. MCKINLAY, S. M. and JEFFERYS, M. (1974). The menopausal syndrome. *Brit. J. Prev. Soc. Med.*, 28, 108.

67. NEUGARTEN, B. L. and KRAINES, R. J. (1965). Menopausal symptoms in women of various ages. *Psychosom. Med.*, 27, 266.

68. PARE, C. M. B., YOUNG, D. P. H. and PRICE, K. (1969). 5-hydroxytryptamine, noradrenaline and dopamine in brain stem, hypothalamus and caudate nucleus of controls and patients committing suicide by coal gas poisoning. *Lancet*, ii, 133.

69. PAYKEL, E. S. (1978). Contribution of life events to causation of psychiatric illness. *Psychol. Med.*, 8, 245.

70. PAYKEL, E. S., MYERS, J. K., DIENELT, M. N. et al. (1969). Life events and depression: a controlled study. *Arch. Gen. Psychiat.*, 21, 753.

71. PAYKEL, E. S., PRUSOFF, B. A. and MYERS, J. K. (1975). Suicide attempts and recent life events: a controlled comparison. *Arch. Gen. Psychiat.*, 32, 327.

72. PERRIS, C. and ESPVALL, M. (1973). Depressive-type psychic reactions caused by success. *Psychiatria Clinica*, 6, 346.

73. PICHOT, P., DREYFUS, J. F. and PULL, C. (1978). A double-blind multicentre trial com-

paring mianserin with imipramine. *Brit. J. Clin, Pharm.*, 5, 87S.

74. PIPPARD, J. (1955). Rostral leucotomy: A report on 240 cases personally followed up after 1½ to 5 years. *J. Ment. Sci.*, 101, 756.

75. POST, F. (1962). *The Significance of Affective Symptoms in Old Age*. Maudsley Monograph No. 10. London: Oxford University Press.

76. POST, R. M., KOTIN, J. and GOODWIN, F. K. (1974). The effects of cocaine on depressed patients. *Amer. J. Psychiat.*, 131, 511.

77. PRICE, J. (1968). The genetics of depressive behaviour. In: Coppen, A. and Walk, A. (eds.), *Recent Developments in Affective Disorders*, Chapter 4. Royal Medico Psychological Association. Ashford: Headley Bros.

78. ROBINS, E., MUNOZ, R. A., MARTIN, S. and GENTRY, K. A. (1972). In: Zubin, J. and Freyhan, F. A. (eds.), *Disorders of Mood*, pp. 33-45. Baltimore: Johns Hopkins University Press.

79. ROBINS, E., MURPHY, G. E., WILKINSON, R. H., GASSNER, S. and KEYES, J. (1959). Some clinical considerations in the prevention of suicide based on a study of 134 successful suicides. *Amer. J. Publ. Hlth.*, 49, 888.

80. ROY, A. (1978). Vulnerability factors and depression in women. *Brit. J. Psychiat.*, 133, 106.

81. RYBO, G. and WESTERBERG, H. (1971). Symptoms in the postmenopause: a population study. *Acta Obstet. Gynaec. Scand.*, 30, 25.

82. SAINSBURY, P. (1978). Clinical aspects of suicide and its prevention. *Brit. J. Hosp. Med.*, Feb., 59.

83. SCHNEIDER, M. and BROTHERTON, P. (1979). Physiological, psychological and situational stresses in depression during the climacteric. *Maturitas*, 1, 153.

84. SELIGMAN, M. E. P. (1975). *Helplessness: On Depression, Development and Death*. San Francisco: W. H. Freeman.

85. SHAW, D. M., CAMPS, F. E. and ECCLESTON, E. G. (1967). 5-hydroxy-tryptamine in the hind brain of depressive suicides. *Brit. J. Psychiat.*, 113, 1407.

86. SLATER, E. and SHIELDS, J. (1953). *Psychotic and Neurotic Illnesses in Twins*. Spec. Rep. Ser. Med. Res. Coun., London, No. 278, HMSO.

87. STENGEL, E. (1964). *Suicide and Attempted Suicide*. Harmondsworth: Penguin Publications.

88. STENGEL, E. and COOK, N. G. (1958). *Attempted Suicide*. London: Chapman and Hall.

89. STENSTEDT, A. (1959). Involutional melancholia: an etiologic, clinical and social study of endogenous depression in later life with special reference to genetic factors. *Acta Psychiat. Scand.*, Suppl., 127.

90. STEWART, W. K. (1977). The middle-aged man who gives up the ghost: Hopelessness following illness in middle age. *Psychosomatics*, 18, 29.

91. TANNER, J., WEISSMAN, M. and PRUSOFF, B. (1975). Social adjustment and clinical relapse in depressed outpatients. *Comprehens. Psychiat.*, 16, 547.

92. TURNS, D. (1978). The epidemiology of major affective disorders. *Amer. J. Psychother.*, 32, 5.

93. VAN KEEP, P. A. and KELLERHALS, J. M. (1974). The imapct of socio-cultural factors on symptom formation. *Psychother. Psychosom.*, 23, 251.

94. VIRKKUNNEN, M. (1974). Suicide in schizophrenia and paranoid psychoses. *Acta Psychiat. Scandina.*, Suppl., 250, 11.

95. WEISSMAN, M. M. and KLERMAN, G. L. (1977). Sex differences and the epidemiology of depression. *Arch. Gen. Psychiat.*, 34, 98.

96. WEISSMAN, M. M. and MYERS, J. K. (1978). Affective disorders in a US urban community. *Arch. Gen. Psychiat.*, 35, 1304.

97. WEISSMAN, M. M., PRUSOFF, B. A. and KLERMAN, G. L. (1978). Personality and the prediction of long-term outcome of depression. *Amer. J. Psychiat.*, 135, 797.

98. WHITLOCK, F. A. (1977). Depression and suicide. In: Burrows, G. D. (ed.), *Handbook of Studies on Depression*. Amsterdam: Excerpta Medica.
99. WINOKUR, G. (1973). The types of affective disorders. *J. nerv. ment. Dis. 156*, 82.
100. WINOKUR, G. (1973). Depression in the menopause. *Amer. J. Psychiat., 130*, 92.
101. WINOKUR, G. and CADORET, R. (1977). Genetic studies in depressive disorders. In: Burrows, G. D. (ed.), *Handbook of Studies on Depression*, pp. 69-77. Amsterdam: Excerpta Medica.
102. WINOKUR, G. and CLAYTON, P. J. (1967). Family history studies 1. Two types of affective disorders separated according to genetic and clinical factors. In: Wortis, J. (ed.), *Recent Advances in Biological Psychiatry*. New York: Plenum Publishers.
103. WINOKUR, G., CLAYTON, P. J. and REICH, R. (1969). *Manic-Depressive Illness*. St. Louis: Mosby.
104. WINOKUR, G. and PITTS, F. N. Jr. (1965). Affective disorder: vi. A family history study of prevalences, sex differences and possible genetic factors. *J. Psychiat. Res., 3*, 113.
105. WOOD, C. (1979). Menopausal myths. *Med. J. Aust., 1*, 496.
106. YOCHELSON, L. (1965). The emotional problems of men in the mature years and beyond. *J. Amer. Geriat. Soc., 17*, 855.

15

ALCOHOLISM IN MIDDLE AGE

PETER M. MIRKIN, M.B., CH. B.

Clinical Director, Alcoholism Treatment Center;
Assistant Professor, Department of Psychiatry;
Research Psychiatrist, Alcohol Research Center;
University of Connecticut Health Center, Farmington

and

ROGER E. MEYER, M.D.

Professor and Chairman, Department of Psychiatry;
Scientific Director, Alcohol Research Center;
University of Connecticut Health Center, Farmington;
Lecturer in Psychiatry, Harvard Medical School

INTRODUCTION

The most useful conceptual model of alcoholism incorporates a biopsychosocial approach. As a biopsychosocial illness, alcoholism includes a genetic, psychological and/or environmental diathesis, as well as biological, psychological and environmental consequences. Such a systems-oriented model substitutes a reciprocal causal model for a simple cause-and-effect relationship. While the alcoholic may appear to be responsible for his illness and undeserving of sympathy, in truth he/she brings a special vulnerability to alcohol abuse (based on genetic, psychological and environmental factors) in a society which countenances alcohol use and is ambivalent about alcohol abuse. In this chapter we shall discuss some of the factors which pertain to alcohol abuse in middle age, outline clinical findings associated with alcoholism in this population, and point out certain aspects which should be considered in treatment.

A SYSTEMS-ORIENTED PESPECTIVE ON ALCOHOLISM

Statistics

It is not possible at present to obtain accurate statistics on the incidence or prevalence of alcoholism in any particular population group because of the lack of a universal definition of the disorder. It is generally accepted that the rate of alcohol-related problems in a population correlates well with the per capita rate of absolute alcohol consumption (31). An NIAAA survey of the late 1960s and early 1970s (9) showed that 31% of the population of the United States had one or more problems related to drinking during the three years prior to the survey interview. The problems identified were: frequent intoxication; binge drinking, symptomatic (withdrawal) drinking; psychological dependence; job-related problems; health problems; financial problems; problems with the law, police or accidents; and belligerence associated with drinking. The modal ages for heavy drinkers among men and women peaked at two age groups: 45-49 and 21-24. A similar population study by Edwards et al. (13) delineated normal drinking patterns and established drinking "trouble" indices for men and women in a South London suburb. His "trouble" index pointed to a high percentage of problems in that community. He replicated some of the American demographic data, but he did not find such a high proportion of heavy drinkers in the middle-aged group.

Typologies of Alcoholism

The average period of drinking prior to treatment is 20 to 22 years and most alcoholics come to treatment during their early forties (62). The data suggest that patterns of abuse are established at an early age, and that this results in the presentation of alcoholism during middle age. While this is true in many cases, it is not the sole clinical profile of middle-aged alcoholics (16, 72). Rosin and Glatt (53) demonstrated two groups of alcoholics in their study of elderly patients. The majority group appeared to have had long-standing alcohol abuse patterns dating back to their youth and early adulthood. They also showed personality profiles similar to younger alcohol abusers, and presented with many medical problems associated with alcohol addiction. This group fits the traditional model of alcoholism put forward by earlier writers (32), and is supported in part by long-term follow-up studies of cohorts (44). Rosin and Glatt found another group of alcoholics (one-third of the sample) who began to drink abusively in their early forties. They had fewer problems in adolescence and young adulthood than the first group, and led fairly stable lives. Their drinking appears to have started as a response to depression, bereavement, retirement, loneliness, marital stress and physical illness. Schuckit et al. (57) identified two similar groups of middle-aged alcoholics. They further differentiated characteristics of male and female alcoholics in the later-onset group. Both men and women started to drink abusively around age 40, with women starting earlier than men on average; the men tended to present for treatment after a 10- to 15-year course during which they initially had driving problems, later had job performance and marital difficulties, and finally presented for treatment because of health problems. Women tended to run a shorter course of two years, during which they quickly had problems with jobs and public intoxication and later had marital difficulties. Women tended to abuse more psychoactive drugs in combination with alcohol.

By focusing on a theoretical diathesis for alcoholism (genetic, psychological or environmental), or by differentiating alcoholics on the basis of the consequences of alcohol abuse (medical, psychosocial, familial, etc.), it is possible to distinguish between "types" of alcoholics and to attempt a problem-centered therapeutic approach. Skinner et al. (61) have described a core-shell approach to the treatment of alcoholism that is loosely based upon this type of formulation.

Psychopathology and Symptomatology

The classification of alcoholics on the basis of psychopathology, psychiatric symptomatology (e.g., anxiety and/or depression) and/or the presence of acute stress has been attempted by a number of authors.* There have been many attempts to classify alcoholics by using clinical and psychometric test data. More recent studies have utilized computer analysis to identify clinically meaningful subgroups (11, 23, 51). In the 1930s Knight separated groups of alcoholics on the basis of the severity of related psychiatric symptoms into "essential" and "reactive" alcoholics (29, 38). Essential alcoholics were those who began alcohol abuse at an early age in association with general immaturity, economic and emotional dependence, personal and social irresponsibility, hedonistic pleasure seeking, an inability to maintain deep or long-lasting relationships, and the need for immediate gratification. Reactive alcoholics were those whose problem drinking began at a later age, usually as a result of some precipitant. They had a greater degree of psychosocial maturity, educational and occupational achievement and responsibility. The two groups bear strong resemblance to the groupings described

---

*Jellinek utilized drinking pattern as a system for classifying alcoholics. This is another form of typology (30).

by Rosin and Glatt (53) and by Schuckit et al. (57). Nevertheless, the term "reactive" may be misleading since, at some stage, all alcoholics are "reactive." In essence, the groupings described by Knight and other authors (53, 57) appear to arrange alcoholics along a continuum according to severity of psychopathology. Clearly psychopathy should be an important differentiating feature in any attempt to classify alcoholics (1). Recent reports that some alcoholics may have suffered from learning and attentional problems suggestive of minimal brain dysfunction as children (66) are consistent with such reports among individuals with the diagnosis of psychopathy in a delinquent population (45).

Familial and Genetic Factors

The work of Goodwin (26), Schuckit et al. (55) and others (34, 71) suggests a genetic diathesis for alcoholism. It is important to differentiate genetic and familial-environmental issues in a theoretical consideration of etiology. Family therapists have written extensively about the families of alcoholics—their parents, spouses and children. Alcoholic men are said to suffer from domineering mothers and stern, distant fathers (54). Alcoholic women are said to have experienced cold, stern, dominating mothers and warm, gentle alcoholic fathers (5, 56). The important intervening variables in a genetic diathesis have been less clearly delineated. Recently Schuckit reported that children of alcoholics manifest higher blood acetaldehyde levels in response to equal ethanol administration (compared with children of non-alcoholics) (59). The etiological significance of this finding (if validated) is not clear. A number of studies have suggested an association between bipolar affective illness and alcoholism (12, 19, 48, 71), and unipolar affective illness and alcoholism (2, 8, 46, 73) in families. Winokur and associates have described a "depressive spectrum" disease in which: female relatives of alcoholics tend to have a higher incidence of depression than alcoholism; male relatives of alcoholics tend to have a higher incidence of sociopathy and alcoholism than depression; and male relatives of depressed females have a high incidence of sociopathy and alcoholism (25, 70, 71).

Depression and Suicide

A problem common to much of the current literature on alcoholism is the difficulty in obtaining a reliable psychiatric diagnosis. This problem generally arises due to variability in the information-gathering process (20, 21) or due to differences in clinical judgment across raters. It is important to differentiate depression as a symptom from depression as a psychiatric diagnosis in a population of alcoholics. Depression as a symptom may be a biological consequence of abrupt abstinence and may disappear readily over days to weeks without need for antidepressant medication. Depressive illness should be more resilient and should require active intervention with medication or electroconvulsive treatment. Unfortunately, most published studies have not differentiated between depression as symptom and depression as illness (35). Where depression symptom rating scales (e.g., Zung, Raskin, Hamilton or Beck rating scales) have been used (28, 47), the frequency of reported depressive symptomatology in alcoholic patients tends to be higher than in studies where such scales have not been employed. Moreover, where these instruments were utilized early on in a patient's hospitalization, depression is more frequent as a consequence of withdrawal and post-withdrawal symptomatology.

At the University of Connecticut Alcohol Research Center, we have dealt with the reliability problem by using standardized research diagnostic criteria (63) for every diagnosis and by using standardized structured interview schedules to gather the necessary information. To determine the reliability of the diagnostic classification of each subject, we compared the diagnoses obtained using one structured interview, the SADS-L (14), with the diagnoses obtained using a different structured interview, the NIMH Diagnostic Interview Schedule. Each subject was interviewed once using the SADS-L and once using the NIMH-DIS. Different interviewers were used on each occasion, and each interview was videotaped. Interrater reliability across diagnostic categories on the NIMH-DIS was quite high, K = .96, while interrater reliability on the SADS-L across diagnostic categories was somewhat lower, K = .83. Our initial unpublished results indicate that agreement from the two interviews for the three most frequent diagnostic categories was good: Alcoholism—100%, Major depressive disorder—75%, and Antisocial personality—72%. The development of standard interviewing instruments (SADS and/or DIS) should help clinicians and researchers to differentiate depressive symptoms from depressive illness.

It is also clear that the concomitant occurrence of depressive illness and alcoholism in some patients (particularly the middle-aged) should be reflected in a high suicide rate in this particular population (6). Over 90% of successful suicides are either depressed or alcoholic or both (4). They are frequently divorced or separated, or have experienced some form of marital stress. Suicide occurs more often in those alcoholics who have been drinking for many years. These individuals are chronically addicted and have many physical sequelae of drinking. They have usually experienced major losses in the form of separation from spouses, families, or jobs (43). Considering

the fact that the likelihood of depression increases with age to a peak incidence between the ages of 45 and 74 (62), it is likely that a significant
percentage of alcoholics who may have begun to drink at that age are primarily depressed. The inconsistent reports of efficacy (7, 69) and lack of
effectiveness of antidepressant medication (27, 60) in the treatment of alcoholism may be due to the failure of the program to differentiate depressive
symptoms from depressive illness. All of these reports antedate the recent
work establishing the correlation between blood levels of tricyclic antidepressant medication and therapeutic efficacy (22, 42). It is unclear whether
alcoholics metabolize these drugs more efficiently than other patients. It is
also unclear whether the effective treatment of a mid-life depression in an
alcoholic will result in the effective treatment of the alcohol problem. Such
studies need to be carried out.

Mid-life Changes

The relationship between alcoholism and mid-life depression may also be
seen in the context of those life changes associated with passage into middle
age. Recent social-psychological investigations suggest that psychosocial development takes place through a series of emotional crises and continues
throughout life. The transitions from one phase to the next may be gradual,
but they are accomplished through painful reevaluation of the meaning and
significance of life.

Levinson et al. (40) believe that there are three tasks at this developmental
stage. First, one must reappraise the past in the face of a heightened awareness of limited time to accomplish dreams. Next, one must modify the
structure of one's life to suit the realities of a de-illusioned future. Men often
make major shifts in marriage, job and life-style at this stage. The final task
is to continue the lifelong process of individuation—the crisis of generativity
vs. stagnation as identified by Erikson (15). Here one is starkly confronted
with an awareness of mortality and must resolve conflicts between a sense
of futile, worthless destructiveness and a creative need to invest in a meaningful future. All of this is accomplished amidst considerable anguish. Usually
one looks toward a special culminating event which will mark the attainment
of hopes and dreams; however, it is seldom sufficient, and the painful reappraisal begins. It is hardly surprising that many resort to alcohol, which
serves as a readily available and socially acceptable means to deal with
frightening disillusionment about the past and anxious trepidation about the
future.

Middle age is not only a time of personal reappraisal, it is also a time for dynamic readjustment within the nuclear family. In the context of that readjustment, alcoholism may develop as an aberrant coping mechanism. Alternatively, shifts in the family structure may unmask previously covert alcohol abuse, resulting in a demand for professional intervention. Children are no longer dependent on the parents in a manner that requires total involvement. The role of the parent is significantly diminished or lost and this requires readjustment to altered roles. In addition, the relationship between the parents requires readjustment. Women may seize upon this opportunity to seek a second career outside of the household; men perceive that they may have "peaked" in their jobs and begin to seek closer involvement with their wives and children at a time when the latter are less involved and seeking distance.

If the man already has a drinking problem which was previously tolerated by his wife, the shifts taking place at this time may precipitate a crisis. If his wife chooses to lavish care on him as a substitute for her absent children, she may demand that he receive treatment. At the same time she may have a hidden agenda that he continue to be dependent. The wife who wishes to have her husband less dependent so that she can pursue her own career may begin to withdraw support, precipitating further compulsive drinking in her dependent spouse. The reverse also applies in the case of an alcoholic wife. Her husband may have been heavily engaged in building his own personal career for most of their married life. As he renegotiates his priorities, he may wish for a closer involvement with his wife. He may become increasingly aware of her long-standing drinking problem. If he has been tenuously involved for many years and seizes upon mid-life to secure a divorce or separation, his tenuously stabilized alcoholic wife may present for treatment as her last source of support is removed.

The family environment may, therefore, serve as a diathesis for problem drinking in the middle-aged adult. Familial problems can also be a consequence of heavy drinking by one of the family members. Whether viewed as an etiological factor or as a consequence, differences in the family support system of the alcoholic appear to be an important prognostic factor. Similarly, the employment situation of the patient can be viewed as risk, consequence or both. Stability of employment has been found to be one of the most important factors in predicting treatment response.

Organic Brain Disease

It has been well-known for many years that prolonged heavy drinking (combined with vitamin deficiency) will cause the opthalmoplegia, memory impairment and neuropathy of the Wernicke-Korsakoff Syndrome. Alcohol is neurotoxic. Newer sophisticated radiodiagnostic and psychometric techniques now reveal more subtle forms of brain damage, especially of the frontal lobes (33, 40, 50, 58). There is a high probability of incurring damage after regular daily consumption of 80 grams of alcohol or frequent heavy binge drinking (24, 67). The frontal lobes affect the ability to perform complex psychomotor tasks, the ability to integrate socially and emotionally appropriate behavior, control of volition and drive, and the ability to make reasonable judgments and observe problems from different points of view.

Middle-aged alcoholics who have been drinking for many years are more likely to have problems in this area. This can manifest as passivity and apathy, lack of drive, inability to change old patterns of behavior, or stubborn denial in the face of concrete rational evidence. This form of brain damage is not detectable by the usual intelligence tests and standard psychometric profiles. It can be suspected in people whose job performance has deteriorated in subtle ways, indicating poor judgment.

What is required to detect frontal lobe damage is a complex series of tasks such as those contained in the Halstead-Reitan battery (17, 18). This examines psychomotor task performance as well as the ability to abstract new concepts from data presented. This may be combined with an EMI or CAT scan to detect evidence of cortical atrophy and ventricular enlargement. Recent reports suggest that if ventricular enlargement in the alcoholic is not severe, it may be relieved by abstinence. Unfortunately, some of the mental ability essential to good jugment and delay of gratification may be impaired by frontal lobe damage.

Drug Abuse

The combination of drug and alcohol abuse in the alcoholic is not uncommon. As the pharmacopaea has changed, so has the pattern of drug abuse in this population. Most alcoholics secure their drugs from physicians rather than from the illicit market. As physician prescribing practices have changed from bromides to barbiturates to benzodiazepines, so has the drug abuse pattern of the alcoholics. Benzodiazepines are currently the most commonly abused group of drugs—particularly in middle-aged women (56, 57, 59, 68). The synergistic interaction of these drugs and alcohol and their greater potency when administered with alcohol* may represent an additional threat to life. Over time some individuals may develop serious mixed addictions.

---

*While not very soluble in water, benzodiazepines are very soluble in alcohol, resulting in a larger dose of drug administered in the presence of alcohol.

Initiating Treatment

Alcoholics frequently present for treatment in a crisis. This often takes the form of threatened job dismissal, separation from spouse and family, arrest for intoxication-related crime or a physical complication of drinking. Whatever the crisis, it offers an opportunity to intervene in the progression of the disease process. The crisis should be seen as part of the disease process and not as an isolated event. Any other position taken will support the denial of the patient and delay treatment. Late onset alcoholics are easier to confront about the need for treatment than others. They often have a history of moderate success in their lives and have less need to use primitive defenses such as denial (39, 74). They often recognize their alcoholic behavior as different from their earlier life-style. Generally, they have built fairly stable family and work relationships, and their families and employers may remember times which were better. With a degree of insight and social support, such people are able to accept their problem and take positive steps to deal with it.

The encounter between the patient and physician may be marked by the wish of both to deny an alcohol problem. Physicians often have difficulty differentiating between pathological drinking and social custom. Any person who has trouble with his health, social relations or work because of drinking should be sympathetically confronted with the facts as they present and advised that help is available for such a problem. If an alcohol problem is denied by the patient, the main therapeutic task is to continue to present a consistent statement of the facts, to advise on the treatment opportunities and to *maintain a relationship* with the patient. In addition, the patient's family should be involved in treatment. Initially, this will give corroborating clinical evidence of alcoholism. The family members may have found ways to stabilize themselves around a clinically intoxicated member. It will be important for them to be able to renegotiate relationships with each other if the alcoholic is to alter his addictive disorder. Family members may need psychiatric help or some sort of counseling.

Treatment Modalities

The severe forms of alcohol withdrawal and the medical complications of alcoholism should be treated by medical personnel in appropriate settings. Following acute medical treatment, the alcoholic should become engaged in long-term rehabilitation. Unfortunately, most rehabilitation programs take a particularistic approach based upon some ideology, rather than on the disease needs of individual patients. A 45-year-old housewife who has been secretly drinking for five years following a divorce has different problems than a 55-year-old construction foreman with cirrhosis who has been drinking a case of beer per day for 35 years (and was referred for treatment following a motor vehicle accident). The former is having trouble dealing with a major loss and associated life changes. She is likely to evaluate her self-worth on the basis of her ability (or inability) to deal with these issues. Her subjective appraisal of her worth will not be enhanced by realizing that she has a socially unacceptable disease such as alcoholism. It will be very important for her to make an alliance with a group that she can experience as empathic and supportive. Disulfiram may be helpful initially to give her a significant period of sobriety to bolster her self-esteem. The foreman, on the other hand, will have to make a major reappraisal of his life-style. It is likely that he will have to give up alcohol as well as change his social life which is built around a drinking pattern. All this will have to be done without recourse to his usual "anti-dysphoriant." He will probably be helped in this by becoming a member of a group such as A.A. and placed on daily disulfiram. Abstinence may be achieved because there will be administrative control exercised through the court system, which will require him to stay in treatment.

Both of the patients described above require a skilled counselor who understands the issues. Psychotherapy with alcoholics has pitfalls which psychodynamically trained therapists tend to neglect. Alcohol has physiological and behavioral concomitants, apart from its symbolic meaning for the patient. The first task of therapy is to help the patient to stop drinking and to help him find ways to stay stopped. The therapist may have to actively help the patient to develop techniques which make alcohol unavailable (such as disulfiram or regular attendance at Alcoholics Anonymous). A detached, "blank screen" approach will not be helpful, especially at the outset of treatment.

Psychoactive Drugs in Treatment

Treating concomitant psychiatric states in alcoholics presents some difficulties because many psychoactive drugs act synergistically with alcohol. Clinicians should have the patient in a controlled setting before instituting treatment with any drugs. Treating depression in alcoholism (or vice versa) reflects some of the diagnostic problems of those diseases. Treatment of a middle-aged depressed alcoholic has other problems. Many treatment programs have a fixed period of inpatient hospitalization—often limited to three or four weeks—and there is pressure not to disrupt the integrity of the program. The doctor may begin treatment without allowing sufficient time to elapse to assess the severity of depression. The prescription of a tricyclic antidepressant to an older patient in a poor nutritional state with potential myocardial disease from vitamin deficiency and alcohol is hazardous. If the patient resumes drinking shortly after discharge, he has an added health risk. One needs to have the patient sincerely committed to follow-up therapy before starting on such a course of treatment. Thus, it is advisable to build a treatment alliance and to begin treatment with disulfiram before starting antidepressant medication. If the patient is not fit for discharge at the expected time because he is still severely depressed, he will probably be better managed on an inpatient psychiatry unit for his own safety.

Disulfiram precludes treatment with monoamine oxidase inhibitors because of drug interaction. The use of lithium carbonate with depressed alcoholics has shown equivocal results (37, 41). If tricyclic antidepressants are employed, it is useful to monitor blood levels. The literature has already established the correlation between blood levels and therapeutic efficacy (22, 42).

There is still controversy about the use of anxiolytic drugs with alcoholics. Phenothiazines can be very effective in treating anxiety of psychotic proportions in those people who use alcohol for that reason. The number of such cases is small. The main problem rests with the use of benzodiazepines. The standard viewpoint is one inherited from people who have experience with A.A.: An alcoholic should not use substitutes for alcohol. This has been further extended to a concern that the patient will become addicted to the substitute, and that his increasing need for the drug will lead him back to drinking alcohol. While studies by Ditman (10), Rosenberg (52) and others (3) have suggested that alcoholics in outpatient treatment who were treated with benzodiazepines stayed in treatment longer, our practice has been to avoid them and to encourage the patient to deal with anxiety in other ways. We tend to feel that anti-anxiety medication can undermine the patient's view that he can remain abstinent and learn to cope without the use of alcohol or other drugs.

SUMMARY

A typological approach to the alcoholic should be treatment-oriented. The identification of depression, mid-life stress, and/or the presence of complicating factors such as cognitive impairment and drug abuse are important to treatment planning and implementation. Familial factors should be considered to the point that family therapy may be an important adjunct to treatment.

Conceptually alcoholism is best viewed as a biopsychosocial illness. Middle age is the time when the majority of patients present for treatment. Alcoholics can be differentiated into "subtypes" on the basis of a possible diathesis or on the basis of the medical and psychosocial consequences of their alcohol abuse. Treatment programs need to consider the diversity of the patient population in formulating effective individualized treatment plans.

REFERENCES

1. ABELSOHN, D. S., and VAN DER SPUY, H. I. J. (1978). The age variable in alcoholism. *J. Stud. Alcohol, 39* (5):800.
2. BAKER , N., DORZAB, J., WINOKUR, G., and CADORET, R. (1972). Depressive illness. Evidence favoring polygenic inheritance based upon an analysis of ancestral case. *Arch. Gen. Psychiat., 27*:320.
3. BAEKELAND, F., and LUNDWALL, L. K. (1977). Engaging the Alcoholic in Treatment and Keeping Him There. In: Kissin, B., Begleiter, H. (eds.). *The Biology of Alcoholism Vol. 5. The Treatment and Rehabilitation of the Chronic Alcoholic*. New York-London: Plenum Press.
4. BARRACLOUGH, B., BUNCH, J., NELSON, B., and SAINSBURY, P. (1974). A hundred cases of suicide: Clinical aspects. *Br. J. Psychiat., 125*:355.
5. BECKMAN, L. J. (1975). Women alcoholics. A review of social and psychological studies. *Q. J. Stud. Alcohol, 36* (7):797.
6. BENENSOHN, H. S., and RESNIK, H. L. P. (1974). A jigger of alcohol, a dash of depression and bitters: A suicidal mix. *Ann. N.Y. Acad. Sci., 233*:40.
7. BUTTERWORTH, A. T. (1971). Depression associated with alcohol withdrawal: Imipramine therapy compared with a placebo. *Q. J. Stud. Alcohol, 32*:343.
8. CADORET, R., and WINOKUR, G. (1974). Depression in alcoholism. *Ann. N.Y. Acad. Sci., 233*:34.
9. CAHALAN, D., and CISIN, I. H. (1976). Drinking Behavior and Drinking Problems in the United States. In: Kisin, B., Begleiter, H. (eds.). *The Biology of Alcoholism Vol. 4. Social Aspects of Alcoholism*. New York-London: Plenum Press.
10. DITMAN, K. S. (1961). Evaluation of drugs in the treatment of alcoholics. *Q. J. Stud. Alcohol*, (Suppl. No. 1); 107.
11. DONOVAN, D. M., CHANEY, E. F., and O'LEARY, M. R. (1978). Alcoholic MMPI subtypes relationship to drinking styles, benefits and consequences. *J. Nerv. Ment. Dis., 166* (8):553.
12. DUNNER, D. L., HENSEL, B. M., and FIEVE, R. F. (April 1979). Bipolar illness: factors in drinking behavior. *Am. J. Psychiat., 136*(4b):583.
13. EDWARDS, G., CHANDLER, J., HENSMAN, C. and PETO, J. (1972). Drinking in a south London suburb. I. Correlates of normal drinking. II. Correlates of trouble with drinking among men. III. Comparisons of drinking troubles among men and women. *Q. J. Stud. Alcohol*, Suppl No. 6, 69.
14. ENDICOTT, J., and SPITZER, R. L. (1978). A diagnostic interview: The schedule for affective disorders and schizophrenia. *Arch. Gen. Psychiat., 35*:837.
15. ERIKSON, E. H. (1963). Eight Stages of Man. In: *Childhood and Society*. New York: W. W. Norton & Co.

16. FILLMORE, K. M. (1974). Drinking and problem drinking in early adulthood and middle age—An exploratory 20-year follow-up study. *Q. J. Stud. Alcohol*, 35:819.
17. FITZHUGH, L. C., FITZHUGH, K. B., and REITAN, R. M. (1960). Adaptive abilities and intellectual functioning of hospitalized alcoholics. *Q. J. Stud. Alcohol*, 21:414.
18. FITZHUGH, L. C., FITZHUGH, K. B., and REITAN, R. M. (1965). Adaptive abilities and intellectual functioning of hospitalized alcoholics: Further considerations. *Q. J. Stud. Alcohol*, 26:402.
19. FREED, E. X. (1970). Alcoholism and manic-depressive disorders; Some perspectives. *Q. J. Stud. Alcohol*, 31:62.
20. GIBSON, S., and BECKER, J. (1973). Alcoholism and depression. The factor structure of alcoholics responses to depression inventory. *Q. J. Stud. Alcohol*, 34:400.
21. GIBSON, S., and BECKER, J. (1973). Changes in alcoholics' self-reported depression. *Q. J. Stud. Alcohol*, 34:829.
22. GLASSMAN, A. H., PEREL, J. M. SHOSTAK, M., KANTOR, S. J., and FLEISS, J. L. (1977). Clinical implications of imipramine plasma levels for depressive illness. *Arch. Gen. Psychiat.*, 34:197.
23. GOLDSTEIN, S. G., and LINDEN, J. D. (1969). Multivariate classification of alcoholics by MMPI. *J. Abnorm. Psychol.*, 74:661.
24. GOODWIN, D. W., HILL, S. Y., POWELL, B., and VIAMONTES, J. (1973). Effect of alcohol on short term memory in alcoholics. *Br. J. Psychiat.*, 122:93.
25. GOODWIN, D. (1977). Alcoholism and depression in adopted out daughters. *Arch. Gen. Psych.*, 34:751.
26. GOODWIN, D. (1976). *Is Alcoholism Hereditary?* New York: Oxford University Press.
27. HAGUE, W. H., WILSON, L. G., DUDLEY, D. L., and CANNON, S. (1976). Post detoxification drug treatment of anxiety and depression in alcohol addicts. *J. Nerv. Ment. Dis.*, 162:354.
28. HAMM, J. E., MAJOR, L. F., and BROWN, G. L. (April 1979). Quantative measurement of depression and anxiety in male alcoholics. *Am. J. Psychiat.*, 136, 4b:580.
29. JACOBSON, G. R. (1976). Essential-reactive alcoholism dimension. In: *The Alcoholisms, Assessment and Diagnosis*. New York: Human Sciences Press, Behavioral Publications, Inc.
30. JELLINEK, E. M. (1960). *Disease Concept of Alcoholism*. Highland Park, N.J.: Hillhouse Press.
31. JELLINEK, E. M. (1959). Estimating the prevalence of alcoholism; modified values in the Jellinek formula and an alternative approach. *Q. J. Stud. Alcohol*, 20:261.
32. JELLINEK, E. M. (1952). Phases of alcohol addiction. *Q. J. Stud. Alcohol*, 13:673.
33. JONES, B., and PARSONS, O. A. (1971). Impaired abstracting ability in chronic alcoholics. *Arch. Gen. Psychiat.*, 24:71.
34. KAIJ, L. (1970). *Alcoholism in Twins*. London: Almquist and Wiskell.
35. KEELER, M. H., TAYLOR, C. I., and MILLER, W. C. (April 1979). Are all recently detoxified alcoholics depressed? *Am. J. Psychiat.*, 136 (4b):586.
36. KELLER, M. (1972). The oddities of alcoholics. *Q. J. Stud. Alcohol*, 33:1147.
37. KLINE, N. S., WREN, J. C., COOPER, T. B., VARGA, E., and CANAL, O. (1974). Evaluation of lithium therapy in chronic and periodic alcoholism. *Am. J. Med. Sci.*, 268:15.
38. KNIGHT, R. P. (1937). The dynamics and treatment of chronic alcohol addiction. *Bull. Menninger Clin.*, 1:233.
39. LAMY, P. P. (1978). Therapeutics and the elderly. *Addict. Dis.*, 3(3):311.
40. LEVINSON, D. J., with DARROW, C. N., KLEIN, E. B., LEVINSON, M. H., and McKEE, B. (1978). *The Seasons of a Man's Life*. New York: Alfred A. Knopf.
41. MERRY, J., REYNOLDS, C. M., BAILEY, J., and COPPEN, A. (Sept 1976). Prophylactic treatment of alcoholism by lithium carbonate, a controlled study. *Lancet, 1* 7984, p. 481.
42. MONTGOMERY, S., McAULEY, R., and MONTGOMERY, D. B. (1978). Relationship between

mianserin plasma levels and anti-depressant effect in double-blind trial comparing single night time and divided daily dose regimens. *Br. J. Clin. Pharmacol.*, 5 Suppl 1, 775.

43. MURPHY, G. E., ARMSTRONG, J. W. JR., HERMELE, S. L., FISHER, J. R., and CLENDENIN, W. W. (1979). Suicide and alcoholism. Interpersonal loss confirmed as a predictor. *Arch. Gen. Psychiat.*, 36:65.

44. NICHOLLS, P., EDWARDS, G., and KYLE, E. (1974). Alcoholics admitted to four hospitals in England. II. General and cause-specific mortality. *Q. J. Stud. Alcohol*, 35:841.

45. PINCUS, J. H., and TUCKER, G. J. (1974). Chapter 2. In: *Behavioral Neurology*. New York: Oxford University Press.

46. PITTS, F. N. Jr., and WINOKUR, G. (1966). Affective disorder VII: Alcoholism and affective disorder. *J. Psychiatr. Res.*, 4:37.

47. POTTENGER, M., McKERNON, J., PETRIE, L. E., WEISSMAN, M.M., RUBEN, H. L., and NEWBERRY, P. (August 1978). Frequency and persistence of depressive symptoms in the alcohol abuser. *J. Nerv. Ment. Dis.*, 166 (8):562.

48. REICH, L. H., DAVIES, R. R., and HIMMELHOCH, J. M. (1974). Excessive alcohol use in manic-depressive illness. *Am. J. Psychiat.*, 131:85.

49. ROBINS, L. N. (1966). *Deviant Children Grown Up: Sociological and Psychiatric Study of Sociopathic Personality*. Baltimore: Williams and Wilkens.

50. RON, M.A. (1977). Brain damage in chronic alcoholism: A neuropathological, neurora-diological and psychological review. *Psychol. Med.*, 7:103.

51. ROSEN, A. (1960). A comparative study of alcoholics and psychiatric patients with the MMPI. *Q. J. Stud. Alcohol*, 21:253.

52. ROSENBERG, C. M. (1974). Drug maintenance in the outpatient treatment of chronic alcoholism. *Arch. Gen., Psychiat.*, 30:373.

53. ROSIN, A. J. and GLATT, M. M. (1971). Alcohol excess in the elderly. *Q. J. Stud. Alcohol*, 32:53.

54. RUDIE, R. R., and McGAUCHRAN, L. S. (1961). Differences in developmental experience, defensiveness and personality organisation between two classes of problem drinkers. *J. Abnorm. Soc. Psychol.*, 62:659.

55. SCHUCKIT, M. A., GOODWIN, D., and WINOKUR, G. (1972). A study of alcoholism in half-siblings. *Am. J. Psychiat.*, 128:1132.

56. SCHUCKIT, M. A., and MORRISSEY, E. R. (1979). Psychiatric problems in women admitted to an alcoholic detoxification center. *Am. J. Psychiat.*, 136:611.

57. SCHUCKIT, M. A., MORRISSEY, E. R., and O'LEARY, M. R. (1978). Alcohol problems in elderly men and women. *Addict. Dis.*, 3 (3):405.

58. SCHUCKIT, M. A., PITTS, F. N. Jr., REICH, T., KING, L. J., and WINOKUR, G. (1969). Alcoholism I: Two types of alcoholism in women. *Arch. Gen. Psychiat.*, 20 (3):301.

59. SCHUCKIT, M. A., and RAYSES, V. (1979). Ethanol ingestion: Differences in blood acetaldehyde concentration in relatives of alcoholics and controls. *Sci.*, 203:54.

60. SHAW, J. A., DONCY, P., MORGAN, D. W., and ROBINSON J. A. (1975). Treatment of depression in alcoholics. *Am. J. Psychiat.*, 132:641.

61. SKINNER, H. A., JACKSON, D. N., and HOFFMANN, H. (1974). Alcoholic personality types: Identification and correlates. *J. Abnorm. Psychol.*, 83 (6):658.

62. SLATER, E. and ROTH, M. (1969). Alcohol and Alcoholism. In: Mayer-Gross, W., Slater, E. and Roth, M. (eds.) *Clinical Psychiatry*, 3rd Edition. London: Bailliere, Tindall and Cassell.

63. SPITZER, R. L., ENDICOTT, J., and ROBINS, E. (1978). Research Diagnostic Criteria. *Arch. Gen. Psychiat.*, 35:773.

64. SUTHERLAND, E. D., SCHROEDER, H. G., and TORDELLA, C. L. (1950). Personality traits and the alcoholic: A critique of existing studies. *Q. J. Stud. Alcohol*, 11:547.

65. SYME, L. (1957). Personality characteristics and the alcoholic: A critique of current studies. *Q. J. Stud. Alcohol*, 18:288.

66. TARTER, R. E., MCBRIDE, H., BUONPANE, N., and SCHNEIDER, D. V. (1977). Differentiation of alcoholics. *Arch. Gen. Psychiat.*, *34*:761.
67. TURNER, T. B., MEZEY, E., and KIMBALL, A. W. (1977). Measurement of alcohol-related effects in man: Chronic effects in relation to levels of alcohol consumption. Part B. *The Johns Hopkins Med., J.*, *141*:273.
68. WANBERG, K. W., and HORN, J. L. (1970). Alcoholism symptom patterns of men and women, a comparative study. *Q. J. Stud. Alcohol*, *31*:40.
69. WILSON, I. C., ALLTON, L. B., and RILEY, L. (1970). Tofranil in the treatment of post-alcohol depressions. *Psychosomatics*, *11*:488.
70. WINOKUR, G. (1972). Depression spectrum disease: Description and family study. *Comp. Psychiat.*, *13*:3.
71. WINOKUR, G., REICH, T., RIMMER, J., and PITTS, F. N. JR. (1970). Alcoholism III. Diagnosis and familial psychiatric illness in 259 alcoholic probands. *Arch., Gen. Psychiat.*, *23*:104.
72. WINOKUR, G., RIMMER, J., and REICH, T. (1971). Alcoholism IV: Is there more than one type of alcoholism? *Br. J. Psychiat.*, *118*:525.
73. WOODRUFF, R. A. JR., GUZE, S. B., CLAYTON, P. J., and CARR, D. (1973). Alcoholism and depression. *Arch. Gen. Psychiat.*, *28* (1):97.
74. ZIMBERG, S. (1978). Treatment of the elderly alcoholic in the community and in an institutional setting. *Addict. Dis.*, *3* (3):417.

16

PSYCHOSOMATIC DISORDERS
IN THE MIDDLE-AGED

STEFAN STEIN, M. D.

Associate Professor of Clinical Psychiatry,
Cornell University Medical College, New York;
Director of Education,
New York Hospital-Cornell Medical Center,
Westchester Division

and

CHARLES A. SHAMOIAN, M.D., PH.D.

Associate Professor of Clinical Psychiatry and Pharmacology,
Cornell University Medical College, New York,
Director of Geriatric Services,
New York Hospital-Cornell Medical Center,
Westchester Division

INTRODUCTION

The portion of the life-cycle commonly referred to as middle age has been defined as the years between the ages of 35 and 55. Until recently, this period had been viewed as rather static and non-dynamic, a time through which one wandered on the way to old age and death. Life was seen as reaching its pinnacle in young adulthood and declining thereafter. The working-through of childhood and adolescent developmental phases was viewed as preparatory for early adulthood, which was characterized as the time for the establishment of career, marriage and family. This view of the mid and late adult years ignored the wisdom of a large general literature pertaining to middle age, particularly works of fiction. Pitkin's *Life Begins at Forty*, Albee's *Who's Afraid of Virginia Wolf?*, Mann's *The Black Swan* and Dodd's

The Job Hunter are just a few examples of writing which characterize the middle adult years as a dynamic period, punctuated by turmoil, with frequent changes in work and family relationships (4).

Clinicians actively pursing the middle-aged patient's physical complaints but not listening attentively for the stressors of this period in the patient's history may miss important cues to underlying problem(s) which accompany various symptomatic manifestations. Unfortunately, until recently, the clinician did not have a readily accessible body of knowledge specifically dealing with the middle years. Psychiatrists, in particular, have largely neglected these years. Erikson began the modern study of the adult life-cycle and commented on the adult years in more detail, but not until recently have the mid adult years been scrutinized more carefully. Levinson (30), Vaillant (56) and others have contributed to a more thorough understanding of this period. The middle years have "come of age" and are now recognized as an important developmental phase of the life cycle (40). Unlike the biological changes of the earlier developmental phases of infancy, childhood and adolescence, which occur rapidly and abruptly, the physiological changes of this period are gradual, and may be manifest in a subjective feeling of "getting old." These biological changes influence one's perception of self, one's ability to function and to relate. Likewise, stress, common to this period, affects the biology of the individual.

THE BIOLOGY AND PATHOBIOLOGY OF THE MIDDLE AGE

Biological aging does not begin at a specific moment, but rather is a continuous process accelerating somewhat during the middle years. The gradual increase in grey hair, the development of presbyopia, and the loss of elasticity of skin resulting in wrinkles are easily observed, objective signs of aging. (44). In a youth-oriented society, these objective signs may be so frightening to some individuals that they may make heroic attempts to hide them with cosmetics or to conceal them with plastic surgery. Feelings about getting older and becoming unattractive may be verbalized openly, or may be disguised in a statement referring to someone else, such as "I'm not attracted to my spouse now that he/she is getting older." Such feelings may lead to extramarital relationships in the hope of proving that one is still attractive to members of the opposite sex. These feelings of becoming unattractive are further accentuated by the relative increase of body fat, with a concomitant decrease in lean body mass in both men and women (5).

Not so noticeable, but also present, is the gradual decrease in muscular strength (5, 18). This is subjectively experienced as a loss of capacity for physically demanding work. The skeletal system supporting the muscle mass also begins to undergo various metabolic and anatomic changes, often experienced as "creaking joints," e.g., painful shoulders, knees, elbows (54). Osteoarthritis gradually makes its appearance. Tossing a ball or playing a body contact sport becomes difficult. This is often a problem for the professional sportsman or athlete who retires at the beginning of the middle years and often must adjust to a new life-style.

The aging process also is reflected by changes in the cardiopulmonary system (27). The vital capacity of both males and females declines with age. Moreover, the residual volume increases with age, especially after 40 years. With increasing age there is also a reduction of the indices of airflow. Smokers suffer increased rates of lung neoplasm and chronic obstructive pulmonary disease. At this age (40-45), deaths begin to occur in contemporaries, which may lead to increased self-concern and a thought such as, "I don't have so much time left."

Simultaneously with the changes within the pulmonary system, the cardiovascular tree undergoes physiological and pathological shifts. Cardiac output falls off at the rate of approximately 1% per year. Likewise, the cardiac index, stroke volume, stroke index and heart work decrease with aging. Also, the volume of the thoracic aorta falls off linearly with aging and there is an increasing stiffness of the arteries related to loss of elasticity and calcification (28). These changes may also lead to sluggishness of the baroreceptor reflexes. Finally, there is an increase in peripheral resistance, with worsening of hypertension.

At this time the mortality from arteriosclerotic heart disease markedly increases. The fear of an acute myocardial infarction during this age span becomes prominent, with such thoughts as "I could die any minute." These events often have dramatic consequences. Wills are drawn, life-styles and marriage are reevaluated and changes in careers may occur. Depression may occur in relation to the realization that one's life goals have not been achieved, and probably will never be fulfilled. Suicide rates, especially in men who have severe medical illness, accelerate during this period. The influence of the biological and pathobiological changes on the psychosocial equilibrium of the individual is considerable. However, the manner in which each individual responds to and copes with these biological stresses is variable.

The genitourinary system likewise undergoes physiological changes during the middle years (15). The glomerular filtration rate, creatinine clearance, and renal plasma flow begin to fall off during this period. The prostrate gradually and slowly hypertrophies with a beginning rise in the incidence of prostatic carcinoma.

Women during this period experience the menopause and its associated physiological sequelae. Moreover, the incidence of mammary carcinoma begins to increase (55). Post-menopausally there is also a significant increase in the incidence of arteriosclerosis and osteoporosis. Thus this period may be traumatic, both psychologically and biologically, for women. Often during this phase, children leave and establish their own families. Women may attempt to reestablish themselves professionally, and begin to realize that not much time is left to accomplish work goals (34). As with the males, the female is especially prone to depression during these years.

In summary, the middle years are a period of constant biological and pathobiological changes in many parameters studied. Because of the gradual increase in pathology and the increase in onset of various malignancies, the middle-aged individual is confronted with the issues of chronic illness and of death and dying. Morever, the presence of elderly parents and the associated problems of the aged constantly confront the middle-aged individual with his/her own future and mortality.

PSYCHOSOMATIC DISORDERS

Earlier studies had suggested that there was a group of illnesses which were primarily psychosomatic in origin. These were believed to be "caused" by specific psychodynamic conflicts and/or psychosocial stresses. Illnesses so considered were peptic ulcer, ulcerative colitis, bronchial asthma, rheumatoid arthritis, essential hypertension, thyrotoxicosis and neurodermatitis. However, more recent study suggests that the concept of psychosomaticity can usefully be applied to all disease states, in that psychosocial elements are contributory to the illness state in general (16). Accordingly, the psyche, environment, etc. may influence the onset and course of the illness. Medical diseases may usefully be thought of as being multifactorially determined. Certain factors are predisposing, others may be described as precipitating, and others as sustaining (59).

Stress, common in our present-day society, has been known for some time to play an important role in the etiology of certain illness. The middle years are indeed such a period of frequent stressful, adverse life events: Parents die, divorces occur, careers are changed, spouses die, chronic illness sets in, etc. Holmes and Rahe have emphasized the importance of adverse life changes as predisposing to illness or death (26). Using the Social Readjustment Rating Questionnaire, and the Schedule of Recent Experiences, which includes large number of life event items (divorce, death of a spouse, loss of a job, etc.) weighted according to their severity (26, 35, 37), Holmes and Rahe studied risk factors in illness onset. These questionnaires do not predict which illness will occur, but rather which individuals will be at risk for developing an illness. Although subject to criticism, the life event studies offer support for the hypothesis that psychosocial factors are important in the development of many medical illnesses (36). Life events are conceptualized as impinging upon a biological organism undergoing physiological changes. These psychosocial factors influence the nature of the underlying biological processes, which in turn affect one's reaction to the environment.

Although the middle-aged individual is prone to a number of different illnesses, only essential hypertension, myocardial infarction and peptic ulcer disease will be reviewed here, i.e., conditions of particular importance in middle age.

ESSENTIAL HYPERTENSION

Accurate incidence and prevalence rates for essential hypertension are not readily available. These statistics are complicated by the inclusion of borderline as well as midrange essential hypertension. Regardless of the severity of the hypertension, about 30 to 70% of the cases have associated environmental, social and psychological factors (41). Borderline hypertension is found in approximately 10% of those in their twenties, while essential hypertension prevalence rates increase with age. By the age of 60, the prevalence rate is 40%. It is found more frequently in men than women below the age of 50. Geographic and cultural factors have also been reported as affecting the prevalence of essential hypertension. For example, patients living in small, protected societies and moving to a more modernized urban type of living manifest an increase in their blood pressure (47). Some believe that social disorganization is associated with an acceleration of the hypertensive phenomenon (6). Race also appears to have an effect on the disease process. For example, blacks are reported as having a higher rate of low-renin hypertension, and a higher mortality rate from hypertensive-related disease than whites (22, 41).

Other factors play an important role in the genesis of this medical condition. "When a society is stable, and when its customs, traditions and institutions are well established and well structured, and its members respond to a predictable sociocultural environment with integrated patterns of psychological adaptation, then blood pressure levels do not become elevated with age. Those who live in a social milieu that is rapidly changing, is unpredictable, dangerous or unfamiliar—so that psychological adaptation to it is difficult or impossible—tend to develop increasing blood pressure levels with age. Not everyone who lives in such a social milieu develops high blood pressure levels or essential hypertension—probably only the predisposed do" (58).

Patterns of coping may be disrupted during the middle years, setting the stage for a rise in blood pressure. New roles and shifts in social or professional status which may occur in the mid-life period require adaptive changes of the individual (40). Hypertensive females are sometimes described as hostile and combative. Their marriages are often fraught with difficulty, they find it difficult to express their angry feelings and they may harbor grudges for long periods of time (23, 46). A genetic component is suggested by some (24).

Life events, whether antecedent or concomitant, play a role in the onset of hypertension. Studies have shown that the beginning of essential hypertension may occur in stress-laden situations, such as the anniversary of the death of an important person (12). Furthermore, other studies have shown an exacerbation of the illness in the face of interpersonal conflicts surrounding issues of dependency and hostility. Two major classes of interpersonal events were thought to be highly correlated with the illness: those resulting in feelings of rage and anger and those in which there was a threat of losing security (8, 39).

Attempts have been made to identify the personality and psychological conflicts of patients with hypertension. These studies, although consistent in their findings, have been criticized on the basis that they are based on subjective impressions. Some, however, have been verified by psychological testing (43). In general, these studies suggest that hypertensive patients have a lifelong conflict about the overt expression of anger, hostility, rage, ambition and/or dependency (2, 52). Many patients cover over these underlying thoughts and feelings by an outward friendliness or by being perfectionistic. They may appear anxious or depressed. Interestingly, one study reported that 50% of the hypertensives had lost a parent during childhood and that the hypertension developed in a situation of bereavement (2). The borderline hypertensive patient, in one study, was described as submissive, introverted, sensitive, suspicious and notably lacking in self-esteem and pleasure in sexual activity (21).

Although psychosocial factors are important contributors to hypertension, they obviously are not sufficient. All individuals subjected to the same psychosocial forces do not develop hypertension. Obviously then, the personal meaning and the ability of the individual to deal with the event are important. Moreover, a genetic predisposition may be necessary for the disease to appear (41). Since essential hypertension is not a homogeneous illness, but rather consists of a number of subtypes of the illness, all statistical generalizations must be viewed with great caution (41).

These findings clearly accentuate the point that eliciting a "medical" history will not be sufficient in properly treating these patients. A personal history dealing with the problems and subjective reactions and adaptations to these must be elicited and evaluated. Studies have consistently shown that a thoughtful, consistent, reliable physician upon whom the patient may depend is of great importance and may be sufficient, at times, to ameliorate the process (33, 45).

ISCHEMIC CORONARY HEART DISEASE

Ischemic coronary heart disease may manifest itself as fatal or recurring myocardial infarction, angina pectoris or sudden death. The middle-aged individual is usually the prime candidate for the acute, sudden myocardial infarction. If not the victim of this disease, the middle-aged person becomes the observer, noticing his friends, fellow workers and colleagues suddenly stricken by this life-threatening process. The thought then becomes, "Am I next?" This simple question surfaces critical issues to be reexamined within the content of how much time does one have left.

Presently, coronary heart disease is also thought to be multifactorially determined. Risk factors implicated include cigarette smoking, elevated serum cholesterol, diabetes mellitus, hypertension, obesity, and stress. Psychosocial factors are now thought to have a more important role than heretofore suspected. In fact, contrary to the earlier anecdotal, uncontrolled case reports, there is presently accumulating a body of objective data supporting this concept (17).

Interestingly, the psychic states of anxiety and depression have also been associated with coronary heart disease and angina (17). Some patients have experienced acute myocardial infarctions upon clinical recovery from the depressive state. Indeed, the infarctions occurred during the hyperactive-arousal state. However, it is not clear whether anxiety and depression are antecedent precursors or immediate precipitants of heart disease. Life events preceding coronary heart disease have also been studied. Groen (17) has found that in all patients studied with an infarction there had been an intense conflict which had special meaning for the patient. Emotional conflictual situations preceding the ischemic attack have also been reported by others (61). The most frequent emotionally laden area centered around conflicts associated with work; the second ranked group of conflicts were associated with family problems (17).

In a study using the Schedule of Recent Experiences to assess stress, patients with or without a previous history of myocardial infarction revealed a higher rate of life event units, indicating stress, occurring within the six months prior to the infarction (38, 51). This was true only for the patients without a previous history of infarction. Those patients with an earlier history of infarction had a large number of life events occurring also preceding the six months. Other studies utilizing similar assessment methods have shown that patients with illnesses prior to the infarction had twice the number of life events as compared to those who developed an infarction but did not have any illnesses just prior to it. These studies strongly suggest the importance of life events as precipitants. As noted, however, the technique and methodology have been criticized (36). One of the major problems has been lack of the individual's own retrospective assessment of distress associated with the event. This latter approach, i.e., patient's self-rating of distress prior to the episode, has been found to be a powerful discriminator between an infarction population and a control group (31). It should be noted here that chronic exposure to stress may have physiological consequences which may have a role in the genesis of coronary heart disease (29).

Not only may life events have a role in the genesis of coronary heart disease, but also certain sociological factors have been associated with a higher incidence of the illness. For example, in certain cultures, the more affluent the individual, the greater the risk. This is especially true for countries outside the United States; in the U.S., the risk appears to be equal among upper and lower socioeconomic classes. Also, certain occupational groups such as "white collar" and "intellectual" have a higher associated risk than those of "blue collar" workers (17). Some investigators have suggested that the greater the degree of incongruity between one's earlier adult life and mid-life social status, the greater the chances of developing ischemic coronary heart disease (17). Others have clearly demonstrated that not only physical and geographical mobility but also social mobility are associated with an increase in the prevalence rate of this illness (13, 50). Based on such findings, the clinician who knows the patient's background well and is aware of the individual's ambitions, goals and drives will be in a better position to determine whether or not that particular patient, in addition to his/her specific clinical data, is at high risk for coronary heart disease. In addition to the coronary heart disease, many are also at risk for suicide, especially after developing an infarction. Suicidal ideation should be actively considered in such patients.

In 1978, Friedman and Rosenman described personality types A and B, the former being predisposed to ischemic heart disease while the latter group was not (14). The type A was described as "an individual who is engaged in a relatively chronic and excessive struggle to obtain an unusually limited number of things from his environment in the shortest period of time even against the opposing efforts of environmental situations or persons. Thus his chronic struggle may consist of attempts to achieve or do more and more in less and less time or a chronic conflict with one or a group of persons. In either case, however, the person afflicted with this behavior pattern never despairs (despite the intensity or duration of the conflict) of losing the struggle. He thus differs sharply, e.g., from subject with a classic anxiety state who, finding or believing his challenges or afflictions overwhelming, seeks solace and reassurance from his physician or his interested friends" (14). These workers subsequently differentiated the group into a number of intermediate types of varying degrees of severity. The original methods used for classifying types A and B have been criticized, and other instruments developed. The Jenkins Activity Survey Questionnaire, for example, delineates the type A personality (3). This questionnaire has revealed that personality factors such as hostility, depressiveness, ambition, sociality, work activity and strivings for independence correlated highly with ischemic heart disease. However, not all investigators would agree that there is a consistent personality structure which predisposes to ischemic heart disease. Some would suggest that the personality factors or patterns are the result of the disease process and not the cause.

PEPTIC ULCERS

Peptic ulcer disease is, in all probability, a group of heterogeneous diseases of differing etiologies and pathogeneses. This model is substantiated by the varied types of lesions and varied anatomical locations. Because of the heterogeneous nature, studies attempting to elucidate the central factors and mechanisms of the illness are subject to criticism.

Genetic factors appear to play some role in predisposing an individual to the disease. Children with duodenal ulcers were shown to have 50% of their family members afflicted with the illness (19). Moreover, the concordance rate for peptic ulcers in monozygotic twins was 54% as compared to 17% for the dizygotics (11). Genetic markers have also been thought to identify those patients who are at risk. For example, patients with blood type 0 have been shown to have a greater chance of developing the illness than those with types A, B, or AB (20). Other such markers reported are: the lack of AB0 blood group antigens in saliva, inherited hyperpepsinogenemia, and the presence of HLA-B5 antigen in white males (57). Thus it would appear that a genetic background may be the setting in which superimposed stressful life events act to precipitate the disease process. Earlier studies documented that emotion-laden situations and stressful environments influence gastric secretion and pH (25). The latter, as well as gastric motility, was also affected by feelings of anxiety, anger and humiliation (32).

Clinical observations and case reports would suggest a relationship between stress and peptic ulcers. This has been documented in the more recent studies of air traffic controllers and men in supervisory roles (9, 10). Moreover, an exacerbation of preexisting ulcer disease has been reported in certain emotional situations (42).

Alexander attempted to define psychodynamic conflicts believed to be centrally important in the etiology of duodenal ulcer (1, 56). These patients were thought to have the major conflict of nondependence versus dependence which ultimately lead to certain personality traits such as an overinflated sense of self-sufficiency, a false sense of independence and a driving ambition. This hypothesis, however, has not been validated and such traits are often found in patients who do not have ulcers. Subsequent studies dealing with the "perforation prodrome" and the "pre-ulcer conflict" have clearly delineated the role of rage, fear and anxiety imminently preceding perforation or onset of the illness (7, 48). Interestingly, an earlier study had made the observation that some of the patients with ulcers had been depressed but none experienced this affective state during an exacerbation of their illness (60). From the foregoing it would appear that emotional states contribute to the genesis and course of peptic ulcer disease. The exact mechanisms, however, remain unclear.

Studies have also been conducted to determine which psychological factors might be used to predict the response to treatment. Using life events and the Schedule of Recent Experiences, a recent study has reported that surgery for duodenal ulcers tends to follow an increase in symptomatic complaints and life changes (49). Moreover, a higher degree of life change post-operatively was associated with a multitude of gastrointestinal symptoms. This is somewhat consistent with a much earlier study which reported that patients who had undergone surgery showed a marked increase in psychosomatic complaints compared to pre-surgery (53).

SUMMARY

There is an important interplay between psychosocial and pathobiological factors in many of the most common illnesses of the mid-adult years. In this chapter, we have reviewed several major developmental events in these decades, and, using three illnesses, presented examples of the relationship between psychosocial factors and illness patterns. The need for a comprehensive approach by the physician is clear, if the patient is to receive treatment that will address the wide range of factors important to short- and long-range improvement.

REFERENCES

1. ALEXANDER, F. (1950). *Psychosomatic Medicine*. New York: Norton.
2. BINGER, C. A. L. et al. (1945). *Personality in Arterial Hypertension*. New York: American Society for Research in Psychosomatic Problems.
3. BORTNER R. W. and ROSENMAN, R. H. (1967). The measurement of pattern A behavior. *J. Chronic Dis.*, 20, 525.
4. BUTLER, R. N. (1975). Psychiatry and psychology of the middle aged. In: Freedman, A. M. et al. (eds.), *Comprehensive Textbook of Psychiatry, Vol. II*. Baltimore: Williams and Wilkins.
5. CALLOWAY, N. O. and DOLLEVOET, P. L. (1977). Selected tabular material on aging. In: Finch, C. E. and Hayflick, L. (eds.), *Handbook of the Biology of Aging*. New York: Van Nostrand Reinhold.
6. CASSEL, J. (1974). Hypertension and cardiovascular disease in migrants: A potential source of clues? *Int. J. Epidemiol.*, 3, 204.
7. CASTELNUOVO-TEDESCO, P. (1962). Emotional antecedents of perforation of ulcers of the stomach and duodenum. *Psychosom. Med.*, 24, 398.
8. CHAMBERS, W. N. and REISER, M. F. (1951). Emotional stress in the precipitation of congestive heart failure. *Psychosom. Med.*, 15, 38.
9. COBB, S. and ROSE, R. M. (1973). Hypertension, peptic ulcer and diabetes in air traffic controllers. *J. Am. Med. Assoc.*, 224, 489.
10. DUNN, J. P. and COBB, S. (1962). Frequency of peptic ulcer among executives, craftsmen and foremen. *J. Occup. Med.*, 4, 343.
11. EBERHARD, G. (1968). The personality at peptic ulcer. Preliminary report of a twin study. *Acta Psychiat. Scand.*, Suppl, 203, 131.
12. FISCHER, H. K. (1961). Hypertension and the Psyche. In: Brest, A. N. and Moyer, J. H. (eds.), *Hypertension—Recent Advances*. The Second Hahnemann Symposium on Hypertensive Disease. Philadelphia: Lea & Febiger.
13. FRIEDMAN, M. et al. (1971). Coronary-prone individuals (Type A behaviour pattern); growth hormone responses. *J. Am. Med. Assoc.*, 217, 929.
14. FRIEDMAN, M. and ROSENMAN, R. H. (1978). *Type A Behavior and Your Heart*. Greenwich: Fawcett.
15. GOLDMAN, R. (1977). Aging of the excretory system: kidney and bladder. In: Finch, C. E. and Hayflick, L. (eds.) *Handbook of the Biology of Aging*. New York: Van Nostrand Reinhold.
16. GOTTSCHALK, L. A. (1978). Psychosomatic medicine today: An overview. *Psychosomatics*, 19, 89.
17. GROEN, J. J. (1976). Psychosomatic aspects of ischaemic (coronary) heart disease. In: Oscar

Hill (ed.) *Modern Trends in Psychosomatic Medicine. (3)*. London, Boston: Butterworths.

18. GUTMANN, E. (1977). Muscle. In: Finch, C. E. and Hayflick, L. (eds.) *Handbook of the Biology of Aging*. New York: Van Nostrand Reinhold.

19. HABBICK, B. F. et al. (1968). Duodenal ulcer in childhood. A study of predisposing factors. *Arch. Dis. Child.*, *43*, 23.

20. HANLEY, W. B. (1964). Hereditary aspects of duodenal ulceration: Serum-pepsinogen level in relation to ABO blood groups and salivary ABH secretor status. *Brit. Med. J.*, *1*, 936.

21. HARBURG, E. et al. (1964). Personality traits and behavioral problems associated with systolic blood pressure levels in college males. *J. Chronic Dis.*, *17*, 405.

22. HARBURG, E. et al. (1973). Socioecological stressor areas and black-white blood pressure: Detroit. *J. Chronic. Dis.*, *26*, 595.

23. HARRIS, R. E. and SINGER, M. I. (1968). Interaction of personality and stress in the pathogenesis of essential hypertension. In: *Proceedings for the Council for High Blood Pressure Research, Hypertension: Neural Control of Arterial Pressure*. New York: American Heart Association.

24. HEIBERG, A. and HEIBERG, A. (1977). Alexithymia—An inherited trait? *Psychother. Psychosom.*, *28*, 221.

25. HOELZEL, F. (1942). Fear and gastric acidity. *Am. J. Dig. Dis.*, *9*, 188.

26. HOLMES, T. H. and RAHE, R. H. (1967). The Social Readjustment Rating Scale. *J. Psychosom. Res.*, *11*, 213.

27. KLOCKE, R. A. (1977). Influence of aging on the lung. In: Finch, C. E. and Hayflick, L. (eds.) *Handbook of the Biology of Aging*. New York: Van Nostrand Reinhold.

28. KOHN, R. R. (1977). Heart and cardiovascular system. In: Finch, C. E. and Hayflick, L. (eds.) *Handbook of the Biology of Aging*. New York: Van Nostrand Reinhold.

29. LEVI, L. (1973). Stress, distress and psychosocial stimuli. *Occup. Ment. Health*, *3*, 2.

30. LEVINSON, D. J. et al. (1978). *The Seasons of a Man's Life*. New York: Alfred Knopf.

31. LUNDBERG, U. et al. (1975). Life changes and myocardial infarction: Individual differences in life change scaling. *J. Psychosom. Res.*, *19*, 27.

32. MITTELMANN, B. and WOLFF, H. G. (1942). Emotions and gastroduodenal function: Experimental studies on patients with gastritis, duodenitis and peptic ulcer. *Psychosom. Med.*, *4*, 5.

33. MOSES, L. et al. (1956). Psychogenic factors in essential hypertension. Methodology and preliminary report. *Psychosom. Med.*, *18*, 471.

34. NADELSON, C. and NOTMAN, M. T. (1977). Emotional aspects of the symptons, functions and disorders of women. In: Usdin, G. (ed.) *Psychiatric Medicine*. New York: Brunner/Mazel.

35. PETRICH, J. and HOLMES, T. H. (1977). Life change and onset of illness. *Med. Clin. of No. Am.*, *61*, 825.

36. RABKIN, J. G. and STRUENING, E. L. (1976). Life events, stress and illness. *Science*, *194*, 1013.

37. RAHE, R. H. (1968). Life change measurement as a predictor of illness. *Proc. Roy. Soc. Med.*, *61*, 1124.

38. RAHE, R. H., PAASIKIVI, J. (1971). Psychosocial factors and myocardial infarction. II. An outpatient study in Sweden. *J. Psychosom. Res.*, *15*, 33.

39. REISER, M. F., et al. (1951). Psychologic mechanisms in malignant hypertension. *Psychosom. Med.*, *13*, 147.

40. ROESKE, N. C. A. (1979). Midlife—Toward a new individuation. *Curr. Concepts in Psychiatr.*, *5*, 18.

41. ROSE, R. M. and LEVIN, M. A. (1979). The role of stress in hypertension, gastrointestinal illness and female reproductive dysfunction. *J. Hum. Stress*, *5*, 7.

42. ROSE, R. M. and LEVIN, M. A. (1979). The role of stress in peptic ulcer disease. *J. Hum. Stress*, *5*, 27.

43. SASLOW, G. et al. (1950). Possible etiological relevance of personality factors in arterial hypertension. *Psychosom. Med.*, *12*, 292.
44. SELMANOWITZ, V. J. et al. (1977). Aging of the skin and its appendages. In: Finch, C. E. and Hayflick, L. (eds.) *Handbook of the Biology of Aging*. New York: Van Nostrand Reinhold.
45. SHAPIRO, A. P. and TENG, H. C. (1957). Technic of controlled drug assay illustrated by a comparative study of rauwolfia serpentina, phenobarbital and placebo in the hypertensive patient. *N. Eng. J. Med.*, *256*, 970.
46. SIFNEOS, P. E. et al. (1977). The phenomenon of "alexithymia": Observations in neurotic and psychosomatic patients. *Psychother. Psychosom.*, *28*, 47.
47. STAMLER, J. et al. (1967). Socioeconomic factors in the Epidemiology of Hypertensive Disease. In: Stamler, J. et al. (eds.) *The Epidemiology of Hypertension*. New York: Grune & Stratton.
48. STENBACK, A. (1960). Gastric neurosis, pre-ulcer conflict, and personality in duodenal ulcer. *J. Psychosom. Res.*, *4*, 282.
49. STEVENSON, D. K. et al. (1978). Life change and the post-operative course of duodenal ulcer patients. *J. Hum. Stress*, *5 (1)*, 19.
50. SYME, S. L. et al. (1965). Cultural mobility and the occurrence of coronary heart disease. *J. Health and Hum. Behav.*, *6*, 178.
51. THEORELL, T. and RAHE, R. H. (1971). Psychosocial factors and myocardial infarction. I. An inpatient study in Sweden. *J. Psychosom. Res.*, *15*, 25.
52. THOMAS, C. B. (1964). Psychophysiological aspects of blood pressure regulation: A clinician's view. *J. Chronic Dis.*, *17*, 599.
53. THOROUGHMAN, J. C. et al. (1967). A study of psychological factors in patients with surgically intractable duodenal ulcer and those with other intractable disorders. *Psychosom. Med.*, *29*, 273.
54. TONNA, E. A. (1977). Aging of Skeletal-Dental Systems and Supporting Tissues. In: Finch, C. E. and Hayflick, L. (eds.) *Handbook of the Biology of Aging*. New York: Van Nostrand Reinhold.
55. UPTON, A. C. (1977). Pathobiology. In: Finch, C. E. and Hayflick, L. (eds.) *Handbook of the Biology of Aging*. New York: Van Nostrand Reinhold.
56. VAILLANT, G. E. (1977). *Adaptation to Life*. Boston: Little Brown.
57. WEINER, H. (1979). Psychobiological markers of disease. *Psychiatr. Clinc. of No. Am.*, *2*, 227.
58. WEINER, H. (1977). *Psychobiology and Human Disease*. New York: Elsevier.
59. WEINER, H. (1977). The Psychobiology of Human Disease: An Overview. In: Usdin, G. (ed.) *Psychiatric Medicine*. New York: Brunner/Mazel.
60. WEISMAN, A. D. (1956). A study of the psychodynamics of duodenal ulcer exacerbations with special reference to treatment and the problem of "specificity." *Psychosom. Med.*, *18*, 2.
61. WEISS, E. et al. (1957). Emotional factors in coronary occlusion. I. Introduction and general summary. *A. M. A. Arch. Int. Med.*, *99*, 628.

17

THE MENOPAUSE AND ITS SYNDROMES

C. Barbara Ballinger, B.Sc., M.B., Ch.B., M.R.C.P., M.R.C.Psych.

Senior Lecturer,
Department of Psychiatry,
Ninewells Hospital and Medical School,
Dundee, Scotland

INTRODUCTION

The word menopause originally referred to the time of cessation of menstrual periods but is now commonly used to describe the years just before and after the cessation of menstrual periods or the time which was previously called the climacteric. Studies of symptoms, including psychological symptoms, in women in the middle years of life have been dominated by references to the menopause, since it is an obvious and easily defined biological change. To some extent this has resulted in neglect of other factors which may be more relevant and the "change" has become the scapegoat for a multitude of complaints. This concentration of attention on the menopause has been emphasized by the introduction of estrogen preparations, which have been promoted as specific treatment for the estrogen deficiency state of the post-menopausal years and therefore specific treatment for all those complaints attributed to the menopause. This approach has great attractions, since attitudes toward "psychological" symptoms and "psychological" treatment still tend to be negative, while "menopausal" symptoms and "hormone" treatment are very much more acceptable.

Another complication of the tendency to ascribe all ills to the menopause is that this event is now looked forward to with great apprehension by many women even before their periods cease. As Barnes (6) has commented, the myth of the menopause may be considerably worse than the reality.

The idea that the time of the menopause is associated with a high risk of mental disturbance was presented as early as 1857 by Tilt (80). In his book, *The Change of Life in Health and Disease,* he took a very pessimistic view of "the evil effects of this time of life." In a series of 500 women said to be "at the change," he stated that "nervous irritability" affected 459 and a hysterical state, including uncalled-for lowness of spirits, affected 146. He claimed that the change of life could be dangerous for those who were always ailing and correlated problems at this time with poor adaptation to puberty and problems with the menstrual periods. Similar pessimistic views were expressed by Merson (52) in 1876 in a study of admissions to a lunatic asylum.

Investigation of the psychological implications of the menopause has continued in various clinical areas with differing approaches. In the gynaecological literature, the emphasis has been on the relationship of symptoms to ovarian failure, with the inclusion of various emotional symptoms in the menopausal syndrome and the use of estrogen preparations to relieve these symptoms. In the psychiatric literature, the concept of involutional melancholia and its possible relationship to the hormonal changes of the menopause has been debated extensively, while the psychoanalytic literature has concentrated on the psychological impact of reaching the menopause and its effect on the production of symptoms at this time.

More recently, several epidemiological studies have been carried out to try and elucidate what symptoms are related to the time of cessation of menstrual periods in women from the general population, as opposed to those attending clinics for gynaecological or psychiatric treatment. There has also been increasing emphasis on the cultural differences in attitudes to the menopause and the influence of environmental factors such as change in family structure at this time of life.

PSYCHIATRIC SYNDROMES AND THE MENOPAUSE

The syndrome which attracted most attention in the psychiatric literature in relation to the menopause was that of involutional melancholia. There was considerable debate about whether such an illness existed as an entity separate from manic-depressive illness and, if it did exist, whether it was related in any way to the endocrine changes of the menopause. The literature has recently been reviewed in detail by Rosenthal (66).

Kraepelin (37) originally described melancholia as a syndrome separate from manic-depressive illness. He stated that melancholia was associated with delusions of sin, poverty and disgrace, that it started at the onset of old age and affected women more than men. He later modified this view (38), including melancholia with manic-depressive illness and stating that, although there was a definite increase in the number of depressives presenting after the 45th year, this was only the continuation of a steady increase in the number of depressive illnesses presenting with increasing age.

Many authors (44, 86, 91) continued to regard involutional melancholia as a separate illness, elaborating on the clinical characteristics of the syndrome and speculating on its relationship to the involutional processes, particularly the menopause. An extreme view of the hormonal aetiology of involutional melancholia was taken by Werner et al. (86). They considered this illness to be only an extreme manifestation of the symptomatology of the menopause caused by the endocrine crisis produced by cessation of function of the gonads. Treatment with ovarian extract was considered specific for this condition. The ovarian extracts used in these early studies were of doubtful potency and an attempt to reproduce this work (59), using stilboestrol with 11 patients treated for three months, produced negative results, as did a study (64) of the use of an estrogen preparation in 20 women presenting with depressive illness at a psychiatric clinic.

The change in attitude towards the concept of involutional melancholia was mirrored in succeeding editions of some standard psychiatric textbooks. In the 8th edition of Henderson and Gillespie's textbook (26), a separate chapter was devoted to involutional melancholia, stressing the clinical features of the first attack occurring in the involution, that is, between 40 and 55 years of age in women and 50 to 65 years of age in men, with depression of mood without retardation and symptoms of anxiety and unreality with hypochondriacal and nihilistic delusions. In the 9th edition of Henderson and Gillespie's book, the position was essentially the same, but in the 10th edition (27) involutional melancholia was included in the chapter on "Affective Reaction Types," with the comment that there were no longer sufficient grounds to distinguish it from manic-depressive psychosis. In Mayer-Gross, Slater and Roth's *Clinical Psychiatry*, involutional psychosis has retained its subheading in the the chapter on manic-depressive illness, with a comment in the 3rd edition (72) that the affective involutional psychoses are a heterogeneous group.

Enthusiasm for maintaining a separate diagnosis of involutional melancholia declined in Britain with the publication in 1934 of a study by Aubrey Lewis (40). He concluded from clinical studies that the depressive syndromes formed a continuum and a separate category of involutional psychosis could not be distinguished on clinical grounds. More recently, attempts have been made to study clinical features or psychiatric illness in a more systematic fashion, using the process of factor analysis. In a study of 1,008 patients, 55 of whom had been diagnosed as suffering from involutional melancholia, Kendell (34) found that on the three variables of symptoms, treatment and outcome, the involutional melancholics were identical with patients with psychotic depression.

Hopkinson (28), in a study of affective illness in patients over 50, compared those who had had previous attacks before the age of 50, the "early" cases, with those whose first attack occurred after the age of 50, the "late" cases. He found the two groups clinically similar except that agitation was more common in the "early" cases, in contrast to the previously held view that agitation was a prominent feature of involutional melancholia which, by definition, should have been found in the "late" cases.

In a study of 307 patients with involutional melancholia "as traditionally described," Stenstedt (75) found the risk for endogenous affective disorder among siblings and parents the same as for a group of manic-depressive patients. He concluded that the group of patients said to suffer from involutional melancholia was made up of late cases of manic-depressive psychosis and exogenous depression. In a detailed clinical study, Stenbäck (74) concluded that there was no evidence for a separate diagnosis of involutional melancholia with a specific aetiology, symptomatology, premorbid personality or course of the disorder.

An endocrinological study of subjects identified as having involutional melancholia on clinical grounds, including time of onset, was reported in 1971 (57). The subjects, aged from 49 to 66 years, were matched with a group with no evidence of mental illness but of the same age and sex; no significant difference was found between the subjects and the matched controls in relation to urinary excretion of gonadotrophins or estrogens.

The results of these studies suggest that there is little evidence to support the concept of involutional melancholia as a syndrome separate from psychotic depressive illness. Also, the limited endocrinological studies carried out so far have failed to show any relationship between psychiatric illness and the hormonal changes of the menopause. There is, therefore, no indication at present that the use of estrogen for the treatment of symptoms at the time of the menopause will have any impact on the prevalence of psychiatric illness at this time of life.

The effects of the menopause on mental health, as measured by admission to mental hospital, have also been investigated by several authors (73, 77, 90).

Tait et al. (77) reported a prospective study of 54 consecutive first admissions to hospital of women between the ages of 40 and 55 years. The mean age of this group of patients was 47 years and 22 of the 54 subjects were post-menopausal. Tait et al. commented on the remarkable absence of the traditional picture of involutional melancholia in the analysis of history of symptoms. The three most common diagnoses were psychotic depression, neurotic illness and late onset schizophrenia. There was no evidence of any direct relationship between the time of onset of the illness and the time of cessation of menstrual periods.

Winokur (90) reported the results of a study of 71 women presenting with an affective disorder requiring admission to hospital. The risk for occurrence of an episode of illness requiring admission to hospital was calculated for the whole group between the ages of 20 and 80 years and then for the 28 post-menopausal women within three years of the age given for the menopause. The risk was expressed as a percentage of the years at risk that were associated with an episode of illness. The risk for the perimenopausal years, as defined in this study, was not significantly different from the risk for the time span of 20 to 80 years. Winokur concluded that there was little value in looking at the menopausal state for clues to the aetiology of affective disorder.

In a study (73) of 880 people admitted to a regional mental health centre in America, all diagnostic groups were included. Nineteen critical life events were defined, including developmental events such as the menopause, menarche and pregnancy, and the occurrence of these events in the year prior to admission was noted. The occurrence of the same events in the previous year was studied in a general population sample of 2,414 people. Reaching the menopause was one of the three items which occurred more frequently in the general population than in the patient group during the one year prior to contact. This finding is directly contrary to the view that the time of the menopause is associated with an increased risk of developing mental disturbance resulting in admission to hospital.

Although psychiatric symptoms are mentioned frequently in accounts of menopausal symptoms, the menopause would appear to have very little impact on psychiatric practice, particularly in relation to the psychoses. From the studies carried out so far, there is no evidence of any increase in affective disorder or mental hospital admissions in general at the time of the menopause, other than as part of the gradual increase seen with increasing age in both sexes.

THE MENOPAUSAL SYNDROME

Controversy about what symptoms constitute the "menopausal syndrome" and which, if any, are related to a fall in estrogen production has continued in the gynaecological literature since Tilt (80) produced his original account. Many gynaecologists were convinced that emotional symptoms were specifically related to the menopause and were caused by estrogen deficiency. As recently as 1971, Williams (88) commented that "most psychiatrists will agree that estrogens are valuable in emotional disturbance at this time."

The group of symptoms originally described as the menopausal syndrome was based on the symptom checklist described by Kupperman et al. (39) for the calculation of the menopausal index. This list of 11 symptoms included such items as nervousness, melancholia, insomnia, palpitations and headache, in addition to the vasomotor symptoms of flushing and excessive sweating. This list was derived from a clinical evaluation of women attending the clinic and the psychological symptoms displayed by these women were accepted as being related to their menopausal status.

The existence of psychological symptoms clearly related to estrogen deprivation at the time of the menopause was argued strongly by Joan Malleson (45, 46) in Britain and Wilson and Wilson (89) in America. Again, their views appeared to be based on the very select group of women who presented at their clinics and the idea of a psychosocial aetiology for symptoms of emotional disturbance at this time was strongly resisted, as if being a criticism of the woman as a person.

In 1951, Donovan (16) challenged the whole concept of the menopausal syndrome, basing his opinion on 110 case histories. He concluded that the temporal relationships between the symptoms and the menopause were not clear-cut and he felt that the frequency and constancy of so-called menopausal symptoms represented a clinical artifact. He pointed out that many of the women presenting at the time of the menopause had done so previously with equally ill-defined symptoms and he even considered that women suffered from sensations of heat and cold before the menopause but these were not called hot flushes or "flashes" until the woman reached middle age.

In contrast to Malleson, Jeffcoate (32) argued that only hot flushes should be called menopausal symptoms and stated that many women in their 40s were told that any minor symptoms were due to "the change," although they were more likely to be due to environmental rather than hormonal changes. He stated that there was no more justification for giving hormone therapy for the emotional symptoms of the climacteric than for giving such therapy for the emotional symptoms of puberty.

Novak (58), English (18) and Rogers (65) all expressed a similar view that the emotional symptoms elicited from women attending their clinics around the time of the menopause were related to factors such as previous personality, marital difficulties and change in family structure, particularly as children grew up and left home. The term "empty nest syndrome" was introduced by Deykin et al. (15) to describe this last factor.

Epidemiological Studies

The assumption that psychological symptoms are specifically associated with the menopause has now been investigated in several surveys using various screening methods. Neugarten and Kraines (55) reported a study of 460 women between the ages of 13 and 65 years. The subjects completed a symptom checklist of 28 items in three groups: somatic, psychological and psychosomatic. The results showed two peaks of symptom frequency coinciding with puberty and the menopause, but whereas the majority of symptoms occurring at puberty were psychological those at the menopause were mainly somatic. A similar increase in somatic symptoms at the time of the menopause was reported by Priest and Crisp (63).

In 1969, Jaszmann et al. (31) reported the results of a survey of 3,000 women between the ages of 40 and 60 years in Holland, using a symptom checklist based on the menopausal index described by Kupperman et al. (39). Complaints of irritability, headache, fatigue, deperession and "mental imbalance" were most frequent in women reporting a change in their menstrual pattern in the previous year and least frequent in post-menopausal women. Women who were menstruating regularly were in an intermediate position. Complaints of dizziness, shortness of breath and palpitations did not show any variation in relation to menopausal status, while hot flushes, excess perspiration and insomnia were reported most frequently by post-menopausal subjects.

In a survey of 226 women between the ages of 40 and 60 on a general practice list, Thompson et al. (78) found that only the complaints of flushing and night sweats showed significant variation with menopausal status, being reported most frequently by post-menopausal women. Ten other complaints, including depression, headache, dizzy spells and tiredness, were reported to the same extent by all women regardless of menopausal status. It was found that complaints of sleeplessness were closely linked with night sweats, being most frequent in post-menopausal women. In a survey (43) of 638 women between the ages of 45 and 54 years of age living in the London area, it was found that hot flushes and night sweats were the only symptoms clearly associated with cessation of menstrual periods. Complaints of headache, dizzy spells, palpitations, sleeplessness, depression and weight increase did not vary with menopausal status but tended to occur together.

None of the studies considered so far used questionnaires specifically designed for detecting psychiatric symptoms. In 1973, Hällström (24) reported a study from Scandinavia involving 800 women in four age strata, 38 years, 46 years, 50 years and 54 years, with detailed psychiatric interviews and physical examinations. There was no significant variation in frequency of onset of mental illness with menopausal status, but women who were defined as perimenopausal, that is, having irregular periods, showed a higher frequency of mental deterioration than pre- or post-menopausal women.

In a study (2) of 539 women between the ages of 40 and 55 years on the list of one group practice, psychiatric screening was carried out using the 60-item General Health Questionnaire (G.H.Q.) as described by Goldberg (23). This self-rating scale was developed for the detection of current emotional disturbance and for use in community surveys. In this survey women who were menopausal or immediately pre-menopausal, that is, between 45 and 50 years of age and still menstruating, had the highest levels of psychiatric morbidity and post-menopausal women the lowest.

None of these surveys indicated any dramatic increase in psychological symptoms in relation to the cessation of menstrual periods and it is unlikely· that vague symptoms of depression, dizziness and headache in women in this age group are directly related to the menopause. However, three of these surveys (2, 24, 31) indicated some increase in psychiatric symptoms in women immediately prior to the menopause who were beginning to display menstrual irregularity and could be defined as perimenopausal. It is known that some changes in hormonal status occur prior to the cessation of menstrual periods and it may be that these changes have some influence on mental health. Recently, a more detailed endocrinological study (11) of women approaching the menopause and presenting at a menopause clinic indicated that those women with vasomotor symptoms showed a significant elevation of L.H. and F.S.H. and significantly lower circulating estradiol levels.

In all these surveys complaints of flushing and sweating increased sharply at the time of the menopause and remained common in the post-menopausal years, whereas the three surveys which have shown any change in psychiatric morbidity with the menopause have indicated an increase in the immediately pre-menopausal years with a fall in the post-menopausal years. This difference in pattern of change of psychiatric symptoms and vasomotor symptoms with the menopause is contrary to the idea that it is the estrogen deficiency of the post-menopausal years that is responsible for the psychiatric symptoms.

The Effects of Patient Selection

As has been suggested previously in this account, the quoted association of psychological symptoms with the menopause has probably arisen because of the highly selected group of patients who attend clinics of any type, but particularly gynaecological and related clinics. Sainsbury (67) found in a survey of several outpatient clinics that women attending the gynaecological outpatient clinic obtained the highest scores for neuroticism, particularly in relation to vague presenting complaints such as menorrhagia.

A study of 217 women between the ages of 40 and 55 years attending a gynaecological outpatient clinic (5) showed that, in comparison with a general population sample from the same city and in the same age range, the clinic attenders had a higher proportion of women with evidence of psychiatric morbidity and significantly more contact with the psychiatric services in the past, as well as in the year following attendance at the clinic. This would suggest that a selected group of women with a higher level of emotional symptoms than women in the general population attend these clinics; the same is probably true of the menopause clinics.

This element of selection probably accounts for the findings reported by Jones et al. (33). They described a menopause questionnaire based on the menopausal index of Kupperman (39) and including such items as irritability, depression, unloved feelings and poor memory. They found that these items grouped together discriminated between a group of post-menopausal patients attending the clinic and a group of normal married pre-menopausal women below the age of 40. They concluded that the difference in meno-pausal status between these two groups accounted for the discriminatory effect, but these items probably discriminate between clinic attenders and non-attenders irrespective of menopausal status. Also, there was more than ten years difference in age between these two groups, so they would not be strictly comparable. It is interesting that the item of "unloved feelings" is included in this questionnaire, since this item may well correlate with the urge for self-referral to a clinic where some interest and attention would be expected.

The issue of selection of women attending the menopause clinics is important in relation to interpretation of clinical findings in these subjects and in applying these findings to the management of women in the general population. It also raises the problem of why people use medical services and why they prefer to use some services rather than others.

Mechanic (51) has described some of the sociological factors relevant to the use of medical services and stated that cultural and social conditions play an important part in determining use of services. At present, menopause clinics are certainly fashionable and promoted in the media and it has been noted (85) that they attract subjects whose complaints are not necessarily related to their menopausal status. Mechanic also described the tendency to present emotional and behavioural problems in the physical guise and the continuing resistance to the concept of mental illness. Menopausal symptoms are more socially acceptable than psychological symptoms.

Vasomotor Symptoms

In several of the epidemiological studies (2, 31, 43, 78), complaints of "hot flushes" and "sweats" increased sharply at the time of cessation of menstrual periods and persisted for some years. In view of Donovan's criticism (16) that the term "hot flush" was used at the time of the menopause for symptoms which had been present long before, this term was avoided in Ballinger's study (2) and the responses to two of the questions from the General Health Questionnaire, "Have you recently been having hot or cold spells?" and "Have you recently been perspiring (sweating) a lot?", were analysed separately. There was a very sharp increase in positive responses to these questions at the time of cessation of menstrual periods and positive responses remained at a high level in women up to five years post-menopausal.

In the gynaecological literature there has been a recent tendency to a more restricted use of the term menopausal syndrome. Both Beard (7) and Utian (83) have expressed the opinion that only the vasomotor symptoms of flushing and sweating and the symptom of dyspareunia in relation to vaginal atrophy and vaginitis can be related directly to reduced ovarian activity and falling estrogen levels. Utian has stated that the psychological symptoms usually ascribed to the climacteric are probably related to psychosocial and cultural phenomena and the changes of aging.

Insomnia

A further item of behaviour which has been included in the menopausal syndrome and studied in relation to menopausal status is sleep pattern.

Although overall psychiatric morbidity shows no dramatic change with the cessation of menstrual periods, insomnia was reported more frequently in post-menopausal women in two studies (4, 31) and found to correlate with the symptoms of night sweats in another (78). It has been shown that complaints of sleeplessness increase with increasing age (42), but in women there is a sharp increase around the age of 50 which is not found in men. A controlled trial of the use of estrogens as a hypnotic in post-menopausal women (79) showed that estrogen did indeed reduce the number of episodes of wakefulness in these women, but the effect on other psychological symptoms was little different from that of placebo. There is, therefore, some evidence to support the view that insomnia may be related to hormonal changes at the time of the menopause. The use of estrogen preparations rather than cerebral depressants as hypnotics at this time is clearly worthy of further investigation.

Sexual Behaviour

Loss of libido was an item frequently included in the menopausal syndrome. Changes in sexual behaviour in middle age and their relationship to the menopause have now been studied in some detail. One sexual problem which is clearly related to the estrogen deficiency state of the post-menopausal years is that of superficial dyspareunia associated with vaginal atrophy and vaginitis.

In a community study of 800 women, Hällström (25) found that relatively few suffered from dyspareunia compared with the number complaining of general diminution in interest in sexual matters. In a menopause clinic group (76), it was found that of 300 women presenting at the clinic, 19 complained of dyspareunia alone, 59 of loss of libido alone, and 58 of both. Vasomotor symptoms were reported more frequently and anxiety and depression less frequently by the group complaining of dyspareunia alone.

The problem of vaginal atrophy in the post-menopausal years has been studied in relation to the vaginal smears and Utian (84) has suggested that the relationship between vaginal cytology and estrogen levels is so clear that the parabasal cell count expressed as a percentage of the total cells present could be used as a cytological index to give an objective measure of response to estrogen therapy.

The symptom of superficial dyspareunia, although not as objective as a vaginal smear, is one of the few symptoms occurring at the time of the menopause which is related to circulating estrogen levels. Hutton et al. (30) found in a group of post-menopausal or oopherectomised women that those women with complaints of superficial dyspareunia and hot flushes had significantly lower estradiol levels than those complaining of hot flushes alone or neither of these symptoms.

The question of loss of interest in sexual contact where dyspareunia is not present is a more subtle and complex issue. Kinsey et al. (36) found that frequency of sexual intercourse in married women declined steadily with increasing age but in single women remained steady until 55 years of age and then declined. Using frequency of intercourse as a measure of sexual drive in women presents some problems, as it is likely to be determined by the sexual activity of the male partner. In a study of sexual activity in a middle-aged group of subjects (60), it was found that women attributed responsibility for cessation of intercourse to their husbands; this was confirmed by the husbands.

In *Human Sexual Response*, Masters and Johnson (50) commented on the belief that many women experience an increase in sexual drive at the time of the menopause and they discussed several possibilities for this change, including freedom from the worry of pregnancy. However, recent studies (25, 60, 63) have not confirmed this belief in an increase in sexual drive.

In an American study (60), it was found that 49% of men and 58% of women had noted a decline in sexual interest by 50 years of age. Priest and Crisp (63) reported a steep rise in positive responses to the question "Has your sexual interest altered?"—from 25% of women in their early 40s to 75% in their early 60s. In Hällström's study (25) of 800 women, there is clear evidence of a decrease in sexual interest and capacity for orgasm in post-menopausal women compared with premenopausal women, independent of the effect of increasing age. Other factors having a significant association with decrease in sexual interest independent of age and menopausal status were low social class, poor marital relationship and the symptom of depression. Hällström (25) makes the interesting suggestion that, although decrease in sexual interest shows a clear relationship with post-menopausal status, it may not be related to the endocrine changes but to women using the menopause as a reason for escaping sexual contact in the setting of a poor marital relationship and previous personality difficulties.

In both the menopause clinic study reported by Studd et al. (76) and the general population study reported by Hällström (25), loss of sexual interest showed a relationship to psychiatric symptoms. Coppen (13) has previously commented on the association of sexual problems with neurotic complaints. In Hällström's study (25), it was depression that was particularly related to loss of sexual interest.

In conclusion, the symptom of superficial dyspareunia is clearly related to estrogen deficiency in the post-menopausal years, but the symptom of loss of interest in sexual matters, although showing some change with menopausal status, is affected by many other factors and does not show any clear relationship to circulating levels of estrogen and gonadotrophins in post-menopausal women.

Treatment

There have been many reports of the use of estrogen preparations and other drugs in the treatment of menopausal symptoms but the results have been very variable (10, 12, 21, 35, 41, 62, 70, 81, 82, 87).

One of the problems in assessing the results of trials of estrogen therapy is the number of symptoms subsumed under the heading menopausal syndrome. This term has been used in some studies as if it were a clear clinical entity with a single aetiology, but it usually includes a diversity of symptoms of differing origin. This confusion is particularly evident in comparative trials of estrogen and psychotropic drugs for the treatment of the menopausal syndrome. In one trial (87), reported from a general practice, menopausal symptoms included fatigue, hot flushes, excessive sweating, insomnia, anxiety, depression, joint and muscle pains, headache and palpitations. It was concluded that opripranol, a tricyclic antidepressant, and stilboestrol were both superior to placebo, but both relieved menopausal symptoms to the same extent. With the symptoms grouped in this manner, these preparations could presumably have quite different effects on different symptoms but produce the same overall change in number and severity of symptoms.

There is also the problem that the relief of symptoms such as flushes and vaginal dryness with estrogen can result in a woman feeling generally better and therefore scoring less for depression and anxiety. Conversely, relief of depression and anxiety with an antidepressant could well lead to increased tolerance of physical symptoms and consequent reduction in number and severity of complaints. It is doubtful if any valid conclusions can be drawn from studies using measures of the menopausal index type.

The problem of different symptoms responding to different types of medication was illustrated by Sheffery et al. (70) in a study of effects of chlordiazepoxide, combined chlordiazepoxide and estrogen, estrogen preparation alone, and placebo on symptoms in women presenting with menopausal problems. The estrogen preparation alone and the estrogen combined with chlordiazepoxide relieved the symptoms of flushing significantly better than chlordiazepoxide alone or placebo. Chlordiazepoxide and estrogen combined were significantly more effective than estrogen alone in relieving anxiety, vertigo and insomnia and significantly more effective than chlordiazepoxide alone in relieving insomnia. Chlordiazepoxide alone was significantly more effective than estrogen alone in relieving anxiety.

Another problem in some of the drug trials is the lack of a placebo group. A large placebo effect in the treatment of menopausal symptoms has been well documented (12). There is little doubt that the consideration and attention received at a clinic can have a considerable effect on a woman's sense of well-being.

Utian (81), in a detailed placebo-controlled trial of oral estrogen therapy, found that it had no effect on insomnia, irritability, depression, palpitations, backache or libido but had a significant effect on vaginal dryness and the hot flush count. He observed what he described as a "mental tonic" effect of estrogen (82) in some patients. This may be due to the relief of those symptoms related to estrogen deficiency, leading to a general increase in well-being.

Campbell (10) reported a double-blind crossover study of estrogen against placebo on a variety of symptoms assessed separately. In the four-month study of 64 patients, the subjects were treated for two months with an estrogen preparation and two months with placebo. In the 12-month study of 56 patients, the subjects were treated for six months with estrogen or placebo and then the crossover took place. A variety of rating scales were used to assess the effects of treatment, including analogue rating scales, the Beck self-rating scale (8), the Eysenck Peronality Inventory (E.P.I.) and the General Health Questionnaire (23).

In the four-month study, estrogen appeared to be superior to placebo in the treatment of insomnia, irritability, headache, anxiety, urinary frequency, memory, good spirits and optimism. It appeared that this was related to considerable fall in frequency of hot flushes, as a change in these symptoms was only shown in women who reported severe hot flushes initially. In the 12-month study, vaginal dryness, flushes and insomnia were significantly improved by the estrogen compound compared with placebo, as was "memory" to a less marked extent. For the other psychological symptoms there was no significant difference between the effect of estrogen and placebo. It is also of interest that, although vaginal dryness responded significantly to estrogen, loss of libido did not, again emphasising the complex issues affecting sexual responsiveness.

In Campbell's study (10), the score on the Beck scale, the General Health Qustionnaire scores and the neuroticism score on the Eysenck Personality Inventory all showed highly significant improvements with both placebo and estrogen but did not differentiate between the two. Campbell makes the observation that these scales are not sensitive enough to monitor changes in women who for the most part do not have any formal psychiatric illness. This would not seem to be a valid criticism, in that all these scales responded sensitively to the improvement produced in all subjects with attendance at the menopause clinic. The marked placebo effect may be considered as an indication of the psychotherapeutic impact of attending the clinic and receiving attention.

The significant improvement in "memory" said to be produced by estrogen in Campbell's study (10) is difficult to interpret. The change in memory function was assessed on an analogue rating scale, previously described by Zealley and Aitken (92) for the measurement of mood. Memory was rated "very poor" at one end of a line of fixed length and "very good" at the other. The subject was asked to indicate how her memory had been in the last four weeks by putting a mark on the line. No formal psychological testing of memory function was carried out and this change in subjective memory assessment as measured on the analogue scale may well be related to concentration change or arousal.

In conclusion, the evidence from drug trials in relation to psychological symptoms at the time of the menopause is confused for two reasons. One is the tendency to group symptoms which are entirely unrelated to each other in the menopausal syndrome and the other is the very marked placebo response. There would appear to be reasonable evidence for the superiority of estrogen over placebo in both Campbell's (10) and Utian's (81) work in the treatment of hot flushes and vaginal dryness, although even this has been questioned (53). There is also evidence to suggest that insomnia responds to estrogen (79) and this may not be entirely due to decrease in vasomotor symptoms. There is no evidence available to suggest that estrogens have any specific effect on other psychological symptoms such as depression, anxiety, irritability or loss of libido. Almost certainly these symptoms, as at any other time of life, are multifactorial in origin and the preponderance of these symptoms in women attending the menopause clinics is due to the element of selection.

PSYCHOANALYTIC OBSERVATIONS ON THE MENOPAUSAL SYNDROME

Psychoanalytic accounts of the problems of women in the years around the time of the menopause have concentrated on the psychological implications of reaching the menopause rather than the physiological impact of the endocrine changes at this time.

Psychoanalytic views on the menopause have been strongly influenced by the opinions of Deutsch (14) in her book, *The Psychology of Women*. Deutsch used the term climacteric rather than menopause and the relevant chapter is headed "Epilogue. The Climacteric," suggesting that this time of life is seen as the conclusion of woman as far as her psychology is concerned.

Deutsch stated that almost every woman in the climacteric goes through a short- or long-term depression, that oddities of conduct occur, and that women are suggestible and display poor judgment at this time. She made no attempt to justify these statements or present evidence to show that these characteristics are any more common at this time of a woman's life than at any other time.

Deutsch (14) discussed the origin of these climacteric behavioural disorders in a detailed and pessimistic manner, in keeping with the idea that the climacteric was the conclusion of life as a woman. Women were said to be losing all they received at puberty in terms of femininity and reproductive potential. This was described as a time of castration, mortification and partial death, when life was pale and purposeless and psychotherapy was difficult, since there was little one could offer. Resignation without compensation was seen as the only solution.

From a study of 100 patients presenting for treatment, and therefore a selected group, Fessler (19) concluded that the condition of the majority of women during the climacteric was not normal. He related many of the difficulties to penis envy, suggesting that while women were menstruating they had a reminder of their reproductive potential which compensated for lack of a penis, but with the cessation of periods there was a return to infantile attitudes of reaction to lack of a penis. He saw disappointment as the core of climacteric depression, but again presented no evidence to support his thesis of depression being more common at this time of life than any other.

The issue of loss in relation to reproductive potential and femininity was frequently stressed in psychoanalytic literature. The relationship of loss to mourning and melancholia was introduced by Freud (22), who suggested that libido from the lost object was withdrawn to the self and then the self was identified with the abandoned object so that loss of the object was experienced as a loss of the ego and mental pain. In the psychoanalytic literature, the loss of self-esteem incurred in the loss of femininity and reproductive potential was stressed in relation to the symptom of depression, which was said to be common in women presenting for analysis in this age group. Deykin (15) also stressed the importance of loss in relation to children leaving home.

Benedek (9) presented a rare optimistic view of the climacteric in psychoanalytic terms. She saw the climacteric not as the conclusion but as a developmental phase and a period of interpersonal reorganisation in women in parallel with the change in hormonal status. She saw the desexualisation of emotional needs as providing the psychic energy for sublimation and integration of the personality. She stressed the importance of previous personality in relation to a woman's ability to adapt to the changes of this time of life.

Other writers (1, 29, 61) stressed the idea that the climacteric or the menopause was a time of emotional crisis. In an introductory discussion of the word menopause, Prados (61) stated that this term was generally used to include "the personality and behavioural changes that women show preceding, accompanying and following this critical age period." However, he, like Benedek (9), was a little more optimistic about the post-climacteric years, saying that this could be a time of stability and satisfaction. He stressed the importance of a woman's previous personality in relation to surviving the menopause. Hoskins (29) discussed the psychosomatic nature of the menopause and considered the physical and mental aspects inseparable. He saw the central feature as anxiety related to the threat to the ego from the loss of reproductive function, which he considered to be a woman's "symbolic token of personal worth."

Achte (1) considered that irritability, sleeplessness, anxiety and emotional instability were common at the time of the menopause and that depression was the most frequent disorder at this time, but he again presented no evidence to support this view. He stressed fear of growing old, loss of femininity and self-esteem, and the importance of past life experience and constitutional factors in the production of psychological symptoms.

In the psychoanalytic literature, the question of personality and ability to cope with stress in the past has often been emphasised in relation to a woman's response to the menopause (1, 9, 61). There is some limited evidence available to support this view. In the study reported by Ballinger (3), women who showed evidence of emotional disturbance between the ages of 40 and 55 years were more likely than matched controls to have been on psychotropic medication in the past and to have visited their general practitioners frequently.

The view frequently expressed in the analytic literature that the time of the menopause is associated with an excess of symptoms such as depression and irritability has not been confirmed by the general population surveys. This discrepancy is probably due to patient selection. Women attending for analysis are unlikely to be representative of the general population; although these patients may be having problems in adaptation to the menopause, it cannot be concluded that most other women are having similar difficulties. However, the descriptive accounts presented in the analytic literature may have considerable relevance to the assessment and management of individual patients presenting with emotional symptoms at this time of life. Also, the issues of loss of femininity and self-esteem may be relevant to the attitudes displayed towards the use of estrogen preparations and the way in which these preparations are advertised and promoted (17).

ENVIRONMENTAL ISSUES AND THE MENOPAUSAL SYNDROME

Increasing attention has been given recently to those environmental factors independent of the menopause which may affect a woman at this time of life, inducing symptoms which may then be attributed to the menopause. Also, those social and cultural factors which influence a woman's perception and anticipation of the menopause and the way these factors may then influence how the menopause is experienced have received more attention.

Family Changes

It has been stated that at the age of 50 years, the median age of the menopause in Western cultures, a woman's parents are aging and her children achieving independence and leaving home. Simon (71) has emphasised the importance of the change in role and status of women as children leave home and the necessity for other outlets for a woman's drive in relation to her emotional adjustment.

There is some evidence to support the view that changes in family structure are relevant to the emotional health of a woman at this time. In a study (2) of a general population sample of women between the ages of 40 and 55 years, a child leaving home or getting married within the last year was associated with an increased risk of emotional disturbance in the mother. It was also found that women with three or more children had a higher risk of psychiatric symptoms than those with two or less. It would appear that many stresses are associated with family; also, the larger the family, the greater the stress. In the same study, there was no evidence to support the view that loss of reproductive potential was an important element in the production of psychiatric symptoms, since women with no children were less likely to display evidence of symptoms than women with three or more children.

As children leave home, a woman's relationship with her husband may become more important in relation to her adjustment. In the epidemiological surveys discussed so far, there was no systematic investigation of this issue, but Hällström's work (25) on sexual responsiveness emphasised the importance of the quality of the relationship between husband and wife in relation to changes in sexual responsiveness at this time.

The effect of death of parents was investigated in the general population survey reported by Ballinger (2, 3), but no significant association between parental death and emotional disturbance in women between the ages of 40 and 55 years was found. However, coping with ill and dependent parents was one of the more frequent issues mentioned by women when they were asked if there had been any problems in the family in the previous year.

The limited evidence at present available suggests that changes in family structure have a considerable impact on the emotional well-being of a woman at this time of life and the symptoms produced may then be attributed to the menopause.

Outside Work

The influence of outside work on the development of symptoms at the time of the menopause shows both cultural and social variation. In a German study (68) of 2,232 subjects, those women who were well motivated for their work and who were relieved of the burden of housework displayed fewer symptoms during the years of the menopause than full-time housewives. In a Belgian (69) study, it was found that for the upper socioeconomic classes working outside the home was always favourable, but this was not true for the lower socioeconomic groups where work outside the home at times added to the stress. Maoz et al. (48), in a study of five ethnic groups in Israel, found that in four of these groups working outside the home was associated with lower level of symptomatology during the menopausal years and for the fifth group the reverse was true. What is not certain from these findings is whether working outside the home actually protects against development of symptoms or whether those women who take up outside work are those who are less likely to develop symptoms. The relationship between outside work and development of symptoms is not straightforward and Maoz et al. (48) warn against advising outside work as a panacea for problems at the time of the menopause.

Cultural Influences

Culturally-determined attitudes towards the menopause may be expected to influence a woman's anticipation and experience of this event. Mannes (47) commented on the problems of adaptation to and acceptance of the menopause against the background of contemporary North American culture, which she described as a youth-worshipping and sex-saturated society. Undoubtedly, the menopause is a very clear reminder of the aging process.

Neugarten et al. (56) reported an interesting variation in expectations of the menopause with age. Younger women, the majority of whom were pre-menopausal, were much more negative in their attitude to the menopause and particularly to the post-menopausal years than were the older women, many of whom were already post-menopausal. This is in keeping with the view that the myth of the menopause is worse than the reality (6). The idea that loss of reproductive capacity or partial death as described by Deutsch (14) is an important issue at the time of the menopause was not supported by Neugarten's findings. Only four out of 100 women considered not being able to have more children as the worst thing about the menopause, compared with 26 who considered not knowing what to expect as the worst thing. Neugarten (54), in a further discussion of the menopause in relation to developmental psychology, concluded that the menopause itself was probably not important in understanding the problems of middle-aged women.

The influence of culturally-determined attitudes on the presentation of menopausal symptoms has been discussed by Flint (20). She presented the findings in a group of 483 women in India, stating that the only problems associated with the menopause in this group were menstrual cycle changes and none of the other symptoms of the menopausal syndrome were detected. She stated that when women achieved their menopause in this culture their quality of life improved in many ways, because they were no longer considered contaminative when they were not able to menstruate or bear children. She described various other cultures where the achievement of the menopause was associated with improvement in status or "reward," as opposed to Western culture where youth is good and aging is bad. She concluded that reaching the menopause is certainly not rewarded in Western society but punished with fall in status in family affairs as children become independent.

In a pilot study of 55 women and their attitude to the menopause, Maoz et al. (49) again found a cultural variation in that women of Oriental-Arab cultures who already had large families had a positive response to the menopause in terms of lack of desire for more children. Women of the other groups did not show this response to the same degree.

Although these studies have only explored some limited aspects of the environment, they indicate that many factors influence the development of symptoms in women in the years immediately before and following the menopause. It may be that the biological change of the menopause is one of the least important factors influencing the development of those emotional symptoms which have been included at times in the menopausal syndrome.

CONCLUSION

Since the menopause is such an easily identified biological event, it has been the focus of attention for many years and a multitude of unrelated symptoms have been attributed to its influence. There is now a substantial amount of evidence available to indicate that only the symptoms of hot flushes, excessive sweating, dyspareunia related to vaginal atrophy and possibly insomnia show a significant change in intensity and frequency at the time of cessation of menstrual periods when estrogen production falls sharply. These are, therefore, the symptoms which may respond to estrogen replacement therapy.

There is no evidence to suggest that the menopause is associated with any change in the prevalence or clinical features of major psychiatric illness and the concept of involutional melancholia as a separate diagnostic entity is no longer generally accepted.

The previous inclusion of various psychological symptoms in the menopausal syndrome probably arose because of the selection process involved in clinic attendance and the erroneous assumption that the clinic group was representative of the general population. There is no evidence of any significant rise in the prevalence of emotional disturbance at the time of cessation of menstrual periods, nor is there any evidence that estrogen preparations have any direct effect on emotional symptoms at this time. Some surveys have shown a slight increase in emotional disturbance in women in the years just prior to the cessation of menstrual periods, when menstrual irregularities are common, but the significance of this finding is not clear.

It has become increasingly obvious that emotional symptoms at this time of life, as at any other time, are influenced by a multitude of environmental and personal factors. One of the critical environmental issues is that of children achieving independence and leaving home. Cross-cultural studies have shown interesting variation in the frequency and severity of menopausal symptoms related to cultural attitudes toward aging and the status of post-menopausal women.

REFERENCES

1. ACHTE, K. (1970). Menopause from the psychiatrist's point of view. *Acta. Obstet. Gynec. Scand.*, *49*, Suppl. 1, 7-17.
2. BALLINGER, C. B. (1975). Psychiatric morbidity and the menopause: screening of general population sample. *British Medical Journal*, *3*, 344-6.

3. BALLINGER, C. B. (1976). Psychiatric morbidity and the menopause: clinical features. *British Medical Journal, 1,* 1183-5.
4. BALLINGER, C. B. (1976). Subjective sleep disturbance at the menopause. *Journal of Psychosomatic Research, 20,* 509-513.
5. BALLINGER, C. B. (1977). Psychiatric morbidity and the menopause: Survey of a gynaecological out-patient clinic. *British Journal of Psychiatry, 131,* 83-89.
6. BARNES, A. C. (1968). Climacteric. *Obstetrics and Gynaecology, 32,* 437-439.
7. BEARD, R. J. (1975). The Menopause. *British Journal of Hospital Medicine,* 631-637.
8. BECK, A. T., WARD, C. H., MENDELSON, M., MOCK, J. and ERBAUGH, J. (1961). An inventory for measuring depression. *Arch. General Psychiat., 4,* 561-571.
9. BENEDEK, T. (1950). Climacterium: A developmental phase. *Psychoanalytic Quarterly, 19,* 1-27.
10. CAMPBELL, S. (1976). Double blind psychometric studies on the effects of natural estrogens on post-menopausal women. In: Campbell, S. (ed.), *The Management of the Menopause and Post-menopausal Years.* England: M.T.P. Press, pp. 149-158.
11. CHAKRAVARTI, S., COLLINS, W. P., THOM, M. H., and STUDD, J. W. W. (1979). Relation between plasma hormone profiles, symptoms, and response to oestrogen treatment in women approaching the menopause. *British Medical Journal, 1,* 983-985.
12. COOPE, J., THOMSON, J. M. and POLLER, L. (1975). Effects of "natural oestrogen" replacement therapy on menopausal symptoms and blood clotting. *British Medical Journal, 4,* 139-143.
13. COPPEN, A. (1965). The prevalence of menstrual disorders in psychiatric patients. *British Journal of Psychiatry, 111,* 155-167.
14. DEUTSCH, H. (1945). *The Psychology of Women—*Vol. 2. New York: Grune and Stratton, pp. 456-487.
15. DEYKIN, E. Y., JACOBSON, S., KLERMAN, G. and SOLOMON, M. (1966). The Empty Nest: Psychosocial aspects of conflict between depressed women and their grown children. *American Journal of Psychiatry, 122,* 1422-1426.
16. DONOVAN, J. C. (1951). The menopausal syndrome: A study of case histories. *American Journal of Obstetrics and Gynecology, 62,* 1281-1291.
17. DRIFE, J. O. (1977). Advertising oestrogens. *Lancet, 1,* 746.
18. ENGLISH, O. S. (1954). Climacteric neuroses and their management. *Geriatrics, 9,* 139-145.
19. FESSLER, L. (1950). The psychopathology of climacteric depression. *Psychoanalytic Quarterly, 19,* 28-42.
20. FLINT, M. (1975). The menopause: Reward or punishment. *Psychosomatics, 16,* 161-163.
21. FOLDES, J. J. (1972). Psychosomatic approach to the menopausal syndrome. Treatment with Opipranol. In: Morris, N. (ed.), *Psychosomatic Medicine in Obstetrics and Gynaecology,* 3rd Int. Congr., London 1971. Basel: Karger, pp. 617-621.
22. FREUD, S. (1917). Mourning and Melancholia. In: *Collected Papers.* Vol. 4, 152-170. London: Hogarth Press 1956.
23. GOLDBERG, D. P. (1972). *The Detection of Psychiatric Illness by Questionnaire.* London: Oxford University Press.
24. HÄLLSTRÖM, T. (1973). *Mental Disorder and Sexuality in the Climacteric.* (Reports from Psychiatric Research Centre, St. Jörgen's Hospital, University of Göteborg, Sweden, 6.) Gothenburg: Scandinavian University Books.
25. HÄLLSTRÖM, T. (1977). Sexuality in the climacteric. *Clinics in Obstetrics and Gynaecology, 4,* 227-239.
26. HENDERSON, D. K. and GILLESPIE, R. D. (1956). *Textbook of Psychiatry* 8th edition. Revised by D. K. Henderson with the assistance of I. R. C. Batchelor. London: O.U.P.
27. HENDERSON, D. K. and GILLESPIE, R. D. (1969). *Textbook of Psychiatry,* 10th edition. Revised by I. R. C. Batchelor. London: O.U.P.

28. HOPKINSON, G. (1964). A genetic study of affective illness in patients over 50. *British Journal of Psychiatry*, *110*, 244-254.
29. HOSKINS, R. G. (1944). The psychological treatment of the menopause. *Journal of Clinical Endocrinology*, *4*, 605-610.
30. HUTTON, J. D., JACOBS, H. S., JAMES, V. H. T. and MURRAY, ,M. A. F. (1978). Relation between plasma oestrone and oestradiol and climacteric symptoms. *Lancet i*, 678-681.
31. JASZMANN, L., VAN LITH, N. D. and ZAAT, J. C. A. (1969). The perimenopausal symptoms: The statistical analysis of a survey. *Medical Gynaecology and Sociology*, *4*, 268-277.
32. JEFFCOATE, T. N. A. (1960). Drugs for menopausal symptoms. *British Medical Journal*, *1*, 340-342.
33. JONES, M. J., MARSHALL, D. H. and NORDIN, B. E. C.(1977). Quantitation of menopausal symptomatology and its response to ethinyl oestradiol and piperazine oestrone sulphate. *Curr. Med. Res. Opin.* *4*, Suppl. 3, 12-20.
34. KENDELL, R. E. (1968). *The classification of depressive illness*. Maudsley Monograph No. 18. London: Oxford Univ. Press 1968.
35. KERR, M. (1970). Amitriptyline in emotional states at the menopause. *New Zealand Med. J.*, *72*, 243-245.
36. KINSEY, A. C., POMEROY, W. B., MARTIN, C. E. and GEBHARD, P. H. (1953). *Sexual Behavior in the Human Female*. Philadelphia: Saunders.
37. KRAEPELIN, E. (1906). *Lectures on Clinical Psychiatry*. Revised & Edited by Johnstone, T. (Authorized translation from the Second German edition). Lecture 1—Introduction: Melancholia. London: Bailliere, Tindall and Cox.
38. KRAEPELIN, E. (1921). *Manic-Depressive Insanity and Paranoia*. Translated by Barclay, R. M., Edited by Robertson, G. M. Edinburgh: E. & S. Livingstone.
39. KUPPERMAN, H. S., WETCHLER, B. B. and BLATT, M. H. G. (1959). Contemporary therapy of the menopausal syndrome. *Journal of American Medical Association*, *171*, 1627-1637.
40. LEWIS, A. J. (1934). Melancholia: A historical review. *The Journal of Mental Science*, *80*, 1-42.
41. LOZMAN, H., BARLOW, A. L. and LEVITT, D. G. (1971). Piperazine estrone sulfate and conjugated estrogens equine in the treatment of the menopausal syndrome. *Southern Medical Journal*, *64*, 1143-1147.
42. McGHIE, A. and RUSSELL, S. M. (1962). The subjective assessment of normal sleep patterns. *The Journal of Mental Science*, *108*, 642-654.
43. McKINLAY, S. M. and JEFFERYS, M. (1974). The menopausal syndrome. *British Journal of Preventative and Social Medicine*, *28*, 108-115.
44. MALAMUD, W., SANDS, S. L. and MALAMUD, I. (1941). The involutional psychoses: A socio-psychiatric study. *Psychosomatic Medicine*, *3*, 410-426.
45. MALLESON, J. (1953). An endocrine factor in certain affective disorders. *Lancet*, *2*, 158-164.
46. MALLESON, J. (1956). Climacteric Stress: Its empirical management. *British Medical Journal*, *2*, 1422-1425.
47. MANNES, M. (1968). Of time and the woman. *Psychosomatics*, *9*, Suppl., pp. 8-11.
48. MAOZ, B., ANTONOVSKY, A., APTER, A., DATAN, N., HOCHBERG, J. and SALOMON, Y. (1978). The effect of outside work on menopausal women. *Maturitas*, *1*, 43-53.
49. MAOZ, B., DOWTY, N., ANTONOVSKY, A. and WIJSENBEEK, H. (1970). Female attitudes to menopause. *Social Psychiatry*, *5*, 35-40.
50. MASTERS, W. H. and JOHNSON, V. E. (1966). *Human Sexual Response*. Boston: Little, Brown.
51. MECHANIC, D. (1968). *Medical Sociology*. Chapter 4: The patient's perspective of his illness: The study of illness behaviour. pp. 115-157. New York: The Free Press.
52. MERSON, J. (1876). The climacteric period in relation to insanity. *The West Riding Lunatic*

Asylum Medical Reports. 6, 85-107.
53. MULLEY, G. and MITCHELL, J. R. A. (1976). Menopausal flushing: Does oestrogen therapy make sense? *Lancet, 1*, 1397-1399.
54. NEUGARTEN, B. L. (1968). Adult personality: Toward a psychology of the life cycle In: *Middle Age and Ageing*. Chicago and London: The University of Chicago Press, pp. 137-147.
55. NEUGARTEN, B. L. and KRAINES, R. J. (1965). "Menopausal symptoms" in women of various ages. *Psychosomatic Medicine, 27*, 266-273.
56. NEUGARTEN, B. L., WOOD, V., KRAINES, R. J. and LOOMIS, B. (1968). Women's attitudes toward the menopause. In: *Middle Age and Aging*. Chicago and London: The University of Chicago Press, pp. 195-200.
57. NIKULA-BAUMAN, L. (1971). Endocrinological studies on subjects with involutional melancholia. *Acta Psychiat. Scand.*, Suppl. 226.
58. NOVAK, E. R. (1954). The menopause. *The Journal of the American Medical Association, 156*, 575-578.
59. PALMER, H. D., HASTINGS, D. W. and SHERMAN, S. H. (1941). Therapy in involutional melancholia. *American Journal of Psychiatry, 97*, 1086-1115.
60. PFEIFFER, E., VERWOERDT, A. and DAVIS, G. C. (1972). Sexual behaviour in middle life. *American Journal of Psychiatry, 128*, 1262-1267.
61. PRADOS, M. (1967). Emotional factors in the climacterium of women. *Psychotherapy and Psychosomatics, 15*, 231-244.
62. PRATT, J. P. and THOMAS, W. L. (1937). The endocrine treatment of menopausal phenomena. *Journal of the American Medical Association, 109*, 1875-1877.
63. PRIEST, R. G. and CRISP, A. H. (1972). The menopause and its relationship with reported somatic experiences. In: Morris, N. (ed.), *Psychosomatic Medicine in Obstetrics and Gynaecology*, 3rd Int. Congr., London 1971. Basel: Karger, pp. 105-107.
64. RIPLEY, H. S., SHORR, E. and PAPANICOLAOU, G. N. (1940). The effect of treatment of depression in the menopause with estrogenic hormone. *American Journal of Psychiatry, 96*, 905-911.
65. ROGERS, J. (1956). The menopause. *New England Journal of Medicine, 265*, 697-703, 750-756.
66. ROSENTHAL, S. H. (1968). The involutional depressive syndrome. *American Journal of Psychiatry, 124*, Suppl., pp. 21-35.
67. SAINSBURY, P. (1960). Psychosomatic disorders and neurosis in outpatients attending a general hospital. *Journal of Psychosomatic Research, 4*, 261-273.
68. SCHNEIDER, H. (1979). Sociology and anthropology of the menopause. Work and symptomatology. In: Van keep, P.A., Greenblatt, R. B. and Serr, D. M., (eds.), *Female and Male Climacteric. Current Opinion 1978*. England: M.T.P. Press pp. 5-6.
69. SEVERNE, L. (1979). Sociology and anthropology of the menopause. Work and symptomatology. In: Van keep, P. A., Greenblatt, R. B. and Serr, D. M., (eds.), *Female and Male Climacteric. Current Opinion 1978*. England: M.T.P. Press pp. 5-6.
70. SHEFFERY, J. B., WILSON, T. A., and WALSH, J. C. (1969). Double-blind, cross-over study comparing chlordiazepoxide, conjugated estrogens, combined chlordiazepoxide and conjugated estrogens, and placebo in treatment of the menopause. *Med. Ann. D.C., 38*, 433-436.
71. SIMON, A. (1968). Emotional problems of women—The mature years and beyond. *Psychosomatics.*, Suppl., pp. 12-16.
72. SLATER, E. and ROTH, M. (1969). *Clinical Psychiatry*. London: Bailliere, Tindall and Cassell.
73. SMITH, W. G. (1971). Critical life-events and prevention strategies in mental health. *Archives of General Psychiatry, 25*, 103-109.
74. STENBÄCK, A. (1963). On involutional and middle age depressions. *Acta Psychiat. Scand.*, Suppl. 169. 14-32.

75. STENSTEDT, A. (1959). Involutional melancholia. *Acta Psychiatrica et Neurologica Scandinavica*. *34*, Suppl. 127.
76. STUDD, J. W. W., COLLINS, W. P., CHAKRAVARTI, S., NEWTON, J. R., ORAM, D. H. and PARSONS, A. (1977). Oestradiol and testosterone implants in the treatment of psychosexual problems in the postmenopausal woman. *British Journal of Obstetrics and Gynaecology*, *84*, 314-315.
77. TAIT, A. L., HARPER, J. and McCLATCHEY, W. T. (1957). Initial psychiatric illness in involutional women. 1. Clinical aspects. *The Journal of Mental Science*, *103*, 132-145.
78. THOMPSON, B., HART, S. A. and DURNO, D. (1973). Menopausal age and symptomatology in a general practice. *J. Biosoc. Sci.*, *5*, 71-82.
79. THOMSON, J. and OSWALD, I. (1977). Effect of oestrogen on the sleep, mood and anxiety of menopausal women. *British Medical Journal*, *2*, 1317-1319.
80. TILT, E. J. (1857). *The Change of Life in Health and Disease*. Second ed. London: John Churchill
81. UTIAN, W. H. (1972). The true clinical features of postmenopause and oophorectomy and their response to oestrogen therapy. *South African Medical Journal*, *46*, 732-737.
82. UTIAN, W. H. (1972). The mental tonic effect of oestrogens administered to oophorectomized females. *South African Medical Journal*, *46*, 1079-1082.
83. UTIAN W. H. (1976). Scientific basis for post-menopausal estrogen therapy: The management of specific symptoms and rationale for long-term replacement. In: Beard, R. J. (ed.), *The Menopause—A Guide to Current Research and Practice*. Lancaster England: M.T.P. Press Ltd pp. 175-201.
84. UTIAN, W. H. (1978). Plasma—oestrogens and climacteric symptoms. *Lancet, 1*, 1099-1100.
85. WANDLESS, I. (1979). Illness seen at menopause clinic. *British Medical Journal, 1*, 1356.
86. WERNER, A. A., JOHNS, G. A., HOCTOR, E. F., AULT, C. C., KOHLER, L. H. and WEIS, M. W. (1934). Involutional melancholia. Probable etiology and treatment. *Journal of the American Medical Association*, *103*, 13-16.
87. WHEATLEY, D. (1972). The use of psychotropic drugs in the female climacteric. In: Morris, N. (ed.) *Psychosomatic Medicine in Obstetrics and Gynaecology*, 3rd Int. Congr., London 1971. Basel: Karger pp. 612-616.
88. WILLIAMS, D. (1971). The menopause. *British Medical Journal*, *2*, 208-211.
89. WILSON, R. A. and WILSON, T. A. (1963). The fate of the nontreated postmenopausal woman: A plea for the maintenance of adequate estrogen from puberty to the grave. *Journal of the American Geriatrics Society*, *11*, 347-362.
90. WINOKUR, G. (1973). Depression in the menopause. *American Journal of Psychiatry*, *130*, 92-93.
91. WITTOSON, C. L. (1940). Involutional melancholia. *Psychiatric Quarterly*, *14*, 167-184.
92. ZEALLEY, A. K. and AITKEN, R. C. B (1969). Measurement of mood. *Proceedings of Royal Society of Medicine*, *62*, 993-996.

18

MALE CLIMACTERIC

FRED O. HENKER, III, M.D.

*Chief, Psychiatry Consultation/Liaison Service,
University of Arkansas for Medical Sciences, Little Rock*

INTRODUCTION

Among middle-aged men there occurs frequently a constellation of symptoms involving disturbances of mood, sexual inadequacy and vaguely defined physical complaints. This syndrome is roughly analogous to female menopause and is most appropriately designated male climacteric. It is subject to considerable controversy, being accepted enthusiastically by some and rejected by others, largely on the basis of failure to demonstrate an abrupt cessation of production of male sex hormones as occurs with estrogen in middle-aged women. Nevertheless, these men experience episodes of disability in the involutional period, not explained on the basis of ordinary demonstrable pathology, and with adequate supportive therapy can be restored to productive gratifying lives for a good many years yet to come.

DEFINITION

Male climacteric is the preferred term though male menopause has appeared in articles from time to time. The latter word is derived from roots denoting "cessation of monthly," and thus can only be applied appropriately to women. On the other hand, climacteric is dervied from a word for ladder, with the connotation of having reached the top with no way to go but down. It is general and thus equally appropriate for use in connection with either men or women. Standard medical dictionaries agree generally on the definition of climacteric as a period of life or a syndrome, occurring at the termination of the reproductive period, accompanying the normal diminution of sexual activity, or between the ages of 40 and 50, manifested by body changes including endocrine, somatic and psychic varieties, applicable to either male or female (3, 11). Another use is occasionally encountered in which the term refers to the late life change into senility (8). In this chapter it denotes a disorder among men at mid-life.

HISTORY

Male climacteric first appeared prominently in the medical literature in the 1930s, at which time it was considered to be a hormone deficiency disorder analogous to menopause in women. Werner, in 1939 (14), described it as a disorder encompassing endocrine dysfunction, autonomic imbalance and psychic disturbances beginning in men between the ages of 48 and 52. Various authors reported diverse symptoms. In 1944, Heller and Myers (5) published an elaborate classification of male climacteric symptoms in five categories: 1. vasomotor, including hot flashes, chills, sweats, palpitation, tachycardia and vascular headaches; 2. psychic, including depression, self-depreciation, crying, suicidal tendencies, insomnia, irritability and paresthesias; 3. sexual, comprising diminished libido and impotence; 4. constitutional, including weakness, fatigue, anorexia, nausea, constipation, weight loss, myalgia, arthralgia and cramps; and 5. urinary, comprising hesitancy, decreased size of stream and decreased force of stream. They confirmed the diagnosis of elevation of urinary gonadotropin produced as a result of the body's reduction in production of testosterone. Superimposed upon the insidious general physical decline noted more or less in all persons past the midpoint in life, various psychological, social and situational factors have been pointed out.

Stieglitz (13) wrote of a slowly developing mental and physical lassitude, determined by the patient's previous personality, leading to depression, reduced sexual potency and diminished libido. The sexual problems, he found, were often ushered in by a transient period of compensatory stimulation of sex drive. Bergler (2) described some middle-aged men as resolving their inner upheaval by retreating into hypochondriasis. Rutherford (12) proposed the perplexing effect of the wife's menopausal symptoms, along with other situational features, as productive of the husband's climacteric. During the last decade much more interest has been shown in the psychological and situational aspects of male climacteric and treatment has included more counseling and psychotherapy than hormone replacement.

MALE SEX HORMONE IN THE CLIMACTERIC

Since male climacteric was conceived of as a hormone deficiency disease, simple testosterone replacement was at first offered as the treatment of choice. In 1945, Werner reported a series of 54 cases successfully treated by means of thrice weekly injections of testosterone (14); the following year he reported impressive results with 273 cases similarly treated (15). In the 1960s, the trend changed to indirect stimulation of gonadal activity by means of weekly injections of chorionic gonadotropin fortified with thiamine and glutamic acid. In 1962, Lindsay reported good results in 70% of 46 men treated with this regimen (7).

Even as the glowing reports of treatment success with hormone injections were appearing in medical literature, a number of papers disputing these findings began to be published. Bauer, in 1944 (1), called the term male climacteric a misnomer, expressing the position that a whole gamut of asthenic and neurotic conditions had been included on insufficient foundation and that response to testosterone shots was likely due to psychologic effect. In 1946, McCullagh (10) took a similar position, pointing out that specific loss of power of production of hormone and sperm by the testes has not been shown to be associated with any period in a man's life span and that impotence was rarely due to testicular failure. In agreement with this stand, Wershub (16), through a study of biopsy and autopsy specimens of testes of elderly men, found them surprisingly normal, and Kent and Acone (6) demonstrated plasma testosterone levels in a group of 68 men between the ages of 20 and 93 to be relatively constant through the eighth decade of life. Thus, in the light of these observations, it became difficult, or even impossible, to reconcile the mid-life constellation of symptoms with an abrupt decline in androgen production. Some reduction in hormone through gradual decline in production could be a contributory factor to these symptoms, but not the total cause.

SYMPTOMS

The diagnosis of male climacteric is made on the basis of history, with the most characteristic feature being onset of disability, within a period of days to weeks, in a previously healthy productive man between the ages of 45 and 60. Otherwise, specific symptoms vary from patient to patient but generally fall into three categories: emotional, physical and sexual. Though all of the symptoms discussed below are not present in all male climacteric patients, most show some disturbances in each of the three categories.

Emotional symptoms include variable degrees of depression, from somber or morose mood with attendant hopelessness, self-depreciation and indecisiveness to depressive withdrawal, variable anxiety and occasional irritability or hostility. The insidiously developing organic brain impairment present to some extent in all middle-aged persons is sufficiently pronounced in a few to lend a quality of lability to the emotion being experienced, thus giving rise to occasional panic episodes, outbursts of rage or crying spells.

In the physical realm are such largely subjective complaints as malaise, lassitude, weakness, easy fatigability, lethargy and poorly defined pain or hypochondriasis. Hot flashes have been reported but are extremely rare (4). These symptoms are seen in the absence of other pathogenic processes which would give rise to them; however, it is conceivable that a patient with some other disease could also develop male climacteric syndrome.

Sexual disturbances include reduction or loss of libido, inadequate erection due to sluggishness, incompleteness or transience, and impotence ranging from occasional to total.

INCIDENCE

The incidence of male climacteric is not exact. Some practitioners diagnose it frequently while others never see it. All men experience some degree of general physical slowing down after mid-life and it is only natural that they feel some regret as they sense that more life is now behind them than ahead. A few become significantly disabled. Actually, men in the climacteric period may be considered as falling on a continuum from the well-compensated, minimally symptomatic individuals to the grossly impaired ones who would be appropriately given some psychotic diagnosis such as involutional melancholia. From some arbitrary point below the minimally symptomatic to another arbitrary point at which the psychotic diagnosis would be applied we have a segment comprising male climacteric. About 5% of the middle-aged male population manifest some degree of troublesome climacteric symptoms, with less than 1% becoming seriously disabled. The incidence would be higher were it not for our cultural belief that men must be strong and not complain, other than about life-threatening disturbances.

PATHOGENESIS

Male climacteric is due to a kaliedoscopic interaction of elements of three categories of dynamic factors: physical slowing down, organic brain impairment and sociocultural aspects of aging. Each influences and is influenced by the other. Sometime around the forties the human body begins a gradual decline. Universally the peak has been reached, growth has stopped, youthful vigor has plateaued or decreased and early signs of deterioration begin to appear. Arteriosclerosis has been developing since the thirties. Testosterone production continues but at a gradually decreasing rate. Temporary or permanent arthritis appears with increasing frequency. Fat deposits mar the previously lithe physique. Assorted latent processes become progressively more evident.

All of this occurs in a sociocultural environment which requires ever more from the individual. Men are expected to show strength, be competitive and manifest virility. Youthful attributes are revered while signs of age tend to be abhorred. Sooner or later the man at middle age begins to take stock of his life. What accomplishments he had hoped for have largely been gained—or the opportunity has now been lost; younger individuals are likely vying for his occupational position; his children challenge his authority. Ahead he sees the inevitable progression of the downward trend. Thus we have physical, psychological and sociocultural factors operating simultaneously in varying proportions; when the sum total of disruptive forces exceeds adaptive reserve, male climacteric syndrome is precipitated.

The insidious physical slowing down is quite logically productive of malaise, lassitude, easy fatigability and vague discomfort, which may yield hypochondriacal thinking. All of these symptoms become especially prominent when amplified by anxiety, lowered mood and attendant fears and feelings of hopelessness, which are products of the patient's reaction to recognition that his sexual attractiveness is deteriorating, that his domestic and occupational superiority is being threatened and that he is headed toward old age, the period spurned by his culture, with no escape but death. These feelings are then accentuated by the loss of well-being associated with the physical slowing down.

A particularly important sector in this general physical decline lies in the brain. Here gradually increasing cerebral arteriosclerosis and varied amounts of assorted other physical insults are beginning to have their effect on the neurones, producing some degree of organic brain syndrome with attendant compromise of adaptive reserve. In addition to the minute but increasing limitation of intellectual functions, we have emotional lability, which may influence emotional expression, leading to occasional panic episodes, crying spells or outbursts of rage. Another effect of organic brain syndrome is the release and accentuation of the basic, previously suppressed, personality. This allows latent traits to become manifest, occasionally in troublesome proportion.

All of these processes are interrelated with each other and with sexual activity. The latter, being a pleasurable process closely attuned to optimal life adjustment, is adversely affected by the general physical slowing down, with its decrease in stamina and loss of overall feeling of well-being, as well as by whatever degree of reduction in male hormone production may be present. Though the hormone supply is rarely depleted enough through natural means to cause sexual inadequacy in this period of life, the gradual decline may be added to other disruptive factors, such as worry, self-depreciation, anxiety and depression, to an extent sufficient to compromise or overshadow the sex drive. Furthermore, panic precipitated by an otherwise isolated sexual failure may produce inhibition persisting months, years or even the rest of the lifetime. Another unfortunate consequence of sexual frustration, coupled with the impaired judgment associated with organic brain impairment, not infrequently affecting climacteric men, is a frenzied search for relief through finding different partners. Although temporary improvement may be obtained, the damages in the form of hurt, divorce, loss of faithful partners, and guilt more often than not outweigh the gains.

The general processes have now been described; however, there is often something more, a precipitating incident, which triggers the disabling process. The following crises, characteristic of mid-life, are often associated with male climacteric:

1. Death, severe illness or menopause of wife. Though outwardly independent, men are often very dependent on their wives and loss of this security produces disturbing feelings of weakness and vulnerability.
2. Business reversal. Most men have great emotional investment in their work so that a loss in this realm represents a great wound to self-esteem.
3. Retirement. Though superficially seen as a time of joy, retirement represents an end to usefulness and control and thus a wound to self-esteem.
4. Children leaving home. When the children go, the man sees the need for him lessened and is confronted with the fact that he is growing old.
5. Serious illness. This destroys the illusion of permanence and also inflicts frustrating handicaps.
6. Death of parents. The man can no longer look up to a higher level; full responsibility rests upon him. It also presages his own demise.

These crises, singly or in combination, occur when coping mechanisms are beginning to be depleted. Thus there are chances of the man's being overwhelmed and experiencing disorganization—male climacteric.

THERAPY

Since the causes of male climacteric are multifaceted, we can only combat it realistically by means of a combined approach. Hormone therapy, psychopharmacology, counseling and psychotherapy all have their places. In the very rare cases in which laboratory determinations reveal clinically low levels of testosterone (normal range, 300-800 ng/dl), replacement therapy is justifiable. Oral buccal tablets and injectable forms are available. Unfortunately, recent results have not have been as glowing as those reported during the 1940s. Physical symptoms improve but depression and anxiety often remain. Thus, there is seldom realistic indication for male sex hormones.

On the other hand, emotional disturbances are prevalent and call for judicious use of psychotropic drugs on a symptomatic basis, even though many emotional problems can be handled through person-to-person conversation. The tricyclic antidepressants are adequate for most depressive symptoms. The more sedating ones, such as doxepin, are better where there is an element of agitation, while suppressed patients seem to respond to the less sedating varieties, such as imipramine. The anxious patient is best treated with a minor tranquilizer like chlordiazepoxide, meprobamate or diazepam, using the smallest dose that will allow reasonable comfort in order not to suppress constructive striving. Due to the propensity for psychological dependency, these drugs should be changed if used longer than a few weeks. The tranquilizer-antidepressant combination preparations enjoy some popularity now in treatment of these cases, but a good many clinicians still prefer the versatility of separate prescriptions.

After emotional reactions have been brought under control, psychotherapy is largely directed at enhancing the use of existing assets in order to return the patient to effective life adjustment. First he must be supported in developing a philosophical view of life which encompasses standards and expectations in harmony with realistic limitations and remaining assets. Conservative reassurance and ventilation are most beneficial and easily within the reach of any family practitioner. These measures reduce the inhibitory effect of doubts, fears and insecurities upon the exercise of adjustment potential. Prestige suggestion, or contact with a benevolent professional, is amazingly beneficial, regardless of what other treatment approach is being used. Direct counseling is indicated in dealing with specific occupational, domestic and community problems. The soonest possible return to a standard daily routine and gainful occupation is best. There is little excuse for: "You've had some tough breaks, you need a nice long rest."

Physical complaints require delicate handling. Though mostly of hypo-chondriacal nature, they may include evidence of coexisting organic pa-thology, which is increasingly common in this age group. Thus, care must be taken to avoid reinforcement of hypochondriasis while concurrently main-taining an inconspicuous watch for serious signs. Phsyical complaints should be received sincerely, evaluated and then deemphasized as tactfully as pos-sible, with attempts at focusing on existing assets, diversion into interesting activity or support in living with physical symptoms. Symptomatic drugs should be used as little as possible lest they strengthen the belief that dangerous pathology exists. When disruptive attitudes and unpleasant emo-tions are relieved, the somatic preoccupation often subsides spontaneously.

Sexual problems can be treated almost exclusively with psychological ther-apy. Since hormone depletion has been shown to have little effect in male climacteric, testosterone preparations are rarely indicated; where they are employed, the response is often due more to suggestion than to physiological effect. Stopping inhibitory drugs and providing reassurance are often enough to relieve the problem. With more resistant cases, conjoint counseling in-volving the patient and his partner is employed. Here a thorough history and examination are performed to disclose any specific defects and then a no demand sensate focus program, as described by Masters and Johnson (9), is initiated, with gradually increasing intensity over a period of weeks, until realistic sexual satisfaction is achieved.

PROGNOSIS

Since male climacteric is not a life-threatening disease, prognosis for life is good. On the other hand, since it is associated with early physical decline, return to life as it was at its prime is unlikely. The more generously endowed the premorbid personality, the more adequate the current situation and the earlier the beginning of therapy, the greater is the chance for return to productive enjoyable life. Conversely, the more detrimental the current situation and the less the interest in therapy, the more likely is the patient to continue in some degree of maladaptation.

REFERENCES

1. BAUER, J. (1944). The male climacteric, a misnomer. *J.A.M.A.*, *126*, 914.
2. BERGLER, E. (1956). The old man act of the middle aged man. *Dis. Nerv. Sys.*, *17*, 230.

3. DORLAND. (1974). *Dorland's Illustrated Medical Dictionary, 25th Ed.* Philadephia: W. B. Saunders Co. 327.
4. FELDMAN, J. M. (1976). Hot flashes and sweats in men. *Arch. Int. Med., 136*, 606.
5. HELLER, C. G. and MYERS, G. B. (1944). The male climacteric—its symptomatology, diagnosis and treatment. *J.A.M.A., 126*, 472.
6. KENT, J. R. and ACONE, A. B. (1966). Plasma testosterone levels and aging in males. *Proc. Symp. Steroid Hormones, 2nd Ed.* Ghent. 31.
7. LINDSAY, H. B. (1962). The male and female climacteric. *Dis. Nerv. Syst., 23*, 149.
8. LIVESLEY, B. (1977). The climacteric disease. *J. Am. Geriatric Soc., 25*, 162.
9. MASTERS, W. H. and JOHNSON, V. (1970). *Human Sexual Inadequacy.* Boston: Little, Brown,.
10. McCULLAGH, E. P. (1946). Climacteric: Male and Female. *Bull. Chgo. Med. Scy., 49*, 193.
11. OSOL, A. ed. (1972) *Blakiston's Gould Medical Dictionary, 3rd Ed.* New York: McGraw-Hill.
12. RUTHERFORD, R. N. (1971). The male and female climacteric. *Postgrad. Med., 50,*125.
13. STIEGLITZ, E. J. (1946). *The Second Forty Years.* Philadelphia: Lippincott.
14. WERNER, A. A. (1939). The male climacteric, report of 54 cases. *J.A.M.A., 127,*705.
15. WERNER, A.A. (1946). The male climacteric, report of 273 cases. *J.A.M.A., 132*, 188.
16. WERSHUB, L. P. (1962). *The Human Testis: A Clinical Treatise.* Springfield: Charles C Thomas.

19

THE BATTERED PARENT AND SOCIAL AND EMOTIONAL STRESSES ON PARENTS

SELWYN O. JUTER, M.D.

Attending Psychiatrist,
Northern Westchester Hospital Center
Mount Kisco, New York

INTRODUCTION

Over the past decade there has been a flood of literature about the battered or abused child (22). More recently, with the rise of feminism and women's rights, there has been a new wave of publications on the battered spouse (15). Finally, we are coming the full cycle of family violence with the realization that parents can also be battered, abused and victimized by their children. The professional literature has traditionally focused on parents and bad parenting as being a major factor in the causation of mental illness. However, clinicians are becoming more aware of a battered-parent syndrome (9). More and more parents are unable to cope with their youngsters. Parents, operating from their own background and knowledge and from current popular psychological mystique regarding child-rearing, often find themselves as much the victims, as the perpetrators, of childhood disorders. The old adage, "there are no problem children, only problem parents," must be reviewed in the light of today's familial, social and cultural trends.

The concept of battered parents refers to the physical and emotional battering of parents within a family, as well as the battering of parents by social forces. The battering can be *direct* or *indirect*. Direct battering can take the form of actual physical assault on parents, verbal abuse, or verbal and nonverbal threats of physical harm. The extreme form of physical abuse

313

towards parents is parricide, i.e., parental murder (22). Indirect battering can be seen in the form of parental neglect, particularly in the case of helpless and dependent elderly parents who have been left uncared for (19), or the psychosocial battering that takes place as the result of various cultural forces. This chapter will attempt to review and discuss these various areas of parent battering in the physical, psychological and social arenas.

PHYSICAL BATTERING OF PARENTS

Literature Review

Despite a recent surge of literature on family violence and conflict, the published data on physical abuse of parents remains extremely sparse (5, 14, 18, 21). A recent library computer search on parent battering through the psychiatric, psychological and sociological literature found few articles concerned with the use of physical force or violence by children towards parents (8, 18). While the published literature on child and spouse abuse is extensive, and research on family conflict and violence is growing (14, 18, 20, 21), the focus has mainly been on the battering of children, siblings, wives, and, more recently, even husbands. Only minimal and indirect references are made about parental abuse.

The first pilot case study of actual assaultive behavior of children towards parents was published in 1979 by Harbin and Madden in the *American Journal of Psychiatry* (9). Steinmetz (19) also recently described a syndrome in which adults neglect and abuse elderly parents who are in a helpless and dependent position on them. The problems of family violence and aggressive behavior between family members have been extensively explored by Steinmetz and Strauss (20). They assert that family life, far from being harmonious, is commonly a source of violent conflict, with the frequent use of physical force between members. Thus, the present literature on battered parents reflects only the "tip of an iceberg" as far as the general subject is concerned. In contrast, the literature on the sociological effects of parent battering and consequent effects on parenting is extensive (4).

Incidence

Due to the lack of statistics, the incidence of assaultive behavior towards parents remains unknown. A comprehensive sociological survey of family violence by Strauss and associates (21) cites the frequency of attacks on parents by children between the ages of three and 18 to be almost 10%. In an unpublished pilot study of middle and high school students, between the ages of 10 and 18, I found the incidence to be closer to 3-4%. Part of the difficulty in establishing incidence lies in the lack of consensus among professionals about what constitutes assaultive behavior. There is some confusion between the use of the term *force*, which is sanctioned by society, and *violence*, which is seen as unacceptable. Goode (5) suggests that "force is the legitimate physical control to effect a positive goal. Violence, however, is the unsanctioned use of physical force that does not have normative legitimization." There is controversy as to whether the definition should be narrow or broad. Does the throwing of a single blow constitute assault or is physical harm or injuries required? A further problem in obtaining good statistics lies in the fact that parents and families are reluctant to reveal incidents of family violence. Parents are particularly loathe to report assaultive behavior toward themselves by their offspring because of feelings of guilt and shame. Also, in reporting such incidents, some parents may fear that they will have to reveal abusive behavior toward their children.

Clinical Data

A recent review of 13 cases of adolescents with histories of parent assault, hospitalized in an acute psychiatric unit of a community general hospital, revealed the following diagnostic breakdown: acute schizophrenic or psychotic reactions—2; adolescent depressive reactions—3, organic brain syndrome with borderline mental retardation secondary to early cerebral palsy—1; alcohol abuse—1; adjustment reaction of adolescence—6. The precipitating reasons for hospitalization were 1. depression with suicidal ideation or attempt; 2. impulsive angry eruptions; 3. behavioral difficulties involving management problems at home or at school; and 4. drug or alcohol abuse.

In all cases there was a history of severe family disturbance. While drug and alcohol abuse was cited as a diagnosis in only one case, there was a history of usage in a majority of cases. An interesting finding was that at least four patients and possibly five showed histories of minimal brain dysfunction. This may account for the poor impulse control and frustration tolerance exhibited by many of the youths. The great majority of these adolescents also had histories of aggressive, antisocial behavior toward others.

A similar survey of 15 adolescents and pre-adolescents with history of physical and verbal parent abuse, drawn from a high and junior high school guidance department, revealed a somewhat different clinical sample. Few of these individuals showed a pattern of violent behavior outside the home setting. Many of these youths tended to be shy and diffident, with poor relationships. The diagnostic picture was frequently unclear from the interview with the adolescent alone. The adolescent had to be seen both individually and with the family in order to clarify his/her functioning capacity.

While the diagnostic term "adjustment reaction of adolescence" is frequently used for adolescent pathology, closer examination of these abusive adolescents, both from the hospitalized sample and from the school sample, showed their personality organization to conform to the diagnostic group termed borderline states. All these persons had in common: 1. weak object relations with a lack of affectional bonds; 2. angry eruptive behavior; 3. lack of consistent self-identity; 4. depressions characterized by loneliness rather than guilt or shame. In addition, they showed the classic object splitting, the inability to integrate love and hate, and primary narcissism of the borderline patient (12, 13). Kernberg (12) states that the borderline person has excessive development of aggressive drives, low tolerance for anxiety and a lack of primary autonomy, characteristics commonly found in these youths.

Family Observations

Many of the findings of the above two samplings correspond to the family data of Harbin and Madden (9). The majority of children who abuse their parents are in the 10-20 age group. The families are in the most cases severely disturbed and show a major degree of family disorganization. Frequently, the parents are divorced. Quite frequently, the abusive behavior occurs in the period just prior to a marital breakup, when the family is under severe stress. Much of family violence occurs when a family is being severely stressed and the coping mechanisms are disturbed or defective. The assaults or threats normally occur at home. In most cases, the abusive youths are living with the parents and dependent on them. The majority of violent adolescents are male, but females have also been involved. The family violence may be a singular impulsive episode or a habitual form of family response. Attacks range from verbal threatening and abusive behavior to destructive outbreaks to property and serious physical attacks on one or both parents. The attacks on parents frequently evolve out of a disagreement or power struggle between parent and child which often involves limit-setting. Most of the attacks reported in these studies occur when the youths are not under the influence of alcohol or drugs.

Family Dynamics

Family conflict

Family life is an inherent source of conflict among members. In their books about violence in the American family, Steinmetz and Strauss attempt to debunk the myth of family non-violence (18, 20). Their statistics portray the family as a battleground of competing power struggles among members, resulting in various degrees of assertive, aggressive and assaultive behavior.

Power struggles between parent and child appear to be the basis of parent-child conflict. With younger children, parents tend to use physical punishment and restrictions of privileges in exerting control. With the adolescent the power struggle tends to become verbal. Adolescents tend to express indpendence in the form of questioning authority, but not necessarily disobeying it. In certain families, however, the verbal struggle can escalate to defiance and verbally insulting behavior, and finally explode into physical violence.

What leads certain children to act out their rage or frustration in a physical way remains the essential question. The use of assaultive behavior towards parents is an expression of the final breakdown of parental authority, and the ultimate violation of deep-seated intrapsychic taboos and restraints.

Hierarchy

Harbin and Madden (9) suggest certain characteristics that seem to render a family susceptible to parent-battering. Among the most common disturbance they cite is a significant disruption in the family hierarchy. In such families the parents feel that the youngsters are in charge. The physical attacks and threats in these families may be an attempt by the adolescent to control the family and replace the ineffective parents. The teenager may want to punish the parents for having exploited him either through permissiveness and lack of leadership or inadequate parenting.

Erosion of parental authority

Conversely, many authorities feel that there has been an erosion and undermining of parental authority due to all kinds of sociocultural changes. Rapid changes in society have "battered" parents, leaving them confused and unsure of themselves. One of these forces is the isolation of the nuclear family due to social and geographic mobility, with the lack of traditional supports from community and generational authority. The emphasis on youth, the neglect of the aged, and generalized lack of respect for authority, both institutional and individual, have had an effect.

The use of libidinal language

An interesting correlation was noticed among the surveyed groups between the occurrence of violent behavior and the usage of pejorative obscene language even in everyday conversation. The frequent use of four-letter swear words (fuck) and other obscene terms usually referring to bodily anatomy, as well as sexual and anal functions, was apparent in the language of both parents and children in these families. While the adolescents tended to use these swear words commonly, in their normal speech, the parents resorted to these terms when frustrated, enraged, or in verbal battles. Sometimes these terms were exchanged between spouses in arguments. One may speculate that the common usage of highly charged terms with "libidinal cathexis," involving sexual and aggressive drive derivatives, must weaken normal taboos and restraints in these families, breaking down inhibitions to acting-out behavior and violence.

Separation

Issues of separation are also important determinants in the occurrence of parent-battering. Separation is one of the normal developmental tasks of adolescence. Traditionally, with the rise of sexual drives in puberty, the adolescent has used his/her sexuality in the development of new heterosexual relations as a way of separating and distancing from the parents. With the rise of peer pressures, the advocacy of equal rights for children, and the increased exposure to cultural violence, especially through television, aggressive, defiant and sometimes assaultive behavior has become more acceptable for many teenagers as a way of expressing their independence.

Reactive battering of parents

Some parent-battering must be considered reactive in nature. The perpetrators of this kind of assault have experienced chronic hatred for a parent they have attacked. The parent in these cases is frequently a sadistic figure with a history of cruel behavior to the child, his siblings or the spouse. The assault is often deliberate, goal-directive and in a sense adaptive. The child who commits this kind of reactive assault is often healthier than other assaultive children. These violent episodes occur because the child is sufficiently autonomous to carry out the assault, but yet too dependent to break away from the parental tyranny or cruelty.

EMOTIONAL FACTORS—STRESS IN PARENTING

The Existential Nature of Stress in Parenthood

Stress is a natural phenomenon, authentic and primary, of parenthood. Traditional psychiatric theory frequently viewed stress and guilt in parenthood as neurotic, usually the result of some maladaptive factors in marriage and family life. When a parent was experiencing distress, it was frequently concluded that he or she was doing something wrong. It is only now being recognized that stress in parenting is perhaps not a sign of pathology or even ignorance, but an inevitable aspect of that state. The resistance to recognizing that parents can be quite normally stressed in their relationship to their children is due to many reasons. One reason is that we all have a strong need to believe in the omnipotent ideal parent—a parent who can gratify all our needs and wishes. According to Freud, this libidinal wish has become sublimated to a belief in God. Another reason is our expectation that parenthood should be smooth and uncomplicated and the family a harmonious state.

There is a tendency in our culture to assume that parenthood should be gratifying and pleasurable, and to de-emphasize the deprivations and restrictions. However, the stresses of parenting exert enormous regressive pressures on parents, re-awakening in them repressed childhood frustrations and deprivations. Parents constantly struggle against this tendency to regress, but frequently find themselves behaving "like children" toward their offspring. Thus parenthood becomes a state of growth and maturational crises, producing stress, just like earlier developmental phases in their lives.

Loneliness

Parents, especially mothers, commonly experience loneliness when their children are in infancy and very young. This feeling of loneliness is frequently aggravated in today's society by the separation of young mothers from their extended families, friends, and communities. The young mother feels disconnected from supportive networks, especially parents and grandparents, which can offer encouragement and reassurance.

Frustration and isolation

Another stress is the enormous frustration felt by a young mother who must spend endless hours interacting with a child who cannot talk or respond to her on any kind of level which is mutually satisfying. She feels further isolated by the restrictions of freedom imposed upon her by her infant and feels cut off from friends, families and neighbors. Some mothers complain of being isolated from the world around them, experiencing a feeling of being hemmed or shut in by their infants, without the option of moving away for even minimal periods of time. Absent fathers who work long hours or travel extensively further contribute to this sense of loneliness and isolation.

Doubt, uncertainty and guilt

Today's parents often express doubt and uncertainty about whether they are doing the right thing. Mothers and fathers in today's "how to cope" culture agonize about how to manage their children. Social changes have increased the options for parents, at the same time that societal and familial supports have faded. This has led to an increase in choices and consequent anxiety for parents.

Associated with the feelings of inadequacy is a strong sense of guilt experienced by many parents. The preoccupation which parents have with thoughts that they have harmed their children on the one hand or not given them certain advantages or opportunities on the other hand is a constant source of stress. There is the anxiety at every stage of their children's development as to how best to handle various situations or to respond to various developmental and maturational crises.

Anger and rage

Anger and rage are frequently experienced in situations where there is a loss of control and can cause great distress. The parents feel angry at themselves for losing control and at the child for causing them to lose control. Every parent has experienced a "no win situation." This usually stems from a power struggle with a child which escalates and deteriorates, no matter what the course of action, resulting in further bad feelings. With older children and adolescents, where parents feel unable to control or influence the behavior of their offspring, the sense of impotence can be transformed to rage. This rage can lead to further self-remorse. Many parents experience enormous lowering of self-esteem due to the feeling that they have lost control and do not know what to do. This anger and rage can be so disruptive to the psyche of parents that it can lead to a breakdown of normal restraints and control, with resulting acting-out behavior. Child abuse is the most extreme expression of this rage. Despite the enormous publicity on this subject, the number of parents who carry out this kind of aggression towards their children remains relatively small.

The capacity to intrude

In the interpersonal sphere, children have the capacity to intrude into or interrupt any experience the parents may want to have alone or together. Parents commonly complain that they never have a moment for themselves or any privacy. If a parent, particularly with young children, wants to read a book, listen to a record, have a conversation, or enjoy any kind of inner experience, the intrusion of a child from minute to minute creates a continuing sense of being interrupted at all times. This feeling of not having any "space" for oneself creates the intrapsychic experience of being "intruded into."

Splitting the parents

The capacity of a child to split and create divisions between parents begins at a very early age. The crying infant and later the intrusive child can effectively impair the parents' sexual life. Very young children learn to play parents against each other. Resentment between spouses can arise out of conflicts over children and competitive rivalry for attention within the family. The breaking apart of the parental alliance can lead to marital strife and divorce.

Vicarious identification and competitiveness

Disruptive feelings of competitiveness and envy can be stirred up in parents. The envy can be directed at opportunities and advantages enjoyed by one's children, but denied or unavailable to the parent when growing up. Or this competitiveness can be expressed through measuring of oneself through the achievement and performance of one's children, because of an unhealthy and vicarious identification with a child. The realization that one may be overreacting to a child's experience because one is reliving a frustration from childhood can in and of itself be stressful to a parent.

Anxiety about future and separation

Finally, there is anxiety and concern about the future. It is natural for parents to be worried about how their offspring will turn out when they grow up and mature. With teenagers and young adults, the question of the child's education, occupation, career and marriage are anxiety-provoking and ommipresent. With separation comes the feeling that the family which one has so painfully put together, and for which one has suffered so many trials and tribulations, is coming to an end.

SOCIETAL FACTORS

Parents are being battered by many forces in our society—social, economic, cultural and traditional.

Rapid Changes in Society

In a culture of rapidly shifting values, parents feel increasingly confused about their role as parents. Illustrating this dilemma of the modern parent, a young father is quoted as saying, "When I was a young boy, *my parents* were angry at me for not being what I should be. Now my children are angry at me for not being what *they* think I should be." The semi-humorous expression, "Insanity is inherited—you inherit it from your children," poignantly emphasizes this point. Thus, the present-day parent feels buffeted from forces on two sides. Battered for the first time by forces and expectations rooted in the past, the parent must now contend with a young generation often in open hostility, rejection and defiance. The parent feels alienated from his past, confused about his role in the present, and rejected by his children. What has struck me most in my clinical work is that, while paper after paper has been written about the value crises (10, 11) and identity problems of youth in a changing society, the parent has been invariably cast as the culprit or the responsible party. Yet time after time the clinical picture is that of confused parents trying to do their best for their children, making sacrifices, but finding themselves overwhelmed, unable to cope, helpless and guilt-ridden.

Increasing Isolation of Nuclear Families

Increased social and geographic mobility has alienated the nuclear family from the extended family, past generations, neighbors, and communities with their traditional values.

The American nuclear family of today is physically and psychologically isolated and therefore devoid of restraining influences. There are no aunts, uncles, or grandparents to interfere or assist in day-to-day living. There is a lack of close-knit ties with the supportive social networks provided by more traditional societies. A consensus viewpoint or value system extending from and reinforced by the church, extended families, and communities no longer exists. Instead we have new communities composed of individuals of varying backgrounds, goals and attitudes.

Peer Pressure and Children's Rights

Today's cultural emphasis on youthful values, with the corresponding neglect of the aged, has contributed to a generalized lack of respect and disregard for authority. The advocacy of children's rights has caused children to expect to be treated as adults, but without adult responsibilities. The philosophy behind some parent education groups is that children are people with equal rights who must be treated with the same respect as adults. The problem is that children, while being mindful of their rights, have to be taught that they also have to be considerate of the rights of their parents, and exercise similar responsibilities and restraints. While parental authority and influence have waned, youth peer groups appear to have strong cohesive bonds. These bonds and strong peer pressures tend to reinforce the values, goals and attitudes of the peer groups, which may not reflect the attitudes of individual parents.

The Mental Health Profession and Child-Rearing

More and more parents are being influenced by popular psychological notions of child-rearing and lean increasingly on child professionals to guide them in the care of their children. Parents have been persuaded that managing children is understood only by professionals, child psychiatrists, psychologists, pediatricians, social workers, etc. Consequently, they feel anxious and guilty when they do not know the "right" way to handle their children's problems. The popular media and many professionals writing child-care books contribute to these feelings by suggesting that parents can raise happy, healthy children simply by following the latest formula. Moreover, they seem to blame the parents whenever things go awry.

The Dilemma of Parenthood

All of these factors have caused parents to be persuaded that there is a right or wrong way for rearing children. However, this is incorrect. Parents are not solely responsible for their children's personality development. Many social and environmental factors beyond the control of the parents also affect the child. The corollary of this statement is that all problems developed by a child are not the sole result of parenting. The G.A.P. (7) issue on the *Joys and Sorrows of Parenthood* talks about the true dilemma theory of parenthood. This is described as the situation where there is no absolute right or wrong way to child-rearing. No matter how much a parent tries, the child may or may not turn out with problems. While we do have choices, *we have no way of controlling the results or consequences of our choices.* This must also be seen in terms of existential philosophy, where Jean Paul Sartre speaks of freedom of choice, but also of our inability to control the consequences of these choices. Furthermore, our psychiatric theories cannot accurately explain why certain children develop problems while others do not. Our current concepts lack specificity or predictability. Psychiatric theories are for the most part retrospective and reconstructive. What determines a chain of events to be linked together to cause a symptom or problem is not yet explained by our current status of ego-psychology. We, as yet, cannot determine why certain events are linked in a chain when the vicissitudes and permeations or possibilities are infinite.

The Problems of Self-Actualization

Another aspect of this dilemma is the conflict parents are experiencing in gratifying their own needs versus gratifying the needs of their children. In recent times increasing emphasis has been placed on the importance of gratifying one's own needs. Cultural factors and personal growth movements have led to an emphasis on the need of the individual to develop his full potential. The rise of feminine awareness has made women question their role as mothers and caused more and more women to seek an identification for themselves outside the role of marriage and parenthood. Family life and rearing children have been de-emphasized as a source of self-esteem.

Recent Social Developments

There are many recent social developments which have profoundly affected family life.

Future shock

What are the effects of rapid change on our value systems and personality? Toffler (2, 23) has coined the term "future shock," meaning that the future is moving in on us so rapidly we are unable to make adequate adjustments. This rapid change causes a fragmentation of the personality, leading to what Toffler calls the modular man. There is also a detrimental effect on our social institutions and personality development. A confusional breakdown syndrome is the result. To what extent, Toffler asks, is abnormal behavior produced by the stresses of high speed change? How much new experience can individuals handle? This is all highly relevant to the present stress on parenthood. It would seem that younger people are more able to cope with change than their parents, who are still rooted in the past.

The generation gap

Until recently the concept of the generation gap has been linked with 1. the adolescent rebellion against parents and authority and 2. the effects of peer pressure. Now the "generation gap" has also to be viewed as a function of rapid change. A rapidly changing society produces an inevitable gap between generations. The values of one generation are outdated by the time the next generation grows up, and therefore they are often seen as irrelevant. In the past it may have taken generations and even centuries for values to change. This meant a certain stabilization of values, allowing time for these to be taught and internalized by the young. The superego, we are taught, is the mental vehicle responsible for the transmission of values from one generation to the next. Thus, the implications and consequences of a rapidly changing value system on superego development are great, and yet to be fully understood. It is probably inevitable that there will be some generation gap in a fast changing society, for child-rearing tends to develop out of the experiences of the parents' own childhood, and is therefore bound to be outdated.

Rise of sexuality and feminism

Parents have also become confused by the rise of sexuality and the new feminism. Society's intense preoccupation with genital sexuality has created both moral and developmental problems for the developing person and confusion within parents as to their own responsibility. Erik Erikson (1), in analyzing the developmental tasks of adolescence and early adulthood, put the development of individual identity before the development of the capacity for intimacy. Thus, we have a generation of adolescents confused about the part sexuality must play in their lives, and parents confused as to how to handle the rise of sexual consciousness. Progressive parents who try to be open-minded and understanding of the new sexual mores frequently find themselves conflicted and embarrassed. Their own sexual attitudes are rooted in the past. On the one hand, they wish to adjust to changing times, while, on the other hand, they are still restricted by their own unconscious attitudes derived from their upbringing.

The rise of feminism has had similar problems for the parents in the demands it places on them. Parents are asked to reexamine their attitudes to meet new social expectations, about which they are ambivalent and uncertain. The new feminism has de-emphasized woman's role as homemaker, compared to that of the career woman with financial indpendence.

A Question of Values

Traditional psychoanalytical thinking has proposed an intrapsychic model as the source of conflict, the resolution of which leads to personality and superego development (3). Subsequent theorists have further elaborated by emphasizing the effect of the interplay of social factors on superego development. Now the existential and humanistic psychotherapies propose that the value systems are not just the result of conflict resolution, but the core of our identity. Identification is derived from an inner core of values to which we make a basic commitment. A functioning society needs a common core of accepted values to give it cohesion and minimal stability. Rollo May (16) has termed this present age "The Age of Emptiness." He says that people not only do not know what they feel, but they also do not know what they believe in. He feels that the chief cause of psychiatric problems is not anxiety, as propagated by Freud, but a feeling of emptiness. Today we try to replace this feeling of emptiness with materialistic goals. In place of a value system, we strive for success, material gains and achievement. Rapid change leads to a confusional breakdown and disruption. However, there are certain essential values which are basic and timeless, and not subject to constant change.

Summary

Parents are being battered by multiple social and cultural forces, none of which they can control. Personality development is as much the result of an interplay of social forces on the psyche as it is the resolution of intrapsychic functions. These social forces must be understood if we are to understand the present dilemma of parenthood. Stress in parenthood is real and not just neurotic or maladaptive. Due to the rapid change in society, parents feel alienated from their past, unsure of the present, and uncertain about the future of the younger generation. Most important, the traditional goals of growth, namely adulthood and parenthood, have become confused and unclear. A generation committed to the goals of self-actualization has elevated the principles of narcissism, self-preoccupation, and immediate gratification, which will increasingly create more difficulties in the future, and make the resolution of adolescence more problematical. The only safeguard against this is a commitment to a value system which gives some stability and coherence to our society. A value system must be ultimately our source of meaning or identity which then becomes the motivating factor of our behavior.

REFERENCES

1. ERIKSON, E. H. (1979). Identity and the life cycle. In: G. S. Klein (ed.), *Psychological Issues*. New York: International Universities Press.
2. ESSMAN, A. H. (1972). Review of A. Toffler *Future Shock*. *Psycho Anal. Q.*, *41*, 143.
3. ESSMAN, A. H. (1977). Changing values—implications for adolescent development. In: S. Feinstein and P. Giovacchini (eds.), *Adolescent Psychiatry V*. New York: Jason Aronson.
4. GARDENER, G. (1957). Present day society and the adolescent. *Am. J. Orthopsychiat.*, *27*, 508.
5. GOODE, W. (1971). Force and violence in the family. *J. of Marriage and the Family*, *33*, 624.
6. GRINKER, R. R. Sr., WERBLE, B. and DRYE, R. C. (1968). *The Borderline Syndrome*. New York: Basic Books.
7. Group for the Advancement of Psychiatry (1973). *The Joys and Sorrows of Parenthood*. New York: Charles Scribner's Sons.
8. HARBIN, H. T. (1977). Episodic dyscontrol and family dynamics. *Am. J. Psychiat.*, *134*, 1113.
9. HARBIN, H. T. and MADDEN, D. J. (1979). Battered parents: A new syndrome. *Am. J. Psychiat.*, *136*, 1288.
10. HARTMAN, H. (1960). *Psychoanalytic and Moral Values*. New York: International Universities Press.
11. HENDIN, H. (1975). *Youth in Crises*. New York: W. W. Norton.
12. KERNBERG, O. (1967). Borderline personality organization. *J. Am. Psychoanalytic Assoc.*, *15*, 641.
13. KNIGHT, R. P. (1954). Borderline states. In: R. P. Knight and C. R. Friedman (eds.), *Psychoanalytic Psychiatry and Psychology*. New York: International Universities Press.
14. MADDEN, D. and LION, J. (Eds.) (1976). *Rage, Hate, Assault and Other Forms of Violence*. New York: Spectrum Publications.
15. MARTIN, D. (1976). *Battered Wives*. San Francisco: Glide Publications.
16. MAY, R. (1973). *Man's Search for Himself*. New York: Dell.
17. SCRATTON, J. (1976). Violence in the family. In: D. Madden and J. Lion (eds.), *Rage, Hate, Assault and Other Forms of Violence*. New York: Spectrum Publications.
18. STEINMETZ, S. K. (1977). *The Cycle of Violence*. New York: Praeger Publishers.
19. STEINMETZ, S. K. (1978). Battered parents. *Society*, *15*, 54.
20. STEINMETZ, S. K. and STRAUSS, M. A. (Eds.) (1974). *Violence in the Family*. New York: Dodd, Mead & Co.
21. STRAUSS, M. A., GELLES, R. J., and STEINMETZ, S. K. (1980) *Behind Closed Doors: Violence in the American Family*. Doubleday/Anchor.
22. TAYLOR, L. and NEWBERGER, E. H. (1979). Child abuse in the International Year of the Child. *New Eng. J. Med.*, *301*, 1205.
23. TOFFLER, A. (1971). *Future Shock*. New York: Random House.

20

THE EMPTY NEST SYNDROME

CRAIG L. ROBERTS, M.E.E.

Department of Home Economics,
Scientific Programmer in the Center for Family Studies,
Arizona State University, Tempe

and

ROBERT A. LEWIS, PH.D.

Head and Professor of the Department of Child
Development and Family Studies,
Purdue University, West Lafayette, Indiana

INTRODUCTION

The empty nest syndrome is clinically defined as the "temporal association of clinical depression with the cessation of child-rearing" (9). It also has been defined as the "sense of loss when grown children leave home" (23). Also associated with the term is the notion of a "profound inability of the parent to cope" (23). Research on various aspects of post-parenthood, however, usually reserves the term "empty nest syndrome" for the severe depression mentioned first. Nevertheless, negative affect associated with the empty nest syndrome is often reported in lesser degrees by mothers and fathers who are not clinically depressed.

THE EMPTY NEST STAGE: A RECENT ADDITION TO THE FAMILY LIFE CYCLE

Few men or women in late nineteenth century America experienced an empty nest, since most children continued to live at home until quite advanced ages or else returned to live with aging parents after having already left home (5). In fact, the proportion of men or women with no children at home never rose above 40% for any cohort between 40 and 75 years. According to United States census data, there has been a dramatic increase during this century in the length of the empty nest (or post-parental) period from an average of two years to an average of 13 (15). This increase, largely a consequence of improved survival rates for both spouses, suggests that couples now spend 16 to 19 years in the post-parental period, more than in any other stage of the family life-cycle (12).

The relatively recent historical emergence of the empty nest period is important, because it clearly identifies one problem of the post-parental transition and the empty nest syndrome—the lack of well established family roles for the post-parental parent, especially the mother (2, 23, 29, 30). According to these studies, post-parental couples find that they cannot easily return to the "honeymoon" roles they had prior to the arrival of children, but instead they must accept the roles which have evolved in the course of their relationship or they must establish new roles for themselves following the departure of children.

THE EMPTY NEST AND FAMILY CRISIS

For many years the transition to the empty nest was seen both in folklore and research as a serious and problematic family crisis or major discontinuity, since it marked the "desertion" of children from the home or their "abandonment" as parents. A number of studies have suggested, for instance, that children's leaving home produces many marital conflicts and results for many parents in a loss of roles which are still highly valued in society. One study found that mothers in the post-parental years reported lower satisfaction with both spousal love and companionship than did mothers in the 15 earlier years of married life (3). Rollins and Feldman (27) discovered that parents who were launching their children reported the least satisfying family life of all.

Mothers were thought to experience more crisis and loss than fathers after children depart from the home, primarily since mothers have depended more upon their roles and position as a parent for a major source of their satisfaction and self-identity (10, 24, 25, 29, 30). Journals frequently run advertisements about antidepressants for women who are experiencing the empty nest syndrome. One study of first admissions to mental hospitals found that 63% of mothers in the empty nest years had high rates of depression (2). A study of women alcoholics found that 21 of 30 women between 45 and 64 began drinking excessively during the empty nest transition (6).

Family crisis at its extreme is evidenced by the divorce of middle-aged couples. The divorce rate for persons in the United States between 45 and

64 has increased 83% from 1960 to 1978, suggesting that the middle years are indeed a time of crisis (31). This increase in the divorce rate does not suggest that earlier divorce rates for persons over 45 were low; in fact, in 1960 and 1970 the divorce rate for persons over 45 was higher than the rate for persons under 45 (31). Some of the crises middle-aged couples experience may be triggered by the departure of children from the home.

FATHERS ALSO EXPERIENCE THE EMPTY NEST SYNDROME

Mothers are not the only persons in families who suffer symptoms of distress and depression after children leave home. Our own studies of parents who had passed through the child launching (18, 19) suggest that just about as many fathers as mothers experienced distress, 23% and 22% respectively. Nearly one-fourth of fathers out of 118 couples chosen randomly in a northeast Georgia county reported unhappiness with their last child's leaving home. These unhappy fathers were found to be also somewhat older men. They tended to have had fewer children. They perceived themselves to be more nurturing persons and yet had poorer marriages. For instance, they reported themselves, after the child launching, to be more neglected by their wives, to receive the least understanding from them, to be the most lonely, to be the least enthusiastic about their wives' companionship, and to have the least empathic wives. We have explained these findings through the principle of *most* interest, i.e., the fathers who reported the most distress were those who had the most to lose with the departure of their last child.

Case study analysis of the fathers who reported the greatest unhappiness suggested a large number of permutations of a small number of themes: fathers discovering that their marriages and friendships had become empty shells about the same time that loved children were leaving; fathers spending their early lives to support their children and wives and later discovering that the other family members now need less of their financial support; and fathers becoming more nurturing at the same time that their wives and children have less need to be nurtured.

The most serious implication of these findings is the possibility that even more men in the future may experience the empty nest syndrome. Such a trend is quite reasonable, if more men are investing time and themselves into child-care and if more men are indeed becoming nurturant with their children. Data to support such trends are difficult to find. However, changing roles for both men and women are giving more options and opportunities for fathers to care for their children (20). Fein (13, 14) has suggested that for some men involvement in physical care-taking of their children is so important that they actually arrange their work schedules to be more often with their children. It would seem, therefore, that, as more men increase their involvement in caring for children, more fathers will eventually experience the empty nest syndrome.

ROLE LOSS AND THE EMPTY NEST SYNDROME IN WOMEN

Tradition has invested the mother with such great responsibility for and involvement in her children that for many mothers the departure of children causes much of the same type and severity of role loss that men experience when they retire (7, 8, 23, 30).

From childhood women are taught that motherhood is necessary for their fulfillment as women, regardless of accomplishments in other parts of their lives. Mothers more often take the major responsibility for care of their children. Mothers more often stay with the children when they are sick and do the major share of cooking and housework resulting from the children's presence. These activities serve to occupy a great deal of mothers' time and energy; thus, when children leave the home the mother loses a major role.

In a study of 40- to 59-year-old women who were admitted into mental hospitals for the first time, the combined analysis of 533 patient records and intensive interviews of 20 women suggested a definite contribution of role loss to the mid-life crisis of these women (2). The role loss was clearly associated with depression. In addition, the depressed middle-aged women were more likely to have suffered maternal role loss than the nondepressed women. Lesser degrees of role loss (e.g., women who still have satisfactory marriages and/or some children remaining at home) and greater degrees of role loss (e.g., women who experience both maternal and additional role losses) had no effect on the severity of the depression. However, post-parental mothers with overinvolvement in their children had a greater rate of depression than non-overinvolved mothers, after children left home.

Reemployment of the post-parental mother might moderate the role loss experienced by the empty nest mothers. Using a sample of 40 graduates of an Eastern women's college, Powell (26) found employed empty nest women to have a significantly lower number of symptoms of psychiatric impairment than empty nest women who were not employed outside the home, as measured by the Twenty-two Item Screening Score (17). Women employed part-time scored an intermediate position.

THE EMPTY NEST PARENT AND ALIENATION

The lack of clearly defined roles for the postparental parent can lead to a sense of alienation, i.e., an uncertainty as to what is "proper" conduct (2). For example, the couple may be unsure as to what kind of relationship they are to have with each other or with their departed children. Parents are admonished by in-law jokes to avoid too binding relationships with their children, at the same time that grandparenthood closes ranks between them and their children's new families (11). Lengthened periods of financial support caused by expensive educations create other tensions, as children and parents may maintain financial ties while seeking other forms of separation and independence from each other.

Duvall (12) has addressed the alienation problems of post-parental parents by identifying and describing the "developmental tasks" for the post-parental wife, the husband, and the entire family of the middle years. However, few of her identified tasks address the parent-child relation *per se*, and none of her tasks for the middle-aged husband address the condition of the post-parental father. Yet, as we have indicated, a sense of loss has been found also for fathers in recent studies (18, 19, 28).

"ON-TIME, OFF-TIME" TRANSITIONS

Individuals have been socialized to accept a developmental perspective of their life course, a perspective in which the individual perceives transitions as clearly marked in time (21). The predictable "on-time" transition events may not be as unsettling to an individual as "off-time" events which usually are unanticipated and unwanted. This concept of "on-time, off-time" has been strongly associated with the empty nest syndrome experienced by some mothers (16, 29, 30). This concept suggests that middle-aged mothers experience greater difficulty when the empty nest transition occurs "off-time," as when children marry earlier than anticipated or when children continue to live at home beyond the time anticipated by the parents.

Spence and Lonner (30) found that "off-time" mothers may adjust by bargaining with their timetable for their children, i.e., to allow time for the "crisis" to resolve itself. Thus, the mother whose daughter remains at home beyond high school may tell herself that the daughter may soon come to her senses and leave home. In the event that the daughter does not fulfill the mother's timetable and expectations, the mother would then need to accept and adjust or, perhaps, suffer even more serious depression. Spence and Lonner, however, doubt that bargaining with one's timetable would ever be as satisfying as "on-time," normative fulfillment of motherhood.

THE EMPTY NEST SYNDROME AND MOTHERS' CONFLICT WITH CHILDREN

The empty nest syndrome may also be associated with a parent's inability to terminate the parent roles, which then may manifest itself in either overt or latent conflict with the already departed children. In an intensive study of 16 hospitalized, equally depressed empty nest mothers, there was almost always some degree of conflict between the mothers and their adult children (9). Seven of the mothers were found to have overt conflict; seven had latent conflict, while two were found to have no conflict.

Overt conflict characterized by frequent, stormy and bitter arguments was found among the less acclimated, foreign-born or first generation mothers who clung to the traditions of their parents' country of origin. Of these seven women, six were widowed or divorced. The conflict became one of the few ways in which they could have contact with their children. The mothers all feared that resolution of the conflict implied silent but lonely peace.

The mothers with latent conflict expressed a vague dissatisfaction with the parent-child relationship, yet intellectually accepted and encouraged their children's independence. These mothers were better educated and more acclimated to American values than the overt conflict mothers. Five out of seven were married and living with their spouses. They had needs for continued closeness with their children which previously had been met (prior to hospitalization) by substitutes, i.e., by friends, work or community activities. The dissatisfaction with the parent-child relationship emerged when contact with the substitute objects was broken by physical illness of the mother or another family member.

TREATMENT OF THE EMPTY NEST SYNDROME

Since the empty nest syndrome involves a number of related emotional symptoms and problems which may affect men and women during the middle years, treatment modes and strategies are multifaceted. In addition, some treatment modes may include not only remedial work but preventive education as well. For instance, treatment may not only include helping dispirited or depressed patients envision more adequate social roles, develop new roles (role-making), and find more adequate outlets for their needs for intimacy, but also encourage patients *before* children leave home to anticipate the changes that children's leaving will produce in their working lives and in their marriages.

Anticipatory socialization is "the process of learning the norms of a role before being in a social situation where it is appropriate to actually behave in the role" (4). Before children begin to leave home, parents can help themselves by anticipating the possible loneliness they may feel and the changes in their family life which may result from fewer family members living in the home.

Anticipating the empty nest years may encourage parents to find emotional substitutes for their children, such as in new friendships, or to seek more rewarding and fulfilling activities in the community, in the workplace, or in the home. Some of these substitutes may bring the same kinds of fulfillments which children earlier brought to parents.

Treatment may also include behaviors which induce positive identification of the patient with the therapist. As role models, psychiatrists can relate their own experiences with child launching, if they have had such, or point out other role models, e.g., parents who have successfully weathered the "crisis of child launching." Group treatment in therapy groups or in women's or men's consciousness-raising groups often produces role models through other parents who themselves have experienced the empty nest transition. Younger fathers can therefore learn from older fathers, as well as from mothers who have learned to adjust to post-parenthood.

In the absence of "successful" role models, therapists may be challenged to help their patients create new roles themselves. Fathers especially may have to innovate new roles, particularly if they have not had adequate models in their own fathers. It is not easy, especially for parents who have been close to children, to adequately release them into the larger society, i.e., to successfully let go of their children and not foster neurotic dependency patterns with them.

Less traditional fathers and mothers should be more successful in role-making treatment, because they are more flexible. Aldous (1) has suggested that the making of new roles demands persons who have high flexibility, interpersonal sensitivity, high self-esteem, and some sense of controlling their own destiny. In sum, therapists who work with patients who have experienced the empty nest syndrome may find themselves having to be role models and to be sensitive to the characteristics of parents who will have more difficulty adapting to the post-parental years.

Patients who express overt conflict with their children might be treated with the aid of *family* therapy (9, 22). Exploration of the expectations of both parents and children can aid greatly in changing expectations from being vague and unrealistic to expressed and possible. Communication patterns within the family can be identified and addressed by the therapist.

Latent conflict between empty nest mothers and their children has been successfully treated by supporting the mother's intellectual acceptance of her children's independence while also aiding the mother's reestablishment of interests in friends, work and other activities (9, 22). Therapy should *minimize* insight development and instead focus on rebuilding the adaptation to the empty nest that the mothers had made prior to the onset of depression.

Finally, Rational Emotive Therapy (RET) can help some patients with the empty nest syndrome by replacing their irrational beliefs with more positive, adaptive ones (23). RET treatment consists of identifying irrational beliefs, teaching the patient to vigorously challenge the irrational beliefs, re-educating the patient to rational beliefs, instituting positive behaviors that are antithetical to depressive affect and focusing the patient upon his/her own life and problems, instead of the children's.

REFERENCES

1. ALDOUS, J. (1974). The making of family roles and family change. *Family Coordinator*, 23 (1):231-235.
2. BART, P. B. (1971). Depression in middle-aged women. In: V. Gornick, and B. K. Moran (eds.), *Women in Sexist Society*, New York: Basic Books.
3. BLOOD, R., and WOLFE, D. (1960). *Husbands and Wives: The Dynamics of Married Living*. New York: Free Press.
4. BURR, W. (1973). *Theory Construction and the Sociology of the Family*. New York: Wiley & Sons.
5. CHUDACOFF, H. P., and HAREVEN, T. K. (1979). From the empty nest to family dissolution: Life course transitions into old age. *J. Family History*, 3:69-83.
6. CURLEE, J. (1969). Alcoholism and the "empty nest." *Bull. Menninger Clinic*, 33:165-171.
7. DEUTSCHER, I. (1964). The quality of postparental life: Definitions of the situation. *J. of Marriage and the Family*, 26:52-59.
8. DEUTSCHER, I. (1969). From parental to post-parental life. *Sociological Symposium*, 3:47-60.
9. DEYKIN, E. Y., JACOBSON, S., KLERMAN, G., and SOLOMON, M. (1966). The empty nest: Psychosocial aspects of conflict between depressed women and their grown children. *Am. J. of Psychiat.*, 122:1422-1426.
10. DIZARD, J. (1968). *Social Change in the Family*. Chicago: Community and the Family Study Center, University of Chicago.
11. DUVALL, E. (1954). *In Laws: Pro and Con*. New York: Association Press.
12. DUVALL, E. (1977). *Marriage and Family Development*, (5th ed.). Philadelphia: Lippincott.
13. FEIN, R. (1974). *Men's Experiences before and after the Birth of the First Child: Dependence, Marital Sharing and Anxiety*. Doctoral dissertation, Harvard University.
14. FEIN, R. (1976). Men's entrance to parenthood. *Family Coordinator*, 25 (4):341-347.
15. GLICK, P. (1977). Updating the life cycle of the family. *J. of Marriage and the Family*, 39 (1):5-13.
16. HAWKINS, E. (1978). Effects of empty nest transition on self-report of psychological and physical well-being. *J. of Marriage and the Family*, 40 (3):549-556.
17. LANGNER, T. S. (1962). A twenty-two item screening score of psychiatric symptoms indicating impairment. *J. of Health and Human Behavior*, 3:269-276.
18. LEWIS, R. A., FRENEAU, P. J., and ROBERTS, C. L. (1979). Fathers and the postparental transition. *Family Coordinator*, 28 (4):514-520.
19. LEWIS R. A., and ROBERTS, C. L. (1979). Postparental fathers in distress. *Psychiatric Opinion*, Nov./Dec.: 27-30.
20. LYNN, D. B. (1974). *The Father: His Role in Child Development*. Monterey: Brooks/Cole.

21. NEUGARTEN, B. (1970). Adaptation and the life cycle. *J. Geriatric Psychiat.*, 4:71-87.
22. NOONAN, R. A. (1973). Depression and the empty nest. Masters Thesis, Smith College of Social Work. Abstracted in *Smith College Review*, 44:41-42.
23. OLIVER, R. (1977). The "empty nest syndrome" as a focus of depression: A cognitive treatment model, based on Rational Emotive Therapy. *Psychotherapy: Theory, Research and Practice*, 14 (1):87-94.
24. PECK, R. (1955). Psychological developments in the second half of life. In: J. Anderson (ed.), *Psychological Aspects of Aging: Proceedings of a Conference on Planning Research*. Bethesda, Maryland, April 24-27.
25. PINEO, P. (1961). Disenchantment in the later years of marriage. *Marriage and Family Living*, 23 (1):3-11.
26. POWELL, B. (1977). The empty nest, employment, and psychiatric symptoms in college-educated women. *Psychology of Women Quarterly*. 2 (1):35-43.
27. ROLLINS, B. and FELDMAN, H. (1970). Marital satisfaction over the family life cycle. *J. of Marriage and the Family*, 26(1):20-28.
28. RUBIN, L. B. (1979). *Women of a Certain Age: The Midlife Search for Self*. New York: Harper & Row.
29. SPENCE, D. L., and LONNER, T. D. (1971). The empty nest: A transition within motherhood. *Family Coordinator*, 20 (4):369-375.
30. SPENCE, D. L., and LONNER, T. D. (1978). Career set: A resource through transitions and crises. *Int. J. Aging and Human Development*, 9 (1):51-65.
31. United States Bureau of the Census. (1979). Marital status and living arrangements. Current Population Reports, Series P-20, No. 388:3. Washington, D.C.: U.S. Government Printing Office.

21

MARRIAGE PROBLEMS AND MARITAL THERAPY IN THE MIDDLE-AGED

Carol C. Nadelson, M.D.,
Derek C. Polonsky, M.D.

*Department of Psychiatry of Tufts New England
Medical Center, Boston, Mass.*

and

Mary Alice Mathews, M.D.

*Department of Psychiatry of the Beth Israel Hospital,
Harvard Medical School, Boston, Mass.*

THE INDIVIDUAL AND MARITAL LIFE-CYCLE

Following Erikson's (10) delineation of stages of adult as well as child development, interest in this area has grown. Gould (15) described several distinct phases of adult development, each of which required mastery of specific tasks. He described stressful transitional periods between the stages, during which the individual redefines his/her goals and self-concept. Levinson (19) from his longitudinal data on men, described eras or developmental stages, and focused on the boundary between self and the interpersonal world. Vaillant (34) using a sample of 95 men studied longitudinally, concerned himself with the processes of adaptation occurring over time.

Neugarten (29, 30) modified the concept of crisis at nodal points and stated that expectable life events are not in themselves crises for most people, but normal turning points which permit changes in self-concept and identity. In her view, there is an increase in introversion in mid and later life and a reorganization of value systems which occurs slowly. Whether or not these turning points precipitate crises depends to a large extent on timing. While psychological change is continuous throughout the life-cycle, in times of rapid social change age norms and the rhythm of the life-cycle are altered. Adulthood has become more fluid, and it is marked by an increasing number of role transitions as well as the disappearance of traditional timetables. There is, instead, a proliferation of roles and a lack of synchrony among age-related roles.

Neugarten further states that the new age-irrelevant society affects the mental health of adults insofar as some of the central issues of the life-cycle for each individual are not entirely predictable or clear. Thus, if timing is central to the individual's self-concept, the change in the concept and relevance of time may engender conflict. On the other hand, as major life events and role transitions have become more irregular, age is less relevant and age norms less limiting than they had previously been. Hence, while adulthood cannot be viewed as an invariant sequence of stages, each occurring at a given chronological age, there is a sequence of developmental tasks and preoccupations that do occur as people grow older. Developmental tasks, however, do not emerge only at given moments to be resolved and put behind once and for all. As lives grow longer, they are more varied and differ from each other based on the experiences and choices of each individual.

It must be noted that data about the life-cycle have largely derived from males. There are no systematic longitudinal studies similar to those of Vaillant or Levinson which have included women. Furthermore, although much attention has been recently paid to the individual developmental process, very little consideration has been given to interactional stresses these precipitate and to the modes of adaptation employed in families or couples over the adult life cycle. Thus, the lack of coincidence of individual and marital development phases has not been adequately addressed. Not only are individuals in a marriage often not in synchrony with regard to their developmental stages, but a change in one partner may be dissonant with the needs of and/or changes in the other. Rates and directions of growth may thus differ. Since there may have been disparity with regard to age, goals or past experience at the beginning, the potential for turmoil and the need for establishing mutually acceptable means of adaptation are enormous.

In order to understand the process of adjustment in marriage, it is necessary to take account of individual developmental and intrapsychic contributions as well as to view the marriage from an evolutionary and interpersonal perspective, since individual and marital development are inexorably intertwined (3, 16, 21, 23).

Marital relationships also evolve through several distinct stages (25). There is an early idealization phase (usually during the courtship and the first one or two years of the marriage) during which negative aspects of the partner are denied and the partner is seen as "perfect," full of unlimited promise. When the realities of day-to-day living make themselves felt, a "disillusionment" phase begins, where the spouses have to come to terms with each other's limitations and compromise on expectations. This may or may not be resolved before the phase of procreativity is confronted—the decision whether or not to have children, and the subsequent role shifts with parenthood. As mid-life approaches, the couple has to deal with parental role shifts, with a variety of losses, and with the separation and emerging autonomy of children. Furthermore, throughout the marriage, the career of either or both partners affects the marriage. Regardless of when a couple marries, whether they are in their twenties or forties, the tasks required in mastering the phases outlined briefly above will have to be confronted.

SELECTION OF A PARTNER

The shifts and stresses a couple experiences cannot become clear unless one begins by considering the dynamic factors involved in the selection of a mate (3, 9, 22). The wishes, longings, projections and life disappointments for each partner affect the choice. Ambivalence is universal and is based on the uncertainty of predicting future events and behaviors, as well as anxiety about the possibility that feelings will change and that, despite attempts at working out the complexities of a relationship, it will fail for unknown or uncontrollable reasons (28).

Freud (13) formulated an individually based theory in which object choices were seen as anaclitically or narcissistically based. The person who makes an anaclitic choice was seen as oriented primarily toward nurturance and protection, and is focused mainly on the gratification of dependency needs. A narcissistic choice is made by a person who sees himself or herself as the object. The person who is chosen represents the ideal self or a projected ego ideal, or is chosen in an attempt to recapture a past self, a projected past object, or a person who was once part of the self.

Part of the process of selection of a mate is based on unconscious signals by which the partners recognize in each other the possibility that they can jointly work through unresolved conflicts which exist intrapsychically in each of them. It can allow for the identification with the loving aspect of parents and parental introjects and relieve rivalries and repressed sexual feelings. It can also fulfill frustrated longings and allow new opportunities for self-realization (28).

At the same time, mutual defenses and collusive "joint resistance" can prevent working-through of conflicts (9) and marriage can become a repository for old conflicts (22). Since the fantasy about the chosen object must come to face reality, each individual can only approach the fantasied goal. Thus, there is a degree of profound unconscious ambivalence in the choice of object. The level of psychological readiness to make a commitment to an intense object relationship is an important factor in the success of a marriage. While some individuals have attained a level of differentiation and individuation which prepares them to cope with the tasks of marriage, others are burdened by unresolved early conflicts, unrealistic expectations (conscious or unconscious) or severe psychological deficits which make the resolution of marital tasks more difficult. Those individuals who enter a marriage in less differentiated developmental stages can grow toward maturity within the marriage. However, those who either cannot cope or cannot resolve infantile desires are vulnerable to disturbances if their goals for the marriage differ from their spouse's.

MARITAL INTERACTION

Sager (32) discusses marital interaction in terms of marriage contracts which, he states, exist at three levels. The first level is conscious and expressed between partners; the second level is conscious but not verbally expressed; and the third is unconscious. It is the unconscious expectations that lead to stress and disappointment in marriage.

Dicks (9), using an object relations model, describes the way in which partners attempt to recreate, with their partners, aspects of their earlier object relationships. In the early idealized phase of the relationship, the negative aspects are denied and the partner is seen as someone who can fulfill many needs. Once this idealization fades, each partner experiences difficulties similar to those experienced with parents, but which have not been resolved. Thus, an understanding of individual dynamics and unconscious wishes and expectations enables us to elucidate the degree to which the spouse does not fulfill these unconscious wishes, and the stress experienced in the relationship.

Marriage must be conceptualized as a dynamic interaction between two people. It cannot be seen in static terms. It can foster development by facilitating the establishment of a close and sexual relationship which offers the opportunity for partners to work through the prohibitions and inhibitions of childhood. Thus, each partner relates on a reciprocal basis. This implies that individual development has proceeded beyond the stage of need gratification and that separation from early objects has occurred. The self must be perceived as autonomous (3).

Marriage does, however, present a paradox, especially for the people who marry before they have resolved the critical tasks of adolescence, separation and identity consolidation. The marital agreement, symbolized in the marriage ceremony, requires that the two become one. Yet the tasks of developing and maintaining a separate identity are important developmental issues. For those whose conflicts around separation-individuation actually precipitated the desire to marry, the need for dependency gratification may be projected onto the partner, who then becomes the parent in fantasy, and the developmental tasks of adolescence are not mastered. If, however, the individual can integrate these opposing forces, a new level of ego control with new opportunities for identification are possible. When this process occurs in the more autonomous environment of adulthood, rather than adolescence, infantile pressures are less intense, and the danger of object loss or identity diffusion is less fearsome. Thus, less anxiety is experienced and greater choice is possible (28).

MARRIAGE AND MID-LIFE

These developmental processes have important implications for the mid-life period (1, 2, 4, 5, 8, 12, 14, 16, 21, 23, 24, 26, 27, 31, 33). Individuals clearly bring their pasts, including their abilities to change, grow and cope, to their interactions with spouses. The way in which the stresses and challenges of mid-life affect a marriage depend not only on the individual histories of the spouses, but also on the capacity of the couple to cope with stresses together, and on the effectiveness of the problem-solving patterns which they have developed over the years. The complexity of the interaction between marital and individual "crisis points" is most apparent at the stage of mid-life transition. If couples differ in their individual life phases, or they have married recently but are both at mid-life, the issues are further complicated.

While mid-life had most often in the past been confined to a chronological period with specific age limits, a more meaningful conceptualization comes from an examination of the role changes and specific issues that are prominent at this life phase, regardless of age. The recognition of the finiteness of time and limited options, with reassessment of goals and achievements and redefinition of roles with respect to parents and children, is important. Furthermore, multiple separations and losses occur and the individual must also find a way to reconcile the physical changes of aging, which may include decreased capacities as well as illnesses or disability. In the interpersonal area there is a shift in emphasis toward companionship, empathy and sharing, and a movement away from a focus on performance and appearance (26, 27).

Recent evidence suggests that changes in personality style may occur during phases of the life-cycle which may differ between men and women, having an impact on the marital relationship (29). Men begin to integrate their more "feminine" self and allow the expression of more warmth, intimacy and empathy. They appear to be more accepting of their nurturing feelings. Women, on the other hand, have been reported to become more assertive and less restricted or guilty. Thus, a reversal of traditional masculine and feminine qualities may occur. Although women have classically been seen as more vulnerable to depression in mid-life because of the "empty nest," it appears that the major factor in mid-life depression in women is role loss when the family structures and responsibilities change. Thus, many time-honored views must be reexamined, and new ideas must take account of the impact of societal change. Erikson further emphasizes this point, when he comments on the need to understand issues of generativity when individuals have not procreated, a factor which he had not accounted for in his original life stage model (11).

The depth of caring and commitment on the part of the couple is tested during the course of a marriage by the shifts in task expectations and dynamics which occur. The mid-life years bring to a marriage many developmental issues which are similar to those the individual faces. It becomes necessary to recognize and integrate success and failure, and to resolve the loss of the fantasy of infinite opportunity. Priorities in relationship shift away from earlier needs for security, performance and role fulfillment towards a desire for greater companionship and understanding. The bonds which maintained the stability of the relationship may be internally generated, shared values, goals and commitments. At times, partners do not define success or failure similarly, nor do complementary shifts occur simultaneously in each of them. The balance of the relationship may shift, leading to re-equilibration and adaptation on another level; or dyssynchrony may ensue and the relationship will be strained or disrupted. A change from the original marital "contract" produces stress unless it is mutually acceptable (26, 27).

In couples who have been married up to 20 years, a general drop in marital satisfaction has been reported (12) with a loss in intimacy, less physical affection and decreased sexual intimacy. The parenting demands brought by adolescent children have frequently been cited as a major factor in marital adjustment during mid-life (14). The pain of separation and the necessity to assume new roles and give up old ones, as well as the revival of early developmental issues for each partner, are important stresses during this time. Chilman (6) reported that children bring mounting pressure and stress to a marriage as they get older. She described two low points in marital satisfaction at nine and 16 years of marriage. These correlated with the stresses of parenting and the anxiety and increased sense of helplessness when adolescents are most concerned about sexual adequacy and freedom of expression. Adolescent intensity and mood swings may cause parents to feel that the family is deteriorating, augmenting their anxieties about their own signs of physical decline and adequacy as parents and people, as well as about missed opportunities, mistakes and failures.

The post-parental or the mid-life period may bring new opportunities as well as conflicts. Freedom from the burdens of financial responsibilities and time constraints may bring couples closer together. They may be able to reestablish past intimacies and enjoy new experiences. They may begin to share new interests and relationships. They may, however, find new sources of conflict and turmoil.

MARITAL PROBLEMS IN MID-LIFE

The sources of difficulty during this period are complex and multidetermined. We will focus on some of the more frequent problems seen in clinical practice.

1. Changes in the Original "Contract"

Since marital partners tend to accept the roles and rules that have been incorporated in the early phase of their relationship, they may experience difficulty if one partner changes and the homeostatic balance of the marital relationship is disrupted. For example, if a spouse is selected primarily for his/her role as the "weaker" partner who maintains the self-esteem of the other, and this partner no longer relates in the same way, then the "stronger" partner may suffer damage to his/her self-esteem. Originally, the "strong" partner may have overvalued performance and achievement and underestimated dependency needs. He/she may have denied "weakness" and projected it onto the partner, who thus became the "weak" one. The strong partner claimed service and care, and the weak one submitted and tolerated the denigration of his/her feelings, needs and opinions. The weak partner felt inferior and did not believe him/herself to be deserving of caring and reciprocity or the right to self-assertion. The growth of the "weak" partner, for whatever reason, thus results in movement away from the assigned role.

The marriage may then become tumultuous, unless the other partner is able to accommodate the change.

Case I

Mrs. A., a woman in her early 40s, requested therapy after her husband threatened to move out to live with another woman. The A's had been married for 17 years and had three children. For years Mrs. A. knew that her husband had extramarital sexual affairs, but she felt that she had to accept the situation because she saw no alternative. She had always believed herself to be incapable of independent functioning and thus she was frightened that she would be left alone.

During the course of therapy Mrs. A. began to move away from the helpless, masochistic position she had so readily accepted for many years, as she became aware of the anxiety she had about independence. She began to see the marriage as a means of both leaving her family of origin and continuing to be dependent.

Whereas divorce was unthinkable many years before, she now entertained the idea. Her friends and family became more supportive of that option. When her husband did leave, she found to her surprise that she experienced relief as well as anxiety and fear. When she found a job, her husband became anxious about her emerging independence and he wanted to return to her. Mrs. A., however, felt that the relationship could not resume as it had existed and she decided to divorce Mr. A.

Mr. A's dependency needs were masked by his wife's greater need to be dependent. He felt secure as long as she remained in that position. When there was a shift in the dynamic, he was confronted with his own unresolved conflicts. Mrs. A's poor self-esteem led her to idealize her husband and to see him as strong, accomplished and self-sufficient. This view enabled Mr. A. to avoid confrontation with his own self-doubts and anxieties. The balance remained unchanged as long as they both played their roles and maintained the equilibrium of the relationship. When Mr. A. threatened to leave, and Mrs. A. began to deal with her own individuation and autonomy, the change confronted Mr. A. in a way that he had not anticpated. The loss of a helpless, dependent wife caused the reemergence of his own unresolved conflicts.

Although the result of treatment was marital dissolution, it is important to emphasize that many marriages may not be viable when a change in balances has occurred. The partners may need to reevauluate the viability of the relationship and they may choose to dissolve their marriage.

While therapists often view separation in a marriage as a treatment failure, because they believe that their task is to resolve differences and promote a closer relationship, it is our belief that when growth occurs in differing directions, a marriage may no longer be viable, or when the partners cannot tolerate the anxiety associated with change together, a separation may be inevitable. Differences in marriage as in any situation cannot always be resolved and reconciled. Furthermore, marital partners may welcome an opportunity to acknowledge and confront the loss more directly.

2. Unfulfilled Goals

The reassessment of goals and achievements may result in disappointment and precipitate problems in a relationship. Disappointment may lead to depression and withdrawal on the part of one or both partners with resultant acting out, such as alcoholism or the occurrence of extramarital encounters. At times it takes the form of a desire to terminate the relationship and seek another partner who is fantasized to be more fulfilling and gratifying. Often the individual is not conscious of the defensive aspects of this response to the loss of a previous ego ideal, and there is much mutual projection and denial which disrupt the relationship.

Case II

Mr. and Mrs. B., both age 50, sought treatment after Mrs. B. discovered that her husband was having an affair. For the previous five years he had been increasingly more withdrawn and had started to drink excessively.

He had become disappointed at his failure to attain his life-long objectives. Because of his recognized brilliance and multifaceted expertise, he had been sought after for many years. Although he had been appointed to important university and government positions over the years, he was never satisfied because he had never been able to reach the level he had desired. He began an affair with a woman 20 years his junior after a colleague received the position he had expected. A short time later, his lover left him for a younger man, after castigating him for his cowardice in not leaving his wife. His wife reproached him for his lack of judgment and loyalty. His children voiced their disillusionment and disappointment in him, and Mr. B. couldn't make sense out of his shattered dreams. He blamed himself and alternately his wife.

His treatment involved working through the disappointment of his expectations about his career as well as his ambivalence about his marriage. Marital therapy promoted a renegotiation of the marital contract.

3. Sexual Problems

Complaints about sexual adequacy and functioning have become more frequent in clinical practice. It is important and often difficult to differentiate the etiology of sexual dysfunctions, especially since these symptoms are often manifestations of marital conflict. Since there has been more open discussion of sexuality and sexual expectations in recent years, couples in their mid-life may feel cheated; they may desire a "last chance" to change an unsatisfactory and ungratifying relationship or to resolve other issues. The "sexual" problem may be used as a way of denying underlying conflicts and focusing on a specific area for which there is a specific treatment approach. The response to pressure toward opened sexuality may lead one spouse to make demands on the the other which are not acceptable.

Case III

Mrs. C., a 38-year-old woman, was causing her spouse considerable distress by demanding an "open marriage" after 17 years. She gave numerous logical "reasons" for her demand. The C's had been high school and college sweethearts and married upon college graduation. Neither had dated anyone else or experimented sexually in any way, and Mrs. C. felt that she was "missing something." Although she claimed to enjoy their sexual relationship, she stated that it was not as exciting or satisfying as she had thought it "should be." Mrs. C. had recently developed a sexual attrraction toward a man with whom she was taking a course. He espoused free sexual expression and was openly seductive in his interaction with Mrs. C. She enjoyed several satisfying sexual encounters with him, and he encouraged her to include Mr. C. When Mr. C was unequivocally negative, Mrs. C. accused him of being "old fashioned." She pressured him and suggested therapy because he was "unable to be sexually free." They were able to resolve their conflicts in conjoint marital therapy where they explored their relationship, including their sexual interaction. They were able to grow into a more mutually satisfying interaction.

4. Procreativity

For couples who either made a decision not to have children or who did not have them for another reason, midlife may be a time during which there is a recrudescence of feeling about this issue. Up until this life phase, the option exists and the fantasy about the future remains open. When the decision not to have children was associated with conflict about parenting, a couple may experience difficulty, either directly or indirectly, experienced as depression or sexual dysfunction, when the option no longer remains.

Case IV

Mr. and Mrs. D. were both 43 when they requested treatment for "frigidity and impotence." They had not had intercourse for the past eight years and adapted to the situation until Mrs. D. found herself in the position of being asked for sexual advice from the younger women in her office. She began to feel that she was missing something. The therapist wondered whether they really wanted to change anything after such a long time. He shared his concerns with the couple but they insisted that they wanted therapy. They were remarkably responsive to treatment, and within four weeks, they were having intercourse.

While on the surface the events which brought them to treatment were related to feelings that time was running out, it became clear that there were other issues. They had managed to avoid open confrontation on the issue of whether to become parents, and at 43 they decided to let "age" make the decision. In part, the success of the sexual therapy could be explained in terms of the resolution of ambivalence about having children. They both felt that they were too old, and that they did not want new responsibilities at this time. While there were many determinants of their expressed fear of being parents, they could bypass these when they felt permitted to make this decision. At mid-life there could be no questioning, so they were able to be sexually active despite their desire to remain childless.

5. Reconstituted Family

The problems of reconstituted families may not be specifically related to the middle years. However, this type of family picture is increasingly more common and one or both partners is often in mid-life. The situation is especially a challenge as couples struggle with differing views about parenting, competition with the divorced spouse, and the strong loyalties and feelings of betrayal that are seen in the children. Unlike couples who divorce before they have had children, couples who are in reconstituted families have an ongoing connection with the "bad" or failed marriage. There is a way in which some resolution may take place with the feelings associated with the failure, but the fact remains that alimony payments continue and conflicts around various logistic arrangements are ever present. Additionally, the spouse may suddenly in mid-life become a stepparent to someone else's children with all the complexities entailed in that role.

Case V

Mr. and Mrs. E. had been married for two years. Mr. E. had two sons, aged 11 and 14, by his first marriage. He was 46 years old, and well settled in his career as a writer. Mrs. E., a 45-year-old physician, had been married briefly and divorced 25 years before. She had an adult daughter who was no longer living with her. Mrs. E. resented Mr. E.'s attention to his sons, and Mr. E. felt that Mrs. E. was never available. When the initial period of romance ended, they each felt disappointment. They had each expected greater commitment from the other and neither had recognized the kinds of compromises they would have to make. Each had blamed the previous failed marriage on the demands of the spouse and both had subsequently lived very indepndent lives. Mrs. E. resented the demands of young children, especially since it had been a long time since she had lived with any. Mr. E. had previously been married to a woman who had no career interests so that he was unable to understand Mrs. E.'s commitment to hers.

The treatment was slow and difficult since each partner maintained a firmly entrenched sense of righteousness. Both of the E's were strong, successful people, who had always made autonomous decisions. They had enormous difficulty learning to listen, to respect their differences and to accept that part of their commitment to each other which necessitated that each relinquish some control.

6. Physical Disability

Illness produces profound shifts in the roles of each partner, with major upheavals for a family. It requires role change and role reassessment, as well as a resolution of the narcissistic assault for the affected person. It is a confrontation with mortality and the finiteness of time and, depending to a large extent on early life experiences, it may bring the anxiety of the threat of abandonment, and it may give rise to a number of adaptive and defensive reactions.

Case VI

Mr. and Mrs. F. were both in their early 50s and had been married for 26 years. The marriage had been relatively stable and happy. They had four children. Mr. F. took great pride in his capacity to be the "provider" and Mrs. F. seemed to be comfortable in her position of homemaker. The shift in their relationship came when Mr. F. sustained a back injury at work, which required a hospitalization. This precipitated in him a severe regression, during which time he seemed to thrive on being a patient in the hospital, and became totally consumed by the pain in his back and the weakness in his legs.

It became clear that his usual counterdependent style had masked enormous dependency needs. When confronted by a "legitimate" reason to be helpless, he seemed to thrive. His wife was quite terrified. She had always leaned on him and had viewed him as a strong, dependable man who would take care of her. She developed somatic symptoms and depression. Attempts were made to help Mr. F. mobilize, but he steadfastly held to the position that he would love to go back to work, but that the pain was so intense as to make it impossible.

Mrs. F. repeatedly "threatened" to get a job herself. Mr. F. initially responded by saying that he could never allow his wife to work. He modified this position, appearing to encourage her to do it, but undermining every step that she took towards this end. She had enormous difficulty with separation and dependency and could not allow herself to appear capable of handling a responsible job. The effect on the family was devastating. Mr. F. now remained at home all the time, and criticized everything that was done. Mrs. F. found this quite disruptive and the children became symptomatic. They fought constantly and began to perform poorly at school.

Family and couple therapy was stormy and taxing. Ultimately, Mrs. F. was able to feel stronger and to get a job. She began to feel much better, somatized less and she seemed to be less depressed. Mr. F. still refused to move, but the strain on the family decreased considerably as they settled into the reversed roles.

While the initial marriage contract was based on Mr. F.; being the strong partner, it shifted when a physical disability radically changed the roles and the dynamic of the relationship. This ultimately forced Mrs. F. to grow toward increased autonomy and to master some of her fears about separation. Mr. F.'s treatment was less successful. He was unable to give up the position of helpless patient, which he discovered enabled him to maintain greater control of his family.

The kinds of problems experienced by mid-life couples also include a variety of other disappointments and losses, including children who fail to live up to expectations and spouses who do not provide what they promised. With each couple the problem of loss and adaptation to change becomes central. While many of these issues have always existed, some demands have changed in recent years because of the changes in societal values, expectations and options. Among these are the changes brought by the women's movement and the return of many middle-aged women to the labor force. Clearly, their expanded horizons affect their families and require other shifts. Therapists frequently see spouses and other family members who find these changes difficult.

MARITAL THERAPY

While some of these considerations apply to marital therapy in general, it is important to risk being repetitive in order to add emphasis. The evaluation of the couple should include an understanding of the presenting problem and the interactional system, as well as the delineation of the psychodynamic contributions of each partner. It is also important that the therapist clarify the reasons for the couple's original union and understand why they remained together. Often, despite what appears to be a long-standing unsatisfactory interaction, there are firm ties.

The therapist must then make the decision about a treatment approach: individual treatment for both partners, with the same or with different therapists; conjoint meetings with two therapists or with one therapist; group treatment, etc. Since a complete description of the advantages and disadvantages of each is beyond the scope of this chapter, let us emphasize that therapists usually are influenced by their own orientation and experience, and there are as yet few clearly established criteria. It is not necessarily the modality which is specifically indicated or contraindicated but rather the skill of the therapist and the motivation of the couple.

What requires emphasis is that the presenting partner may be mistakenly identified as the patient or that couples therapy will not be considered either because it was not requested or because the therapist may not be oriented in this direction despite the evidence that it is the most successful treatment modality for marital problems (17). The therapist must be aware of the potential for projection and externalization, and of the value of seeing the spouse, if only in evaluation, to better understand the situation. The fact that couples are often stuck in roles of collusive mutual projection and that the "bad" part of the self may be split off and projected onto a spouse makes it important that the therapist clarify whether this is indeed the situation.

In evaluating these problems, the current literature on adult development is particularly useful for the clinician. While it is difficult enough for a couple when both partners are roughly the same age, and are dealing with more or less the same developmental issues, it is even more so where there is a wide divergence in the ages. Each partner may have great difficulty in understanding and being empathetically attuned to the issues of the spouse. The therapist must be aware of the differences and be able to facilitate recognition and work in this area.

REFERENCES

1. BART, P. and GROSSMAN, M. (1978). Menopause. In: *The Woman Patient: Medical and Psychological Interfaces*. C. Nadelson and M. Notman (eds.), New York: Plenum Press.
2. BERMAN, E. M. and LIEF, H. I. (1975). Marital therapy from a psychiatric perspective: An overview, *Am. J. Psychiat.*, 132:538-592.
3. BLANCK, R. and BLANCK, G. (1968). *Marriage and Personal Development*, New York: Columbia U. Press.
4. BRADBURN, N. M. and CAPLOVITZ, D. (1965). *Reports on Happiness*, Chicago: Aldine Press.
5. BURGESS, E. W. and WALLIN, P. (1968). The middle years of marriage. In: B. Neugarten (ed.), *Middle Age and Aging*. Chicago: University of Chicago Press.
6. CHILMAN, C. (1968). Families in development at midstage of the family life cycle, *The Family Coordinator*. 17:4, 297-312.
7. CLAYTON, R. R. (1975). *The Family, Marriage and Social Change*, Lexington, Mass.: Health and Co.
8. DEUTSCHER, I. (1968). The quality of postparental life. In: B. Neugarten (ed.), *Middle Age and Aging*. Chicago: University of Chicago Press.
9. DICKS, H. V. (1963). Object relations theory and marital studies. *Brit. J. Med. Psychol.*, 36, 125.
10. ERIKSON, E. (1950). *Childhood and Society*, New York: Norton.
11. ERIKSON, E. (1979). The Life Cycle. Presented at International Psychoanalytic Meetings, New York, N.Y., August.
12. FELDMAN, H. and ROLLINS, B. C. (1970). Marital satisfaction over the family life cycle, *J. Marriage and Family*, 32:26.
13. FREUD, S. (1958). *Observations on transference love* (1914), *Standard Edition*, 12, 157-172, London: Hogarth Press.
14. GLENN, N. D. (1975). Psychological well being in the postparental stage: Evidence from national surveys. *J. Marriage and the Family*, 37:1, 105-110.
15. GOULD, R. (1972). The phases of adult life: A study in development psychology, *Am. J. Psychiat.*, 129:5, 521-531.
16. GRUNEBAUM, H. and CHRIST, J. (1976). Marriage and society. In: H. Grunebaum and J. Christ (eds.), *Contemporary Marriage: Structure, Dynamics and Therapy*. Boston, Mass.: Little, Brown.
17. GURMAN, A. (1978). Contemporary marital therapies: A critique and comparative analysis of psychoanalytic, behavioral and systems theory approaches. In: T. J. Paolino and B. S. McCrady (eds.), *Marriage and Marital Therapy*. New York: Brunner/Mazel.
18. JACQUES, E. (1965). Death and the midlife crisis. *Intl. J. Psychoanal.*, 46:502-513.
19. LEVINSON, D. J. (1977). The mid-life transition. *Psychiatry*, 40:109-110.
20. LEVINSON, D. J. with DARROW, C. N., KLEIN, E. B., LEVINSON, M. H., and McKEE, B. (1978). *The Seasons of a Man's Life*. New York: Knopf.
21. LURIE, E. (1974). Sex and stage differences, in perceptions of marital and family relations. *J. Marriage and Family*, 36:2, 260-269.
22. MAIN, T. F. (1966). Mutual projection in marriage. *Comp. Psych.*, 7, 5.
23. MARTIN, P. (1976). *A Marital Therapy Manual*. New York: Brunner/Mazel.
24. MARMOR, J. (1974). The crisis in middle age. In J. Marmor (ed.), *Psychiatry in Transition*.

New York: Brunner/Mazel, pp. 71-76.

25. NADELSON, C. C., POLONSKY, D. C., and MATHEWS, M. A. (1979). Marriage as a Developmental Process. Read at workshop called "Contemporary Marriage," June 15, 1979, Psychotherapy Institute of Beth Israel Hospital and Harvard Medical School, Boston, Ma.

26. NADELSON, C. C., POLONSKY, D. C., and MATHEWS, M. A. (1979). Marriage and midlife: The impact of social change. *Journal of Clinical Psychiatry, 40*:(7) 292-315; 298-321.

27. NADELSON, C. C., POLONSKY, D. C., and MATHEWS, M. A. (1978). Marital stress and symptom formation in midlife. *Psychiatric Opinion, 15*:(9) 29-33, Sept.

28. NADELSON, C. C. (1978). Marital therapy from a psychoanalytic perspective. In T. J. Paolino and B. S. McCrady (eds.), *Marriage and Marital Therapy*. New York: Brunner/Mazel.

29. NEUGARTEN, B. L. (1968). *Middle Age and Aging*. Chicago: University of Chicago Press.

30. NEUGARTEN, B. L. (1979). Time, age and the life cycle. *Am. J. Psychiat., 136*:7.

31. PINEO, P. C. (1968). Disenchantment in the later years of marriage. In: B. Neugarten (ed.), *Middle Age and Aging*. Chicago: University of Chicago Press.

32. SAGER, C. (1976). *Marriage Contracts and Couple Therapy*, New York: Brunner/Mazel.

33. THURNHER, M. (1976). Patterns of personality development in middle aged woman: Longitudinal study. *Intl. J. Aging Hum. Dev., 7*:2, 129-135.

34. VAILLANT, G. E. (1977). *Adaptation to Life*, Boston: Little, Brown.

22

THERAPEUTIC WORK WITH STEPPARENTS

EMILY B. VISHER, PH.D.

President, Stepfamily Association
of America, Inc.
Palo Alto, California

and

JOHN S. VISHER, M.D.

Adult Services Chief,
San Mateo County Mental Health Services
Daly City, California

INTRODUCTION

Family patterns are shifting with the tides of social change and clinicians need to be aware of the characteristics and dynamics of these new families. With the escalating divorce and remarriage rate, a new type of family, the stepfamily, is demanding recognition and acceptance.

In the United States it is estimated that over 35 million adults are stepparents, and one child in six under the age of 18 is a stepchild. Until recently, parents and stepparents generally were dropped into the same conceptual box although stepparenting is not the same as parenting. Stepparenting is different from parenting not so much because of the non-blood relationship, but rather because of cultural myths surrounding the stepparent, and because there are structural differences between biological families and stepfamilies. If these differences are unrecognized by clinicians, individuals in remarriage families who seek professional help often feel misunderstood and unsupported, and therefore unhelped. Understanding and validation of stepfamily feelings and experiences are necessary for successful therapy to take place. In addition, procedural guidelines are emerging to assist clinicians in their work with stepfamilies.

CULTURAL MYTHS SURROUNDING STEPFAMILIES

There are three major cultural myths that create difficulty for stepfamilies:
a) The wicked stepmother myth.
b) The myth of "instant love" (6) or "instant adjustment" (2).
c) The myth that stepfamilies are the same as biological families.

Children in most cultures grow up with stories of wicked stepmothers. A Chinese man said recently, "There are many wicked stepmother stories in Chinese literature, and it's true that stepmothers are wicked, though I knew a nice one once." A young American stepson said to his stepmother, "You can't be my stepmother beacuse you're not mean enough!"

While mothers at times believe themselves to be mean, Cinderella, Snow White and Hansel and Gretel influence the self-image of many stepmothers by producing discomfort and internal conflicts which often lead to external conflicts as well (5); negative cultural expectations lie beneath the feelings expressed by one stepmother when she said, "I feel as though everyone is watching over my shoulder waiting for me to screw up."

While there are cruel stepfathers in literature, they occur primarily in stories for adolescents and adults and the psychological impact is apparently not as significant.

In direct opposition to the wicked stepmother myth is the expectation of instant love or adjustment. Simply stated, this is the expectation that un-related individuals coming from different family backgrounds will immedi-ately develop a harmonious, loving, and cohesive relationship. Quite the opposite is the rule.

Stepparents feel guilty because of their failure to experience instant har-mony. Children are more realistic in their expectations, but adult pressure to fit in and "love" new stepparents and stepsiblings is in opposition to their awareness that all relationships take time to develop. As a result guilt and anger build up and impede or even obliterate any semblance of cohesiveness.

Closely related to the myth of "instant adjustment" is the expectation that a remarriage with children recreates a nuclear family. Particularly in the United States the "ideal" family is the close-knit, one unit, nuclear family. Although to the anthropologist this is a relatively recent family type, it is the "family" to which all other families are compared—and found inferior. Having grown up in this tradition, adults in remarriage families very frequently embark upon the impossible and often psychologically damaging task of forcing the stepfamily into a nuclear family mold. Unfortunately, they are often pressured to do so by friends and relatives and at times by mental health professionals. Because several major structural characteristics of step-families are different from those of nuclear families, clinicians need to be able to incorporate this new family pattern into their thinking so they will be more helpful to individuals in stepfamilies.

STRUCTURAL CHARACTERISTICS OF STEPFAMILIES

The two most important goals for families are the creation of autonomous children and the stabilization of parental personality and competence (4). The tasks which must be performed to reach these goals are different for stepfamilies than they are for nuclear families because of major structural differences between the two types of families. Six major structural differences which distinguish stepfamilies from nuclear families are discussed below.

1. A Stepfamily is A Family Born of Loss

Even when there has not been a death, after a divorce a love relationship has been lost, parents and children have been separated, and numerous other losses may have taken place, i.e., the loss of friends, relatives, or a familiar community. The dream of a marriage uncomplicated by former spouses and instant children is also lost, and for the children a remarriage means the loss of an exclusive relationship with the remarried parent.

The first task of stepfamilies is the need to finish the mourning of earlier losses, and to accept a family different from the one of former dreams and expectations.

2. All Individuals Come Complete with Family Histories

Not only do the adults carry with them baggage from their family of origin, but they may also carry baggage from previous marriage families and former single-parent households. All the children, particularly half-grown individuals, come equipped with expectations and "givens" from previous families, rather than arriving unburdened, unformed and helpless as they were at birth. Only children may be dropped into a gang of several stepsiblings, laissez-faire rule may clash with martial law, and the myriad of daily activities may bog down in the mire of unanticipated differences. It is essential to negotiate and renegotiate differences between all members of the stepfamily. In this way a new tradition or a new "sentimental order" (7) for this particular family has its beginning. Family meetings can often be a means to this end, though for some stepfamilies such meetings are productive only when a clinician is present.

3. Parent-Child Relationships Precede the New Couple Bond

It is the quality of the relationship between the couple that determines the life of the stepfamily and this is a new and tender relationship compared to existing parent-child relationships. There are many forces at work which pull at this new relationship, among them lack of cultural and institutional supports, parental guilt at forming a primary relationship with a new spouse, and jealousies between various members of the stepfamily.

Stepparents, stepchildren, and stepsiblings as well are suddenly attempting to work out their relationships. If different groupings of family members (e.g., stepparent-stepchildren, parent-child, stepparent-one stepchild) plan satisfying times together, the older relationships can begin to merge with the newer ones and stepfamily integration results.

Parents and stepparents often need considerable help in nurturing their new relationships and they may seek professional guidance because of their lack of unity. Clinical intervention can be extremely beneficial in providing information regarding stepfamily characteristics, together with support for a strong couple alliance.

4. There is a Biological Parent Somewhere Else

When the other biological parent has died, the adults may have fewer feelings of helplessness, and there may be less ambiguity in their deadlines regarding family plans. However, the former spouse may become an idealized ghost, thereby producing loyalty conflicts for the remaining parent as well as for the children, and intruding in many ways into the midst of the remarried family.

When there has been a divorce, the need to share children may create a sea of pain. All too often the children become pawns and messengers between their two biological parents. A parent without custody often withdraws from contact with the children because the emotional climate and the frequent good-byes are so painful.

Helping parents and stepparents accept and respect the parenting skills of all the parental adults in the children's lives is of profound importance. If this can materialize, then the children are free to relate to stepparents as well as to both biological parents, and more cohesiveness and satisfaction are possible for each family unit.

5. The Children Are Often Members of Two Households

Because the children are swinging back and forth between two households which are likely to be very different from one another, there are transition periods that produce strains for everyone involved. When the children arrive, there are fights as adjustments to the new environment are made, and before they leave the children may become unruly. As one 12-year-old said, "I can be bad then because there won't be any time to really punish me because I'll be leaving right away."

In addition, saying "hello" and "good-bye" symbolizes uncertainty and change and as such produces anxiety. For the adults as well as for the children, these shifts in family organization are difficult. There is no stability to the family system: As soon as Suzy warms up to the family dog, learns to slide down the slide with her stepsiblings, and wants her stepmother to read her a bedtime story, she is gone for two weeks. Or in another stepfamily, just as Martha and Tom have learned how to juggle their lives so that they can go to work, play with the three children, and snatch a few hours for themselves, the din subsides and the children have left. And like the tide this process keeps repeating itself.

Even when the adults are willing to accept differing family systems as simply being "different" and not "right" and "wrong," the constant shifting of the family organization can create a sense of living in a home built on quicksand. If the couple forms a stable and satisfying couple relationship, this can provide the necessary continuity and family stability. This alliance and security also allow the couple to feel less threat from outside their own four walls, so that the children have the freedom to come and go. Although managing the family is like playing an accordion, the instrument itself remains intact as its shifting shape produces rich and melodic music.

6. There Is No Legal Relationship between Stepparents and Stepchildren

The fact that stepparents have no legal relationship to their stepchildren leads some stepparents to maintain considerable emotional distance between them and their stepchildren. They wish to avoid the pain that would accompany a change in custody arrangements allowing them less contact with their stepchildren, or the loss that would follow the death of their spouse or another divorce which would leave them with no legal rights to be with their stepchildren.

This is a legal area in which the law lags behind. The laws are being interpreted and changed in the direction of more custody and visitation rights for stepparents, but there remains a long road ahead for this legislation.

More pervasive and nagging are the less dramatic daily inconveniences which produce a sense of non-existence for stepparents—not being recognized as a person able to sign the permission slip for a stepchild's school camp-out; not being recognized as a person able to sign for medical and dental procedures (except in life and death situations in which the responsibility actually rests with the medical profession); not being included in court investigations of a custody change that will bring a stepchild to live in the stepparent's household. Such invisibility is not faced by biological parents with custody, though at times biological parents without custody face similar legal discrimination.

When there are minor children in the home, clinicians at times need to advise stepparents of these legal problems. Lawyers can provide legal agreements to be signed by the biological parents giving the stepparent (or at times where necessary, the non-custodial parent) the right to sign for the children. At times the custodial parent is unwilling to relinquish this control to the stepparent or the non-custodial parent refuses to sign such a document. In these cases, the custodial parent may be willing to sign a general agreement giving such authority to all persons responsible for the children, such as school personnel, family attorney, or medical practitioners.

Summary

Although the goals of all families are similar, because of different cultural myths and different family characteristics, the paths to these goals are different for stepfamilies than for nuclear families. Stepparenting is different from parenting.

Because of the complexity and stress, an increasing number of individuals in stepfamilies are seeking professional guidance. Clinicians can provide valuable support as they help remarried parents and stepparents recognize the challenges they face and assist them in their mastery of the necessary tasks for family growth and integration.

THERAPEUTIC HELP WITH STEPFAMILY TASKS

Procedural Considerations

In order to achieve their goals there are four major stages, or tasks, for stepfamilies to master. While these can be listed in a chronological order, in reality stepfamilies deal with components of all stages simultaneously and as a result all tasks need addressing in various stages of therapy.

The tasks may be categorized in the following manner:
a) Mourning various losses.
b) Negotiation of previous traditions and development of new stepfamily traditions.
c) Development of new interpersonal relationships and preservation
   of older parent-child relationships.
d) Family integration and personal individuation.

In helping remarried parents and stepparents with these tasks, it is important for clinicians to consider the fact that remarried couples have had
no time to adjust to one another or consolidate their relationship before
there are ex-spouses phoning at inconvenient times, and children banging
on the bedroom door and bouncing on the bed, or unexpectedly arriving on
the doorstep suitcase in hand to move in with the parent and new stepparent.

Difficulties with the children are the most common reasons for remarried
parents and stepparents to seek professional help. The relationships are often
very tenuous and the feelings may be violent and unacceptable to the individuals themselves, as well as to the other stepfamily members. As a result,
nearly all verbal expression is blocked until the adults feel some security in
their relationship. When this occurs, the adults are then better able to
tolerate negative feelings from the children and from one another in regard
to the children.

Even when couples have been married for many months, they may never
have achieved a sense of couple solidarity. In biological families a strong
couple alliance is necessary for optimal family functioning (3); with the added
relational complexities of stepfamilies, such a bond seems vital.

Clinicians can support couple unity by seeing the couple together, unless
this approach seems inadvisable, and not including the children until there
is enough emotional glue to hold the couple together. Even when children
need to be seen, they can be seen separately from the adults.

Clinicians can often be helpful by providing education and direct feedback
and concrete suggestions at the beginning of therapy contacts with stepparent
couples. Sharing information about the characteristics of stepfamilies with
the couple or with the individual adult, if both are not present, can be
extremely productive. Articles and books on stepfamilies or referral to stepparent groups are helpful for many adults, as these reduce the sense of
isolation and personal failure.

Very often the couple needs direct guidance in establishing a few essential
limits at home so that chaos can be replaced by enough stability to deal with
the tasks outlined previously. For example, Mary and Charles agree that
they will leave food for Charles' 16-year-old son, Bill, to heat for himself

when he arrives home three hours later than he has promised—rather than waiting for Bill to arrive, all the time growing more hungry and irritable and erupting into the daily battle of "I know more about child-rearing than you do."

Providing options and an atmosphere in which alternatives can be discussed is at times crucial, because stepfamily pressures often appear completely overwhelming. Helplessness and a sense of panic are common to stepparent couples as they feel trapped in a web of circumstances. It is freeing and calming for them to hear that the children will survive staying with a sitter for a few days, attending boarding school, or continuing to live with the other biological parent, so that family relationships can be explored and worked out, and further decisions made.

At times, therapists and counselors are willing to see together all of the parental adults in a child's life. This is usually done in an attempt to free the child from being a tale bearer, messenger, or pawn between angry ex-spouses. Ex-spouses are not ex-parents, and many times they are willing to accept parenting abilities in each other.

Raising the possibility of such a meeting (once the new couple has attained adequate couple security) is often enough to produce direct contact between the parental adults outside therapy. While there are a few stepparents who feel comfortable leaving such discussions to the two biological parents, in most instances stepparents need to be included with their spouses in these interviews. This is one more message as to the importance of couple unity in their involvement with the children. In such contacts, with or without the presence of a therapist, the focus is on the welfare of the child, not on understanding and repairing severed interpersonal relationships.

As is true with all types of families, working with the adults may be all that is necessary to bring about needed changes. With older children in many stepfamilies more contact is needed with them and with the family as a whole to work out satisfactory stepfamily relationships.

Countertransference may be a particular problem in working with step-parents. A therapist may find it easy to listen to a woman describe her jealousies towards fellow workers in a fortune cookie factory, yet find many deep feelings stirred by listening to a stepmother describe her jealousies towards her husband and his children. Whereas the therapist has no experience with life in a fortune cookie factory, he or she has a wealth of experience with biological families, both personal and professional, and so the territory feels familiar. As a result, the stepmother's strong reactions seem bizarre, or at least revealing of deep personal problems. While there are certainly stepparents with severe intrapsychic difficulties, many garden-variety stepparents are frequently seen as villains, and important interpersonal elements are overlooked by clinicians as they identify with the biologic parent. It is difficult at times to avoid this trap, and when this negative countertransference does occur, the stepfamily situation can deteriorate further as the stepparent attempts to become a member of an existing group, which includes the therapist as well as the biological parent and children. A contrasting example would be one in which the therapist is a stepparent, and as such over-identifies with the stepparent in the family being seen. In this situation objectivity and sound clinical judgment may be lost because of the strong positive countertransference. As a result, the stepfamily may find the therapist pushing in directions that are not helpful for this particular family. Familiarity with the literature on stepfamilies (8) can help clinicians deal with their countertransference feelings.

Stage I. Mourning Various Losses

Any choice requires giving up something else, and any marriage involves losses—a family of origin, a familiar community, or a circle of friends. Remarriage with children, however, is born from many very painful losses. The intensity of the loss goes unrecognized by many, and as a result there is often incomplete mourning and non-acceptance of the sadness of other stepfamily members.

Clinicians can help individuals relinquish long-held dreams and expectations of marriage and family. There is pain and grief at these losses and therapeutic sensitivity to the feelings of adults is important. Therapists and counselors working with children in stepfamilies are usually more empathetic to the child's sorrow and anger at total or partial separation from a parent, or from a familiar school and friends. They are also understanding of the child's added sense of loss when a parent remarries and must now be shared with another adult and perhaps with other children. It may be more difficult to recognize the pain that accompanies the death of a dream or a fantasy.

An initial hour with one young woman is illustrative of the psychological pain involved:

Sally sought help because she was about to be married to a man with two children aged eight and 11. She had not been married previously and she wanted to talk about ways in which to work into the family unit as smoothly as possible.

Sally had read books on child development and she asked many perceptive and pertinent questions. She was also familiar with the characteristics of stepfamilies and she talked about fears of her future in this new family situation.

Towards the end of the hour Sally spoke of feeling much more reassured, and also of wanting to cry. She could think of no reason why she felt like crying, but when asked about her dreams of marriage she burst into tears. The remainder of the time was full of sorrow as Sally began to recognize and also let go of her dreams of a honeymoon in Hawaii followed by evenings with her husband in a cozy little apartment all their own.

Identification of her losses and understanding of her sorrow made it possible for Sally to later turn her attention to the gains that lay ahead for her.

When a first marriage family has failed to live up to cherished expectations, a remarriage family is often besieged by even greater expectations. To some adults it seems like a last chance to realize longed-for family happiness. Giving up a cherished fantasy and accepting the stepfamily for what it is may take time. If therapists push too hard, a wall of resistance may be the only result.

The losses are many, and often severe. Grandparents in their own hurt and anger may have disowned their grandchildren, or be unaccepting of stepgrandchildren; stepmothers may have left supportive jobs to stay home and be "full-time" mothers and stepmothers; remarried fathers may withdraw from their children because of the pain of separations; friends and a familiar community may have been replaced by hostile neighbors and a strange environment. And above all, no matter how hard the adults struggle, a stepfamily cannot be poured into the "ideal" biological family mold. It is a different type of family and acceptance of its uniqueness is a necessary prerequisite for appreciation and joy in its richness of experience and relationship.

Professional guidance through the many rejections and losses they experience may be one of the greatest needs of adults in stepfamilies.

Stage II. Negotiation of Previous Traditions and Development of New Stepfamily Traditions

When any two organizations merge, traditions and ways of doing things previously taken for granted suddenly pop into awareness. In stepfamilies all individuals come together from diverse backgrounds. An important task becomes that of negotiating and working out a new stepfamily system.

In first marriages the "givens" that must be negotiated come from the parents' families of origin. Not so with remarriages. There have been one or more "marriage family patterns," and children also have a pattern from their birth family. The way the house is cleaned, the car washed, the spaghetti made is different in every household, and in the merging of individuals from differing family backgrounds clashes are inevitable. Resolution of these differences is basic to stepfamily unity.

Discipline problems lurk around every corner because the adults have already worked out separate parenting styles in former marriage families. A stepparent with no children has only a fantasized parenting style unmodified by the mundane realities of child-rearing. Thus it becomes important for the life of the stepfamily to help the adults accept that "givens" are "emotionally" rather than "rationally" based (the "sentimental order" of Stern (7)), and therefore not "right" or "wrong," but simply "different" ways of doing things.

A sense of family comes from shared experiences, and stepfamilies can begin new traditions from the day of the remarriage. It is important, however, for clinicians to help the adults include input from the children in the negotiations, particularly when the children are preteen or teenagers.

Stage III. Development of New Interpersonal Relationships and Preservation of Older Parent-Child Relationships

An essential task, and a difficult one for stepfamilies, is the development of new interpersonal relationships. Stepparents and stepchildren are dealing with added relationships which lack the freedom of choice of other relationships. Unfortunately, there is often a great deal of pressure for stepparents and stepchildren to love one another, a demand that leads to guilt and anger. Relationships take time to develop, and clinicians can act to slow down the adult's mad rush to achieve instant adjustment and caring relationships between stepparents and stepchildren.

A child raised by someone else cannot possibly reflect a stepparent's training, and in many families stepparents get locked into power struggles with stepchildren as they attempt to force their values on the children.

In first marriages, when a child is born there is a time of nurturance prior to the need for training and limit-setting; in a stepfamily there is a need for a friendly relationship between stepparent and stepchild before the child is willing to accept the values of the stepparent. Stepparents need to back away and let the biological parent deal with the child while building up a friendly and trusting relationship.

Stepparents and stepchildren can often relate well when the biological parent is not present. Encouragement of quality sharing times together to build this new relationship can work towards stepfamily integration. In addition, children's fears of losing their biological parent to stepparent and stepsiblings can be lessened by their having time alone with that parent.

Helping the new couple nourish its own relationship is a key issue for many stepparents. While the presenting problems are focused on the children, the basic difficulty may have to do with a lack of commitment the stepparent feels from his or her spouse. Ex-spouses seem to come first, or grandparents of the children who do not accept the stepparent, or friends from the previous marriage who reject the new partner. Joan and Eric represent one type of situation where a lack of couple unity was precipitating a new family breakup:

Joan and Eric came to a counselor because Eric's 15-year-old son, Rick, was causing so much tension in the home that the couple was about to separate. Rick was uncooperative, surly and disobedient. He swore at Joan and Eric alike and precipitated many fights between the couple over his behavior.

Joan found Rick's behavior unacceptable and was furious with him. Eric felt guilty that Rick was living with them because Rick's mother had rejected him, and Eric was angry at Joan's constant complaints about Rick. Eric spent a great deal of time talking with his son, while Joan felt isolated and miserable, and Rick continued his undisciplined behavior.

When Eric suddenly realized that he was going to need to make a choice between moving out with Rick or forming an alliance with Joan, he gave Joan a strong commitment to the marriage. Immediately Joan's isolation evaporated, as did her anger at her stepson and Eric's anger at her.

Rick continued his undisciplined behavior at first, and then slowly began to change because he no longer was able to divide the couple and bring his father running to his side.

Stage IV. Family Integration and Personal Individuation

As losses are accepted, new traditions negotiated, and stepfamily relationships strengthened, integration takes place. For more complete integration and personal growth, there is an added element: the necessity of dealing with ex-spouses or "other parents."

Children are part of two parents and, with a few exceptions, if there is space for them to relate to both of their biological parents, it appears that they are more self-confident and secure (9). Having access to both parents also enables children to accept stepparents more readily since they feel less need to choose sides. If there is cooperation between the children's two households, paradoxically the stepfamily is more integrated and unified. When this cooperation is not present, or even at times when it is, teenagers separate from both families at a younger age than do adolescents in biological families. Perceiving this as a teenager's natural response to a remarriage helps both parents and stepparents feel less personally involved and rejected.

With the passing of time, the healing of memories takes place, and as the children mature and become independent they are able to form independent relationships with parents and stepparents alike, provided relationship doors have remained open to them.

Even when lack of cooperation and strained relationships continue to exist between ex-spouses, and the sharing of children remains painful and difficult, if the stepparent couple is emotionally close the stepfamily remains intact. The children have the experience of a functioning couple to use as a model for their own adult lives.

No perfect models are yet available for stepfamilies or therapists and counselors working with them. Therefore, it is a temptation for clinicians to retreat to biological family models when confronted with the array of stepfamily systems. Compared to biological families, viable stepfamily systems appear to be infinite in number. Children in stepfamilies grow and join their peers from biological families, arriving at similar places, albeit by different routes (1, 10), and adults in stepfamilies grow and achieve personal stability within a myriad of kaleidescopic patterns.

REFERENCES

1. BOHANNAN, P. J. and ERICKSON, R. J. (1978). Stepping in. *Psychology Today,* Jan. :53.
2. JACOBSON, D. S. (1979). Stepfamilies: Myths and realities. *J. of the National Association of Social Work,* 24:202.
3. LEWIS, J. M., BEAVERS, W. R., GOSSETT, J. T., and PHILLIPS, V. (1976). *No Single Thread.* New York: Brunner/Mazel.
4. LEWIS, J. (1979). Personal communication.
5. NADLER, J. H. (1976). Unpublished doctoral thesis on psychological stress of the stepmother.
6. SCHULMAN, G. L. (1972). Myths that intrude on the adaptation of the stepfamily. *Social Casework,* 49:131.
7. STERN, P. N. (1978). Stepfather families: Integration around child discipline. *Issues in Mental Health Nursing,* 1:50.
8. VISHER, E. B. and VISHER, J. S. (1979). *Stepfamilies: A Guide to Working with Stepparents and Stepchildren.* New York: Brunner/Mazel.
9. WALLERSTEIN, J. S. and KELLY, J. B. (1976). The effects of parental divorce experiences of the child in later latency. *Am. J. Orthopsychiat,* 46:256-269.
10. WILSON, K. L., ZURCHER, L. A., MCADAMS, D. C., and CURTIS, R. L. (1975). Stepfathers and stepchildren: An exploratory analysis from two national surveys. *J. of Marriage and The Family,* 37:526-536.

23

SCHIZOPHRENIA IN MIDDLE AGE

JOHN S. STRAUSS, M.D.

Department of Psychiatry,
Yale University School of Medicine
New Haven, Connecticut

INTRODUCTION

Schizophrenia was originally called "dementia praecox" because the cases so identified involved mental deterioration that started earlier than most other dementias. Some of the first cases, such as Morel's patient with "démence précoce" (which probably was actually a case of syphilis), were found in adolescence and young adulthood, giving rise to the frequent misconception that the onset of schizophrenia occurs almost exclusively in those ages. In fact, most studies (e.g., 2) show a fairly gradually diminishing incidence curve for schizophrenia between the ages of 15 and 54. Slightly over half as many patients have the onset of schizophrenia in the age group 25-35, as between ages 15-24. About the same number have the onset between ages 35-54 as between 25-34. Several schizophrenia incidence studies use first hospitalization data to define onset, but even recognizing that first psychiatric admission may occur somewhat later than onset of disorder (23), it is clear that the onset of schizophrenia in middle age is hardly rare.

In considering schizophrenia in middle age, another group of patients besides individuals with recent onset consists of those with the disorder starting earlier, in whom it has persisted. Although schizophrenia is neither as "praecox" nor as "dementia"—in the sense of invariably chronic—as was originally believed, still the prognosis for anyone with the disorder must be at least somewhat guarded. Thus, individuals with an onset of schizophrenia in adolescence and young adulthood, in whom recovery is not complete, make up a second large group of middle-aged schizophrenics.

Does the existence of these two groups of schizophrenics have any par-

366

ticular clinical importance? Is the age factor worth noting, or is only the presence of schizophrenia the significant element? Judging by the minimum amount of literature written on the topic, the importance of middle age in these patients would seem to be negligible. A search of abstracts and textbooks reveals no systematic clinical stuides focusing on the importance of the age variable for theory or practice, other than epidemiologic studies primarily cataloging incidence and prevalence figures at various ages. Perhaps this is because developmental aspects of middle age in general have only recently been widely recognized (10, 20), so that in many contexts the characteristics of this age period have been viewed as unimportant. Since absence of data or references does not necessarily indicate absence of importance, however, this report will explore whether the two groups of middle-aged schizophrenics, the recent onset and more chronic patients, are of particular interest because of age-related factors, in terms of understanding etiology and prognosis and in providing treatment for them and working with their families.

ONSET IN MIDDLE AGE AND THE ETIOLOGY OF SCHIZOPHRENIA

The onset of a significant number of cases of schizophrenia in middle age could reflect four possibilities—random distribution, late-occurring organic vulnerability, causal patterns of psychosocial stress, or some combination of these. In considering any of these four hypotheses, it is also important to include another replicated finding—the age of onset male/female correlation. In practically all epidemiologic studies of schizophrenia, the mean age of onset in men is about ten years earlier than the age in women. Even careful studies to rule out artifacts of diagnosis produce the same results (11). Perhaps because epidemiologic data are so often not considered in clinical research and practice, this repeated finding has generally not been incorporated into these aspects of psychiatry or theories that emerge from them.

Unfortunately, at the same time the age/sex findings do not provide any definitive answers. The one conclusion that can be drawn from epidemiologic data on age/sex patterns in schizophrenia onset is that no simple etiologic explanation seems adequate. Adolescent hormonal changes or separation from parents clearly do not account for the large percentage of schizophrenic disorders beginning between ages 30 and 50. Nor does the average age at onset/sex difference allow for a simple theory of vulnerability caused by organic-maturation. Rather, the wide age range of onset, the significant number of new cases in middle age, and the age/sex differential suggest some more complex contribution of these factors to etiology (e.g., 5). One possible pattern of complex causation is that the differentials in age/sex of onset and the wide range of onset distribution reflect an interaction of environmental stress and organic vulnerability. For example, organic vulnerability to schizophrenia might cause a decompensation when the individual is faced with certain stresses. Men might be more stressed by demands for autonomy during ages 15-24 and women might be more stressed by family responsibilities between ages 25-35. Such a hypothesis could be formulated in more detail and preliminary tests of it could be carried out with methodologies now available (12, 16).

Perhaps more about middle age onset schizophrenia and its implications for etiology can be learned by considering clinical reports suggesting that schizophrenia arising in mid-life is often different in symptoms and prognosis from schizophrenia with an earlier age of onset. In the past, reports emphasized the poorer prognosis and more disorganized clinical pictures presented by patients with earlier onset schizophrenia. In fact, many questioned whether the more organized clinical pictures of delusional psychosis occurring in mid-life could accurately be considered as schizophrenia, and alternative labels such as "involutional psychosis" were sometimes used for these patients. Although clinical impressions about the validity of these observations persist, the newer, more reliable methods of descriptive and epidemiologic psychiatry have not yet been used to test them in detail.

If one assumes that mid-life onset schizophrenia does often have a particular clinical picture, then several implications follow. Individuals who get through their childhood, adolescence, and early adulthood without becoming schizophrenic might be viewed as having or acquiring the organic and/or psychosocial and developmental strengths to provide a firm foundation of basic social skills. These skills might mitigate the impact of schizophrenia or assist in recovery from it. Thus, age of onset in these clinical observations relates to the vast literature on premorbid adjustment (13). The better the premorbid adjustment (more probable at later ages of first onset), the less virulent the disorder is likely to be. The nature of such an interaction between premorbid adjustment and type of disorder is still largely unknown. However, it is commonly believed that later onset schizophrenia is more likely to be of a paranoid subtype, in which many areas of thinking, affect, and social function are left generally intact and deterioration is not a marked feature (5).

The new diagnostic approaches using a multiaxial structure may help to test these clinical impressions. Multiaxial diagnoses classify a patient in terms of several labels or "axes" rather than just one—such as "schizophrenia." The new APA diagnostic manual, DSM-III, for example, uses five axes:

syndrome, personality, physical illness, psychosocial stressors, and social competence. If these axes are systematically and reliably used, it will be possible by a review of records—or, even better from a sampling perspective, a community survey—to determine the degree to which the relationships among premorbid social adjustment, syndrome type and age of onset are valid.

In reviewing the implications of mid-life schizophrenia for etiology, we thus arrive at more disconfirmation of previous supposed answers than at a final resolution. The interaction between age of onset and sex is too solid a finding to be ignored. It suggests that a complex causal view rather than a simple maturation or leaving home type model of cause be adopted. Perhaps a model of organic or developmental vulnerability interacting with the peak stress periods characteristic of certain life phases is the best way to speculate about the age/sex incidence findings. The possible existence of a different clinical picture supposedly more common in mid-life than in early adulthood and adolescence, with better premorbid function and more organized delusional symptoms, further complicates an understanding of etiology. In spite of the unfortunate complexity involved, it might be most accurate to suppose a four-way interaction between syndrome type, premorbid adjustment, age, and stress that accounts for the patterns of mid-life schizophrenia. There is evidence that such a pattern does exist (13), although the data have not always fit as neatly as might have been hoped.

One hypothesis that may best synthesize the existing information, including the wide range and variations in age/sex and the particular clinical characteristics involved, would state that schizophrenia—especially in terms of positive symptoms such as delusions and hallucinations—is a relatively nonspecific response to severe stress. The likelihood of such a response appears to have a small but significant genetic contribution. Another contribution might be from developmentally influenced patterns of information-processing, coping mechanisms, and personal definition of what situations are stressful. Decompensations created by combinations of these factors can and do come at any age. The specific way and degree to which the person decompensates within various potential patterns of schizophrenia would be influenced by the strength and type of coping mechanisms he has.

This is not a simple view, and more operational definition of the variables involved may make it less so. But then it is often surprising how in working with psychiatric phenomena we still hope for even relatively simple answers, whereas many other branches of medicine have long since given up such a hope. Understanding mechanisms involved in hypertension, for example, requires consideration of about 18 variables related by interacting patterns forming a network of systems. Are the etiologies of schizophrenia likely to be less complex?

THE PROGNOSIS OF SCHIZOPHRENIA IN MID-LIFE

As noted earlier, there are two groups of patients with schizophrenia in mid-life, those with recent onset and those whose disorder, starting at a younger age, has persisted. This distinction is particularly important for prognosis. As described in earlier reports, the prognosis of schizophrenia is not homogeneous (17). Even if diagnostic criteria are used that include indices such as social relations functioning or prior duration of disorder, which in themselves are prognostically valid for a variety of psychiatric disorders, the range of patient outcomes is considerable. Rather than expecting any diagnosis to provide the ultimate in defining prognosis, available evidence now suggests that prognosis may best be considered as several semi-independent processes or axes. These are social relations function, symptom severity, symptom type, occupational function, and need for hospitalization. Each of these characteristics appears to be the best predictor of its own level at follow-up, although in most instances there is also a significant but weaker predictive power across variables as well.

Considering these basic principles of prognosis, it is clear that mid-life schizophrenics who have been dysfunctional for some time will have a worse prognosis than patients with more recent onset. Thus, regardless of factors like developmental level that may be associated with specific age of onset, if one takes a population of patients at any given age, those who have had the disorder for an extended period are more likely to continue to have chronic disorder in the future. One study that controls for this potential artifact by selecting patients at varying ages of onset and following all for the same duration does not find age of onset in itself to be a significant predictor of outcome (19).

It must also be remembered that no prognostic indices, alone or in combination, can be counted on to predict outcome definitively for the individual patient. At best, the correlations of predictors with outcome sometimes reach as high as $r = 50$. Even at that level, the predictor or predictors account for only one-fourth of the variance in the outcome measure.

Thus, systematic studies suggest both the value and limitations of several prognostic indices. This fits with reports of Bleuler (4) and others describing chronic schizophrenics who late in life begin to recover dramatically. In fact, prognosis in mid-life schizophrenia may be of particular interest because at that time a process must exist in even some of the most chronic patients that paves the way for or at least permits later improvement.

It seems most likely from available information that there is nothing special in the prognosis of mid-life schizophrenia. Patients with a long history of disorder or poor social or work function have a worse prognosis than those with recent onset and good pre-illness functioning. If, as seems likely, most mid-life first-episode schizophrenic patients are in the good prognosis group, and if first-episode patients in this age range actually do recover fairly consistently, it may be "only" because they follow the more general rule.

TREATMENT OF MID-LIFE SCHIZOPHRENIA

Much has been learned about the treatment of schizophrenia in general and perhaps mid-life schizophrenia in particular. This learning has involved what not to do as well as what treatment programs should be used. Perhaps most certain is that the patient should not be isolated in a monotonous, long-term, no-expectation, custodial treatment environment. The tendency to "put away" severely disturbed schizophrenic patients, causing them to lose any social or occupational skills they had, sever ties with their family and community, and lose motivation has been revealed as an important source of chronicity (3, 22). Beyond this, the use, singly or in combination, of medications, milieu, individual, family or group psychotherapy, behavior modification, occupational and social skills training programs may be helpful. For some types of treatment, such as antipsychotic medications and goal-oriented group and milieu programs, effectiveness, at least with some patients, has been rather definitely shown (14). For other types of treatment and treatment combinations, clinical experience suggests they can be valuable, but systematic evidence to support the impressions has not been generated. Given this state of affairs, perhaps the best solution is to proceed with treatment planning on the basis of clinical judgment, informed where possible by available data and the most likely conceptual formulations. It is, as always, important to avoid being blinded by current treatment styles to the extent of ignoring what the patient is saying and demonstrating in terms of specific treatment needs.

In choosing among the various conceptualizations, one possibility is to view schizophrenia as a disorder with many aspects, each of which may need to be dealt with. The multiaxial structure described earlier for diagnosis and prognosis provides a framework for such a view of treatment. A treatment program can be designed that attempts to note problems with symptoms, styles of coping, stressful life events, social relations, occupational function, and family and living context (18). The use of medications, psychotherapies, milieu, management of environmental and family problems, interpersonal skills training, and occupational programs can be considered and focused in terms of those needs revealed by the comprehensive patient assessment necessary for multiaxial diagnosis.

But besides specific programs for specific problems, another essential part of the treatment for such patients is the clinician working with the patient in a continuing way. The need for such a person and his or her precise role is disputed widely and practice varies all the way from treatment in some medication clinics, where no such person exists, to psychoanalysis. But whether the clinician providing a center and a continuity for treatment is a "case manager" or a psychotherapist, considerable skill is required, and for clinicians with limited training, supervision is essential. Such a person is needed not only to coordinate the various treatment efforts, but to continue to assess areas of stress and competence, and to help the patient and family deal with the problems involved and understand them to the degree possible.

For treating schizophrenia, a clinician as the center of treatment is also required because the disorder tends to persist. Such persistence has two implications: The features of the disorder and treatment needs may shift over time, and the course of the disorder plays a part in the development of the individual and his family. Although the specifics of adult development and stages of family evolution are still being argued, there is increasing belief that important development in these areas does exist. As such development takes place, the demands and support characteristics of the environment change, the expectations on the patient shift, conflicts may lessen or resolve, and disabilities may come to have fewer harmful effects. Perhaps it is by such a process, possibly combined with hormonal and other organic shifts, that the unexpected remissions noted by Bleuler in his long-term follow-up studies of schizophrenic patients can be explained. In any case, only the central role provided by a skilled clinician can tailor treatment to these changing characteristics of the disorder, the person, and the environment.

THE ROLE OF THE FAMILY

Although many persons with mid-life schizophrenia have no families, many others do. In this age group, the impact of the disorder on spouses and children and reciprocal impacts on the patient may be especially profound and should not be ignored by treatment providers interested in affecting the course of disorder in the patient and in the welfare of the family. It is important to emphasize this point because so often the scarce resources available for working with the more severely disturbed patients are used for the patient alone in order to meet the needs of all those coming for care.

Such a focus may often be self-defeating, as suggested by recent evidence about the family's impact on the course of the patient's disorder and the patient's impact on the family. Studies by Vaughn and Leff (21) suggest that certain patterns of "expressed emotion" in families may contribute to recurrence of symptoms in schizophrenic persons. Intrusive and demeaning patterns of relations appear to be especially important in this regard. Attempts to treat these types of communication are now under way to see if changes in them will improve the course of disorder in patients living with such families (7).

Another important part of the patient-family interaction is the frequently neglected phenomenon of the impact the patient has on the family. Many reports have described this impact as a burden that the symptomatic patient puts on family members (9). Such a burden may actually be only one component of a more complex interactive system. Clausen (6) and Freeman and Simmons (8) have shown ways in which spouses respond to the onset and course of disorder in their mates. Patterns of support, denial, derogation, demand, and neglect are as complex as would be expected when families of different types and in different states, made up of people with various pesonality styles and coping mechanisms, collide with a severe, often frightening, disorder with such a wide range of manifestations and beliefs about it.

When the patient is middle-aged, children are often involved in the problems of the family. For such children, the difficulties are apparently especially severe if the schizophrenic disorder is manifested in some partial, erratic, or non-florid way (1). Given the mutual impact of patient and family members, it is impressive how relatively few treatment settings still do not (in some instances, cannot) attend to the family context of the schizophrenic patient.

Clearly, it is important for treatment settings to help meet family needs for the benefit of all concerned. There are several methods proposed for working with such families, including counseling and conjoint family psychotherapy using interpretive, role-playing, or other techniques. Although it is not yet clear which of these is effective and how this effectiveness is influenced by the type of family involved, avoiding the issue by ignoring the family situation seems the least defensible practice of all.

CONCLUSION

Considered together, the etiologic, prognostic, treatment, and family implications of schizophrenia in middle age are reminiscent of many of the issues raised in discussions of involutional melancholia. Is it a separate disorder? What are the etiologic roles of organic and psychosocial factors? What specific treatment needs are involved? For schizophrenia in middle age, many of these questions can be answered only by a combination of data, clinical judgment, and speculation. One solution that may be most reasonable is to view middle age as one of several biopsychosocial contexts in which schizophrenia occurs. This context and its shifts over time probably involve certain types of organic and psychoscial stresses, supports, demands, and rewards that help to determine the occurrence of schizophrenia, its prognosis, and optimal treatment planning, and in turn are influenced by the disorder in an interactive way. In this complexity, with its mixture of knowledge, ignorance, and speculation, the multiaxial approach can lend structure to approaches for assessment, conceptualization, and treatment. Hopefully, such a multidimensional approach will also provide a clearer foundation for a more comprehensive theory of schizophrenia in mid-life. A systems theory using clearly-defined concepts may be the most accurate to explain the findings that are emerging (15). Perhaps with an approach of that kind, the understandable but somewhat aggravating ambiguities and lacunae of our current knowledge in the field will begin to be resolved.

REFERENCES

1. ANTHONY, E. J. (1970). The impact of mental and phsyical illness on family life. *Am. J. Psychiat.*, 127(2):138-146.
2. BABIGIAN, H. (1975). Schizophrenia, epidemiology. In: A. Freedman, H. Kaplan, and B. Sadock (eds.), *Comprehensive Textbook of Psychiatry II*. Baltimore: Williams & Wilkins, pp. 860-865.
3. BARTON, R. (1959). *Institutional Neurosis*. Bristol: Wright.
4. BLEULER, M. (1974). The long-term course of the schizophrenic psychoses. *Psychol. Med.*, 4:244-254.
5. BOWERS, M. B., STEIDL, J., RABINOVITCH, D., BRENNER, J. W. and NELSON, J. C. (1980). Psychotic illness in mid-life. In: W. H. Norman and T. J. Scaramella (eds.), *Mid-Life: Developmental and Clinical Issues*. New York: Brunner/Mazel.
6. CLAUSEN, J. (1975). The impact of mental illness: A twenty-year follow-up In: R. Wirt, G. Winokur, and M. Roff (eds.), *Volume 4, Life History Research in Psychopathology*, Minneapolis: University of Minnesota Press.
7. FALLOON, I. and LIBERMAN, R. Personal communication.
8. FREEMAN, H. and SIMMONS, O. (1963). *The Mental Patient Comes Home*. New York: Wiley.
9. GRAD, J. and SAINSBURY, P. Evaluating a community care service. In: H. Freeman and J. Farndale (eds.). *Trends in Mental Health Services*.
10. LEVINSON, D. J. with DARROES, C. N., KLEIN, E. B., LEVINSON, M. H., and McKEE, B.

(1978). *The Seasons of a Man's Life*. New York: Knopf.

11. LEWINE, R., STRAUSS, J. S., and GIFT, T. E. Sex differences in age at first hospital admission for schizophrenia: Fact or artifact? Submitted for publication.

12. MYERS, J. K., LINDENTHAL, J., PEPPER, M., and OSTRANDER, D. (1974). Life events and mental status: A longitudinal study. *J. Health & Soc. Behav., 18*:398-405.

13. PHILLIPS, L., BROVERMAN, I. K., and ZIGLER, E. (1968). Sphere dominance, role orientation, and diagnosis. *J. Abn. Psychol., 73*(4):306-312.

14. STRAUSS, J. S. (1979). Psychosocial treatments for schizophrenia: New directions for practice and research. Report to NIMH.

15. STRAUSS, J. S. (1979). Towards an operational systems model for psychopathology: I. Basic principles as suggested in the relationship between work and symptoms. Presented at the McLean Symposium in honor of Alfred Stanton, June.

16. STRAUSS, J. S. (1980). The prevention of chronicity. *Psychiatric Annals, 10* (9):23-29.

17. STRAUSS, J. S. and CARPENTER, W. T. (1974). Characteristic symptoms and outcome in schizophrenia. *Arch. Gen. Psychiat., 30*:429-434.

18. STRAUSS, J. S., DOCHERTY, J. P., and DOWNEY, T. W. (1980). Towards comprehensive understanding and treatment of schizophrenia. In: J. Strauss, M. Bowers, T. Downey, S. Fleck, S. Jackson and I. Levine, (eds.), *Psychotherapy Treatments for Schizophrenia*, New York: Plenum.

19. STRAUSS, J. S., KOKES, R. F., RITZLER, B. A., HARDER, D. W., and GIFT, T. E. (1979). Is social competence a valid axis for DSM III? Presented at the 1979 Annual Meeting of the American Psychiatric Association.

20. VAILLANT, G. E. (1977). *Adaptation to Life*. Boston: Little, Brown.

21. VAUGHAN, C. and LEFF, J. (1976). The influence of family and social factors on the course of psychiatric illness. *Br. J. Psychiat., 129*:125-137.

22. WING, J. and BROWN, G. (1970). *Institutionalism and Schizophrenia*. Cambridge: Cambridge University Press.

23. ZERBIN-RUDIN, E. (1963). *Zür erbpathologie der schizophrenien: Mitteilungen der Max Planck Gesellschaft*, pp. 87-101.

24

THE MENTALLY RETARDED IN MIDDLE AGE

J. M. BERG, M.B., B.CH., M.SC., F.R.C. PSYCH., F.C.C.M.G.

Director of Genetic Services and Biomedical Research,
Surrey Place Centre, Toronto, Canada;
Professor of Psychiatry and of
Medical Genetics, University of Toronto

and

A. J. DALTON, PH.D.

Director of Behavioural Research, Surrey Place Centre;
Research Associate, Department of Physiology,
University of Toronto

> *. . . . For age is opportunity no less*
> *Than youth itself, though in another dress . . . .*

Henry Wadsworth Longfellow, 1875, *Morituri Salutamus*

INTRODUCTION

There are two particular widely applicable circumstances which have made the mentally retarded adult, as he or she advances from young adulthood to middle age and beyond, a focus of increasing attention in recent times. First, improved life expectancy, among the handicapped as well as in the general population, has resulted in the presence of greater numbers of retarded persons of advancing years. Second, growing interest in the natural

376

history and in the quality of life of these individuals, with advocacy of active rehabilitative (as opposed to passive custodial) arrangements for them, has led to more frequent appraisal of their characteristics and needs. Such appraisals have involved various disciplines, including biomedical, psychological, social and educational ones. Nevertheless, study and documentation of the retarded adult are still much less extensive than that of the retarded child. For the reasons indicated, a reasonably comprehensive review seems timely in the context of the present volume. An attempt to do so is presented in this chapter.

BIOMEDICAL CONSIDERATIONS

Life Expectancy

Considerations bearing on life expectancy in the mentally retarded were presented by Richards (45) in a previous volume in this series concerned with old age, and therefore need not be dealt with in detail here. Richards noted, in studies of mentally retarded persons admitted to an English institution, that the death rate of these persons was appreciably higher than that of the general population at all ages. The excess mortality, for both sexes, was greatest below 20 years, with quite rapid diminution of this excess as adult age advanced. Furthermore, excluding Down's syndrome, he found that the more severe the degree of mental handicap, the less the chance of survival. Interestingly enough, in view of evidence of relatively early onset and increased severity of Alzheimer's disease in Down's syndrome (see page 387), the extent to which the death rate of adults with the syndrome exceeded that of other adults with similar mental levels increased at ages above 40 years.

Observations on life expectancy, based on large samples of retarded individuals, have been reported during the 1970s from other countries also, for instance by Forssman and Akesson (21) in Sweden and by Balakrishnan and Wolf (3) in Canada. Though sample composition and methodological approaches have varied, overall findings are quite similar to those described above. In addition, it is apparent from these investigations that life expectancy for the intellectually impaired in general has increased in recent times, as indeed it has for the population at large. The improved prospect of retarded persons reaching middle age and older years and differential mortality rates amongst them are relevant considerations in determining the nature, and planning the extent, of suitable rehabilitative and other measures.

General Physical Health

The incidence of physical abnormalities and poor general health is relatively high among the mentally retarded, particularly among those whose retardation is severe. As in the population as a whole, mentally retarded persons with major congenital defects of internal organs, such as the heart, are likely to have a lower life expectancy than those without such defects. A significant number of the former do not reach middle age, so that serious congenital abnormalities of vital organs is a concern largely at younger ages. On the other hand, less life endangering defects, such as sensory and motor ones, are compatible with long life and are to be expected in many middle-aged retarded individuals. Callison et al. (10), for example, demonstrated greater impairment in near vision, visual field functions, auditory acuity and grip strength in a longitudinal study of relatively mildly retarded middle-aged individuals, compared to chronic schizophrenics and to mentally normal controls. Such impairments are very likely to be even more frequent in more markedly retarded persons, a consideration which is illustrated by the study of Reynolds and Reynolds (44). In a large sample of mentally retarded adults (mean age = 35 years) living in community residential facilities in New York State, they found a greater prevalence of both speech and hearing problems in those with lower, as opposed to those with higher, mental levels.

Additionally, though comprehensive information on the subject is practically non-existent, it may well be that efficient functioning of various body systems, such as the endocrine, gastro-intestinal and genito-urinary ones, does not continue for as long a time as in the general population. A further consideration is that many who are mentally retarded live in comparatively adverse physical environments with such characteristics as overcrowding, poor hygiene and improper diet, resulting in both increased exposure and less resistance to infections and the like.

Because of the increased probability of health problems referred to above, and because mentally retarded individuals are less likely than others to complain about symptoms indicative of ill-health, periodic medical check-ups (say annually), which have become a feature in many countries for middle-aged persons in general, seem especially desirable for the mentally retarded. This has been a sensible practice for long years in institutions and group homes for the retarded, though often in too cursory a format to be entirely effective.

It would be remiss not to refer also to the question of dental health. The distressing, even appalling, dental state of many residents in mental retardation institutions was exemplified in a report by MacFarlane (35). Though written some 20 years ago, it is unlikely that the picture has changed dramatically since then. In a survey of 1941 residents, of all ages and grades, in two English retardation institutions, he found that only 7.9% were dentally healthy and needed no treatment. All the rest required prostheses, scaling, gum treatment and/or extraction. Though age-related data were not provided, it can be anticipated that the state of the oral cavity in those not encouraged to practice dental hygiene and not provided with dental services will worsen as age advances. The middle-aged retarded individual in these circumstances, whether in an institution or in the community, has additional burdens of oral pain, discomfort and infection, as well as aesthetic unattractiveness, all largely preventable, heaped upon his or her other disadvantages.

Mental Health

In general, disturbed behaviour, ranging from relatively minor peculiarities to frank psychosis, occurs among middle-aged mentally retarded persons with many similar clinical manifestations to those found in others of like age. The subject is largely neglected in psychiatric journals and books. When reference to it is made, it is usually in the context of institutionalized populations. Such populations very often contain an overrepresentation of the mentally disturbed and ill, partly because aberrant behavior can present itself as incompetence and is frequently a reason for admission, and partly because institutional environments can precipitate pressures and frustrations which may lead to such symptoms as withdrawal, negativism, aggression, sexual deviations, stereotypies and mannerisms.

In most instances, behavioural disturbances and other evidence of psychiatric ill-health have an onset before middle age and persist till then and later. The causes are no doubt as varied, and often as obscure, as in the rest of the population. In some cases, as mentioned above, environmental stresses may be aetiologically crucial. In others, there appears to be a direct causal link with the underlying cerebral pathology which also was responsible for the mental deficit. Tuberous sclerosis (Bourneville's disease) is an example. Many, though by no means all, adults with this autosomal dominant disorder tend to be hyperactive and self-injurious or otherwise destructive, and distinct psychotic features are not unusual. Critchley and Earl (14) regarded a primitive type of catatonic schizophrenia as an "inextricably intertwined" accompaniment of mental defect in tuberous sclerosis; various other psychoses also have been described, for instance by Herkert et al. (28).

Aberrations of the sex chromosomes, such as a supernumerary X or Y, provide examples of a different kind of biological defect in which there is an association, both in children and adults, with mental illness, as well as with usually relatively mild mental deficit. Both women (51) and men (1) with an extra X chromosome appear to show an increased incidence of various psychiatric disturbances, and males with an extra Y chromosome frequently have been reported to have antisocial and violent propensities of different degrees of seriousness (7). It is as well to add a word of caution that accounts of such cases may create impressions of a characteristic behavioural stereotype for each of these chromosome disorders, which is demonstrably invalid in many instances (6). This reservation is perhaps particularly applicable in regard to the so-called XYY syndrome because of a considerable literature linking the additional Y chromosome with crime.

With reference to criminality in the mentally retarded in general, there is conflicting evidence of a possible relationship of mental deficit with certain types of criminal offences (42), whether such crime is considered to be a manifestation of mental illness or not. Such attention as the subject has received usually has been in relation to adolescents and young adults rather than the middle-aged. A relevant consideration in this sphere is the prospect that retarded offenders are more likely to be apprehended than brighter ones.

The problems of recognizing and differentiating various types of mental illness in retarded adults are well exemplified by studies of Penrose (41) and, more recently, of Reid (43) and of Heaton-Ward (27). They each undertook investigations in large mental retardation institutions in Britain. Psychiatric disorders found in such institutions are, to some extent, classified differently by different observers. Furthermore, prevalence figures for these disorders in institutions are almost certainly not representative for mentally retarded adults in general for reasons indicated above and because of the influence of varying admission and discharge policies and practices. In addition, associated mental deficit, particularly in the most gravely retarded patients, can modify, or even mask, manifestations of psychiatric disturbance. In the profoundly retarded at least, inability to communicate adequately increases the difficulty of delineating mental ill-health, and divergent views about diagnostic criteria add further pitfalls.

Despite these dilemmas, the studies mentioned provide instructive data on mental illness in retarded adults. Penrose (41) found psychopathy (defined broadly as psychosis, psychoneurosis, and such forms of behaviour disorder as alcoholism, perversion and delinquency) more often in patients of higher, than those of lower, mental level. Of the two main forms of psychosis described, schizophrenia was commoner than affective disorder, the latter

being particularly unusual in patients with I.Q. below 50. Reid (43) concluded that manic-depressive, schizophrenic and paranoid psychoses could
be diagnosed on usual clinical grounds in relatively less markedly retarded
patients, but that such diagnoses were more difficult, if not impossible, in
profoundly and some severely retarded cases because of communication
barriers. Heaton-Ward's (27) findings were rather similar.

Among conclusions which may be drawn from the observations of these
investigators is that psychiatric disturbance in mentally retarded adults is
at least as widespread and varied as in the general population, with different
prevalence rates at different mental levels, and with special diagnostic difficulties in the most gravely retarded. It may be added here that Reid's and
Heaton-Ward's texts include helpful observations on the efficacy in retarded
adults of traditional forms of physical treatment (drugs, electroconvulsive
therapy) for various psychoses. In essence, such treatment appears to be
about as beneficial as in psychotic patients generally, though it is difficult
to draw definite conclusions.

Observations bearing on the question of dementia in some retarded adults
have been reported over a number of years. In particular, it has been noted
that neuropathological findings of Alzheimer's disease are substantially more
common, and more marked, in older Down's syndrome adults than in similarly aged persons with other varieties of intellectual defect. Malamud (36)
described these findings (mainly consisting of senile plaques, neurofibrillary
tangles and granulovacuolar changes in a diffusely atrophic brain) over the
age of 40 years in 35 out of 35 (100%) Down's syndrome individuals and in
31 out of 225 (14%) miscellaneous patients with other types of mental retardation; in large samples of adults below 40 years the corresponding per-
centages were 1.6% and 0%, respectively. The exact effects of such
pathology, or its precursors, on mental function in surviving persons is not
entirely clear. However, clinically apparent intellectual and emotional deterioration leading to dementia certainly occurs in some, and precise neu-
ropsychological tests, such as those of short-term visual retention, have
shown greater deficits in Down's syndrome adults over 44 years old compared
to younger ones (16). These defects have been correlated with computerized
transaxial tomography (CTT scan) evidence of cortical atrophy and ventricular
enlargement (15). One wonders whether various psychoses, which are pe-
riodically reported in adults with Down's syndrome (49), may be at least
partially explicable in terms of the cerebral pathology referred to above. It
may be added here, parenthetically, that age-related tissue changes in
Down's syndrome adults, differing in frequency, time of onset and extent
from like changes in other retarded adults, are not confined to the central

nervous system. Sylvester (50), for example, found that fenestrations of the aortic and pulmonary valves occurred much more often, and probably earlier and more severely, with increasing age after 30 years, in Down's syndrome individuals than in controls with other types of mental deficit.

Sexuality and Reproduction

Concerns about sexual inclinations and habits of mentally retarded persons usually are based on fears that they may be sexually deviant or, more commonly, that they will have children who are abnormal or for whom they cannot provide adequate attention and care. Though such concerns are focused mainly on younger, rather than older, adults, some reference to the subject in the context of the present chapter seems appropriate.

Sexual deviations and perversions do occur, of course, among mentally retarded adults as they do in others, including very intelligent individuals. It is by no means clearly apparent, however, that such occurrences are more prevalent among retarded persons than among others of comparable age and sociocultural background. Penrose (42) referred to failure of concealment and less restrictive canons of behaviour in the backgrounds of many retarded persons as factors which could influence views about prevalence. It may be added that institutional environments, involving deliberate or inadvertent barriers to heterosexual contacts and relationships, also would serve to encourage alternative sexual activity which might be regarded as aberrant. Ironically enough, therefore, those who would inhibit or prevent heterosexual pursuits for retarded adults for fear of sexual misconduct are in effect encouraging, however unintentionally, aberrant sexual behaviour. It is a consideration which requires close attention in making provisions for the well-being of the retarded, including those of middle age.

With regard to reproduction, a distinction between potential parents who are relatively severely (say I.Q. below 50) and relatively mildly retarded is useful. Most of the distinct genetic disorders (specific gene defects and autosomal chromosome abnormalities) connected with mental retardation, which frequently involve high risks to offspring, are usually associated with severe retardation. In these circumstances, a potential parent, if he or she survives to adulthood, is often infertile or even sterile. For instance, reproductive incapacity certainly accounts to a large extent for the facts that only a couple of dozen fully affected Down's syndrome females have been reported to have been mothers and that no non-mosaic Down's syndrome male is known to have been a father (49). By contrast, many midly retarded adults are about as fertile as adults in general and their children tend to be retarded or intellectually dull also, though commonly less so than their parents (47). Often more heat than light is generated in the long-standing debate as to the relative contributions of nature and nurture to the mental level of these children, a subject beyond the scope of the present chapter. There is concern also, quite properly, about the psychological stresses which raising children may impose on some parents whose capacity to cope with substantial responsibilities is limited.

Whether it is genetically or socially wise to have children or not is a matter for individual decisions (often advantageously assisted by appropriate counselling) in individual couples, be they retarded, of average intelligence or bright. No "across-the-board" edicts on reproduction for a particular group, who constitute as varied a segment of society as the retarded, are, in our view, justified. Certainly, heterosexual relationships and marriage in fertile retarded adults, including the middle-aged, are not precluded by a conclusion that child-bearing should be avoided, particularly in the light of increasing availability of birth control measures which are largely simple and secure and likely to become more so in the future.

PSYCHOLOGICAL CONSIDERATIONS

Intelligence

A clear understanding of how intelligence develops and changes with increasing age in mentally retarded adults has significant implications in planning for their needs. A long-standing, conventional view is that intellectual capacity of mentally retarded persons gradually deteriorates with age. Recently, however, this view has been vigorously disputed.

Conflicting results have been obtained by using one or the other of two traditional modes of investigation, namely the cross-sectional or longitudinal method. The cross-sectional approach requires that several groups of subjects of different ages be tested at the same time, whereas the longitudinal approach necessitates re-testing of the same group of individuals on different occasions spread over an extended period. Most cross-sectional studies have supported the notion of intellectual decline with age, while longitudinal investigations have usually indicated that intellectual abilities either do not decline or show continued improvement well into middle age (4). The principal methodological problem with the cross-sectional method is that differences in I.Q. which seemingly are due to age may actually be due to generational or cohort differences. The longitudinal method, by contrast, can have the disadvantage of selective loss of subjects over the years, as, for example, when brighter participants are absorbed into the general population. The difficulties inherent in both methods have been overcome partly in studies which combine features of each in so-called "semi-longitudinal" (17) or "cross-sequential" (25) investigations, thus resulting in a more accurate picture of age-related developmental changes in intellectual abilities.

Bell and Zubek (5) tested 100 mentally retarded adults employing the Wechsler-Bellevue Intelligence Scale (Form I), and re-tested the same individuals five years later. The sample was composed of five different age groups, each group consisting of persons with similar backgrounds and environments. The results unequivocally indicated that each age group, except the oldest (over 50 years), showed significant gains in I.Q. scores on retest. The gains ranged from 4.4 points to 9.1 points, and corresponded well with those reported earlier by others (12, 13). The largest I.Q. gains were registered by "young" (aged 25 to 34 years) and "middle-aged" (35 to 44 years) adults. Those over 45 years old showed I.Q. scores which did not hold up well with age, and the I.Q. scores of those in the over-50 age group were significantly lower than those of any of the other age groups studied. I.Q. scores, uncorrected for age, were lower for the older groups at the outset of the study, possibly reflecting the effect of cohort differences. The usual "age correction" provided in the Wechsler manual for intelligence testing would automatically obscure this difference.

Fisher and Zeaman (19) conducted a large archival study involving I.Q. test and re-test records of 1,159 mentally retarded persons living in institutions and ranging in age from childhood to over 75 years. Stanford-Binet mental age scores constituted the basic data for each case studied semi-longitudinally. They concluded that mental age (MA) continues to grow at least until the late 30s and that a tendency to decline occurs only with advancing age after 60 years. Furthermore, they reported that, at similar levels of retardation, sex and diagnostic category had little effect on the growth of intelligence with age. In a partial replication of Fisher and Zeaman's study, Demaine and Silverstein (17) examined 189 individuals with Down's syndrome ranging in age from four to 50 years (20 cases were 30 to 40 years old and six were 40 to 50) and a second group of 189 persons with other varieties of mental retardation. All had been tested at least twice with the Stanford-Binet. They found a strong linear increase in MA from four to 16 years after which MA tended to level off with little or no differences between the subjects with and without Down's syndrome. The authors suggested that age-related changes in MA may be the same for all retarded persons, whether they had Down's syndrome or not.

Conflicting findings on the relationship of age to intellectual functioning could be due to various factors. For example, commonly employed tests of intellectual capacity, such as the Stanford-Binet and Wechsler tests, have not been standardized with residents in institutions, so that apparent age-related changes in I.Q. may reflect an unknown contribution of the institutional environment. Most of the relevant research has focused on children and young adults with little participation of middle-aged adults. The discharge policies of many institutions often result in the release of brighter, younger residents. This "brain drain" may produce an impression that older institutionalized retarded persons are duller than younger ones. Such a possibility was examined recently by Goodman (25), who consistently found an increase in I.Q. scores with age when the selective effect of subject "attrition" was eliminated. She also noted substantially higher I.Q. scores on the Wechsler Adult Intelligence Scale in 144 mentally retarded adults released to the community, compared with 140 still-institutionalized persons of comparable age and years in the institution. Kramer et al. (31) previously had observed a similar phenomenon. They reported that more than half of the retarded adults who were released from an institution to community-based residential facilities were persons with I.Q. scores above 50, thus resulting in a bias favouring lower I.Q. scores with age if only those who remained in the institution were studied.

In recent years, a promising approach to the study of intellectual changes with age has focused on investigating the developmental growth of specific capabilities rather than on tracing the course of intelligence considered as a single global capacity. Thus, Goodman (24) has suggested that "fluid intelligence" (that is, functions such as attention span and ability to change a set and to resist distraction, which can be measured by the Porteus Maze and Raven's Progressive Matrices tests) takes a different developmental path for retarded adults than for non-retarded ones in the age range of 26 to 43 years. Furthermore, she reported that older retarded adults did better on tests of fluid intelligence than a comparable group of young retarded adults aged 19 to 25 years. These results are particularly significant since fluid intelligence normally is expected to be highly vulnerable to the aging process in comparison to "crystallized intelligence" (that is, abilities such as verbal comprehension, general knowledge and social awareness, which can be measured by vocabulary, information and language comprehension tests).

In a different sphere, attempts to determine relationships between intelligence and various parameters of electrical activity of the brain in retarded persons merit mention, even though nearly all studies have been conducted on children or young adults. For example, a correlation has been found between I.Q. score and visual evoked potentials (20). From a review of the literature by Ellingson and Lathrop (18), a less convincing relationship is apparent between the frequency of electroencephalogram alpha rhythm and intelligence. These authors, in an investigation of their own, found no significant differences between Down's syndrome individuals aged 13 to 42 years, non-retarded psychiatric patients and healthy university students. Nevertheless, with improvements in recording, analytical and computational methods, this avenue of investigation may yield important new insights in the future.

Adaptive Behaviour

There is currently a major endeavour, in many countries, to achieve greater participation of the mentally retarded in as many facets of general community life as possible. For such participation to be effective, a certain level of personal and social competence is necessary. The prospects of achieving this understandably have appeared much more realistic for relatively midly or moderately retarded persons than for severely or profoundly retarded ones. In the former cases, provided that behaviour is not disturbed or otherwise bizarre, that demands made and responsibilities are not beyond the capacities of those affected and that supportive social and vocational resources are available, satisfactory adaptation in the general environment is very often attained. Indeed, the large majority of mildy retarded or mentally dull adults function adequately in society, without specific intervention by any agencies, if the fact that they do not come into conflict with authority or their neighbours is used as a yardstick.

Until recent years, there seemed little hope of producing significant changes in the behavioural competence of severely and profoundly retarded individuals. However, in the past few decades, new teaching and training methods, often based on operant conditioning techniques, have engendered greater optimism. For example, a thorough review of 565 published papers, largely concerned with progress in this sphere from 1955 to 1974, indicates an impressive array of socially advantageous behavioural achievements in markedly retarded persons (8). Most operant conditioning studies have involved children. However, successes with seriously retarded adults now are being reported increasingly in teaching such simple, but useful, skills as, for instance, using a telephone (34) or bus (29) and in modifying disruptive behaviour (30), with consequent increase in functional independence.

Developmental changes throughout life in various aspects of adaptive behaviour of retarded persons, with different intellectual levels and living in different circumstances, have been studied by a number of investigators.

The Adaptive Behaviour Scale of the American Association on Mental Deficiency, developed by Nihira et al. (40) in California, has been widely used for these purposes. Using this Scale, Nihira (38, 39), for example, documented changes with age in the behavioural dimensions of personal self-sufficiency, community self-sufficiency and personal-social responsibility in a large number of retarded individuals, including many adults.

One of us (A.J.D.), in collaboration with S. M. Cibiri and L. J. Jackson, investigated 581 institutionalized retarded adults (Down's syndrome excluded) aged 20 years and over, employing a 320-item behaviour rating schedule called the Basic Life Skills Scale (BLS) (11). About 10% of the subjects were mildly retarded and the rest were distributed approximately equally thoughout all lower intellectual levels. Figure 1 provides a preliminary analysis of these data for five different adult age groups. The performance ratings for the eight behavioural skills assessed, designated A to H in the Figure, were undertaken by residential counsellors familiar with the persons they rated. These BLS performance ratings, or scores, were on a six-point scale from 0 to 5, ranging from total inability (lowest scores) to competent ability (highest scores) at performing the skills in question. The figure shows mean differences, which are statistically significant, for these values in different age groups. The explanations for this are elusive and require further detailed study in regard to such age-related social and medical variables as, for instance, selective admission and discharge policies and sensory defects, respectively. For the present purpose, however, these findings, like the above-mentioned observations of Nihira, convey the important message that, in general, retarded adults of various ages (including those with marked mental defect) show adaptive behaviour capacities which substantially exceed the very limited expectations usually held out for them in the past.

Despite the complexities, well-designed studies aimed at better understanding of age-related changes in intellectual and adaptive behaviour capacities in the mentally retarded certainly are desirable, all the more so as efforts increase to develop beneficial living, teaching and vocational arrangements for them. Wise decisions about such arrangements, and their evaluation, depend to a significant extent on knowledge of potentials, and limitations, at different ages in different types and degrees of mental deficit. Retarded adults in particular, especially older ones, have to date received less attention in these respects than they deserve.

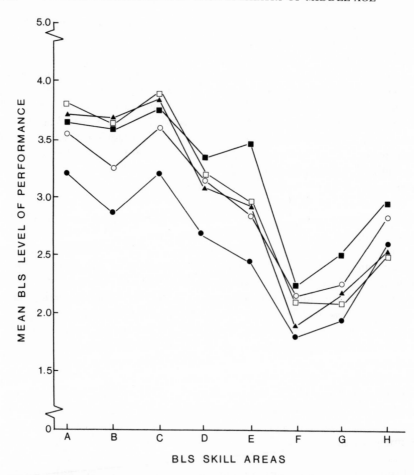

Figure 1. Profiles of basic life skills as a function of age, in retarded adults, based on performance rating scores employing the Basic Life Skills Scale (BLS).

Note: Skill areas measured are indicated by letters (A = Motor; B = Perceptual; C = Self-
care; D = Communication; E = Social; F = Community Living; G = Academic;
H = Personal-Social).

Age groups: ● = 20-29 (n = 336); ○ = 30-39 (n = 134); ■ = 40-49 (n = 43); □ = 50-59
(n = 32); ▲ = 60 and older (n = 36).

SOCIAL CONSIDERATIONS

Living Arrangements

Perhaps the most significant recent trend in many countries, with respect to living arrangements for retarded persons, has been the growing advocacy of the proposition that accommodation in small units or homes in the general community is more advantageous for them than life in large, often relatively isolated, institutions. These views are being expressed in relation to the retarded of all ages and mental levels, and middle-aged adults, among others, increasingly are being housed alongside mentally normal neighbours. The trend is in many ways laudable in that its rationale is derived from the premises that the intellectually impaired do not constitute a menace to society and that rehabilitative measures are preferable to mere custodial ones.

However, a generous outlook and honourable intentions by themselves are not enough; there remains a need for constructively critical research and evaluation as to what kinds of accommodation and associated arrangements are most suitable for whom. This involves a better understanding of the capacities linked with the many types of mental retardation at various ages, as well as of the large number of variables in the environment (including public attitudes and the availability and quality of supportive services) which may enhance or detract from these capacities. Among other considerations, stereotypes of "institutions" as invariably deleterious and of "community homes" as necessarily meritorious should be abandoned. It could well be, for instance, that some gravely retarded persons (particularly those with concomitant handicaps) are better off in an institution, and that some community residences lead to virtual imprisonment within narrow confines because of concerns about, say, passing traffic or upsetting neighbours. Several substantial reviews, covering many facets of the whole subject, have been published recently, among which those of Baker et al. (2), McCarver and Craig (37), Rosen et al. (46) and of Heal et al. (26) may be referred to as instructive sources of information.

As mentioned earlier, a high proportion of mildly retarded or intellectually dull adults manage their affairs adequately largely on their own without special intervention by others, and many are reasonably competent in such major respects as maintaining their own homes, establishing stable personal relationships, participating in satisfying social pursuits, and achieving useful vocational goals. Others can do so with support from responsible community agencies or relatives. At the other end of the scale, the problems of the profoundly retarded are often compounded by physical disabilities, and they need extensive protection and supervision throughout life.

The few attempts that have been made to measure and assess various living arrangements for the mentally retarded of middle age have been concerned mainly with those whose mental levels fall between the extremes of borderline or mild and profound intellectual deficit. Even in these studies, the middle-aged usually are part of a larger sample of persons with a wide age range. Examples of recent studies of this type are those undertaken by Schroeder and Henes (48) and by Birenbaum and Re (9). Schroeder and Henes compared 19 persons (mean chronological and mental ages were 29 and five years, respectively), who had been discharged up to two years previously from an institution to group homes, with a matched sample of residents who remained in the institution. Those in the group homes progressed significantly more in communication skills, but less so in self-help and socialization skills, than the controls. Birenbaum and Re reported on 63 adults, with an average I.Q. of 50, who had left institutions at the mean age of 32 years to live in a community residence in a large United States city. After almost four years, some had advanced in the direction of more independent living, others had been returned to the original institution apparently because of behavioural problems, and the majority remained in the group home in what the authors called "a prosaic routine of sleep, work and at home recreation of a passive nature" not too different, they felt, from that of marginally employed or unemployed non-retarded individuals.

The findings in such investigations have been diverse and even contradictory, which is not surprising in view of the large array of personal and environmental variables which influence outcome. The mentally retarded of middle age are certainly among those on whom methodologically sound further study is necessary to determine the impact of these variables, for better or worse, on their prospects. All the more reason for doing so is the fact that large numbers of retarded persons are surviving to middle age and beyond. Furthermore, because of advancing years, death or incapacity of their parents deprive many of them of close attention and concerned interest in parental homes which frequently are significant bulwarks and supports in the lives of more youthful intellectually impaired individuals.

Vocational Aspects

Many of the considerations raised in regard to living arrangements for mentally retarded adults apply also to vocational matters. The two circumstances usually are closely linked when provisions for these individuals are being contemplated and made. As in other respects, retarded adults differ greatly in their vocational capabilities, with a range from practically complete helplessness to able and responsible performance of quite complex and sophisticated jobs. Where a particular individual fits in this wide specturm depends on many factors, including intellectual level, adaptive capacity, degree of emotional stability, and type of training. Work prospects are dependent also on the economic and social climate in any society, in that these circumstances largely determine availability and competition for employment, as well as attitudes of potential employers, fellow-workers and the general public.

It is important to emphasize that even markedly retarded adults can function well in some jobs if they are reasonably stable, motivated and appropriately taught. An illustrative example concerns a severely retarded middle-aged man who had spent much of his life in an institution where he learned to operate a machine which transformed strands of wire into fencing. He much enjoyed his work, performed it with great efficiency, and liked to encourage visiting dignitaries to try their hands at it because he was amused by the frequently incompetent efforts on their parts! Gold (22, 23) is among those who have been active proponents of the proposition that persons with severe retardation are substantially more capable of mastering work complexities and achieving levels of productivity than they traditionally have been given credit for. In the light of this consideration, appropriate vocational training and opportunities are eminently desirable, because suitable productive pursuits, as opposed to enforced and tedious idleness, are emotionally advantageous to the individual and of practical benefit to the community as a whole.

In reality, only a minority of those under consideration are satisfactorily employed. In Britain, for example, it has been noted that less than 5% of the approximately 32,000 trainees in community-based Adult Training Centres (mainly severely and moderately retarded adults) are so employed, despite reliable estimates that more than double that percentage of trainees could succeed in open employment and a further 25% in sheltered work settings (52). A study of a rather brighter, and probably older, sample in the United States points in the same direction (32). In this instance, only 17 out of 75 moderately or midly retarded adults, aged 40 years and over, living in Ohio communities were found to be employed, 11 competitively in salaried or wage-paying positions and the remaining six in workshops. If this is the situation in relatively affluent and developed countries like the United Kingdom and the United States, the position is almost certainly even less satisfactory in most, if not all, poorer developing nations.

Kriger, who conducted the last-mentioned study, is one of the few investigators who has paid special attention to aging and aged retarded adults. Her enquiries and observations on the subject (32, 33) are illuminating, and include findings which strongly suggest that such persons, even though housed in the community, generally appear to participate minimally, if at all, in community life. Furthermore, she pointed out that few, if any, guidelines or criteria are available about them with regard to appropriate and necessary services, programmes and facilities. This applies as much to vocational concerns as to other aspects of rehabilitation. Clearly, it is necessary to devote much more effort than heretofore to the characteristics and needs of the mentally retarded of middle age and older years.

CONCLUDING REMARKS

Middle age, however defined, merges imperceptibly with earlier and later periods of life. Its boundaries, like many of those between countries, are largely man-made, arbitrary and prone to modification. Furthermore, there are few, if any, features of mentally retarded persons which are confined exclusively to the middle-aged and which do not manifest themselves earlier and/or persist later. Observations in the present chapter, therefore, though focused on middle age, inevitably are concerned to some extent also with younger and older individuals.

It is important to emphasize that the middle-aged retarded, like those in other age groups, do not constitute a unitary, circumscribed entity about whom sweeping generalizations are valid. They differ widely, of course, in such respects as aetiology, mental levels, behavioural manifestations and physical findings. Thus, methods of investigation and assessment, no less than biomedical, psychological, social and educational measures for their well-being, may be appropriate for some, but not for others.

Middle-aged retarded individuals constitute a substantial proportion of the intellectually handicapped, with numbers which have grown as mortality in younger years has declined. A recurrent theme in this chapter has been evidence of the relative paucity of data available about them, and hence the necessity for more intensive study of their characteristics and needs. This is a vital prerequisite in helping them to function in as optimal a manner as possible, with consequent benefits not only to themselves but also to the communities in which they live.

REFERENCES

1. AKESSON, H. O., FORSSMAN, H., WAHLSTRÖM, J., and WALLIN, L. (1974). Sex chromosome aneuploidy among men in three Swedish hospitals for the mentally retarded and maladjusted. *Brit. J. Psychiat.*, *125*, 386-389.
2. BAKER, B. L., SELTZER, G. B., and SELTZER, M. M. (1974). *As Close as Possible: A Study of Community Residences for Retarded Adults*. Cambridge, Mass.: Behavioural Education Projects.
3. BALAKRISHNAN, T. R., and WOLF, L. C. (1976). Life expectancy of mentally retarded persons in Canadian institutions. *Amer. J. Ment. Defic.*, *80*, 650-662.
4. BARTON, E. M., PLEMONS, J. K., WILLIS, S. L., and BALTES, P. B. (1975). Recent findings on adult and gerontological intelligence. *Amer. Behav. Scientist*, *19*, 224-236.
5. BELL, A., and ZUBEK, J. P. (1960). The effect of age on the intellectual performance of mental defectives. *J. Geront.*, *15*, 285-295.
6. BERG, J. M., and LOWY, F. H. (1975). XYY syndrome: A comment. *Mod. Med. of Canada*, *30*, 692-693.
7. BERG, J. M., and SMITH, G. F. (1971). Behaviour and intelligence in males with XYY sex chromosomes. In: D. A. A. Primrose (ed.), *Proceedings of the Second Congress of the International Association for the Scientific Study of Mental Deficiency*. Warsaw: Polish Medical Publishers, pp. 135-141.
8. BERKSON, G., and LANDESMAN-DWYER, S. (1977). Behavioural research on severe and profound mental retardation (1955-1974). *Amer. J. Ment. Defic. 81*, 428-454.
9. BIRENBAUM, A., and RE, M. A. (1979). Resettling mentally retarded adults in the community—almost 4 years later. *Amer. J. Ment. Defic.*, *83*, 323-329.
10. CALLISON, D. A., ARMSTRONG, H. F., ELAM, L., CANNON, R. L., PAISLEY, C. B., and HIMWICH, H. E. (1971). The effects of aging on schizophrenic and mentally defective patients: Visual, auditory, and grip strength measurements. *J. Geront.*, *26*, 137-145.
11. CIBIRI, S. M., and JACKSON, L. J. (1976). *Basic Life Skills Scale: A Method for Evaluation of Developmentally Handicapped Persons' Functional Independence*. Toronto: Ontario Ministry of Community and Social Services.
12. CLARKE, A. D. B., and CLARKE, A. M. (1954). Cognitive changes in the feebleminded. *Brit. J. Psychol.*, *45*, 173-179.
13. CLARKE, A. D. B., CLARKE, A. M., and REIMAN, S. (1958). Cognitive and social changes in the feebleminded—three further studies. *Brit. J. Psychol.*, *49*, 144-157.
14. CRITCHLEY, C., and EARL, C. J. C. (1932). Tuberose sclerosis and allied conditions. *Brain*, *55*, 311-346.
15. DALTON, A. J., and CRAPPER, D. R. (1977). Down's syndrome and aging of the brain. In: P. Mittler (ed.), *Research to Practice in Mental Retardation*. Vol. 3. Baltimore: University Park Press, pp. 391-400.
16. DALTON, A. J., CRAPPER, D. R., and SCHLOTTERER, G. R. (1974). Alzheimer's disease in Down's syndrome: Visual retention deficits. *Cortex*, *10*, 366-377.
17. DEMAINE, G. C., and SILVERSTEIN, A. B. (1978). MA changes in institutionalized Down's syndrome persons: a semi-longitudinal approach. *Amer. J. Ment. Defic.*, *82*, 429-432.
18. ELLINGSON, R. J., and LATHROP, G. H. (1973). Intelligence and frequency of the alpha rhythm. *Amer. J. Ment. Defic.*, *78*, 334-338.
19. FISHER, M. A., and ZEAMAN, D. (1970). Growth and decline of retardate intelligence. In: N. R. Ellis (ed.), *International Review of Research in Mental Retardation*. New York: Academic Press. Vol. 4, pp. 151-189.
20. FLINN, J. M., KIRSCH, A. D., and FLINN, E.A. (1976). Correlations between intelligence and the frequency content of the visual evoked potential. *Physiol. Psychol.*, *5*, 11-15.
21. FORSSMAN, H., and AKESSON, H. O. (1970). Mortality of the mentally deficent: a study of 12,903 institutionalised subjects. *J. Ment. Defic. Res.*, *14*, 276-294.

22. GOLD, M. W. (1973). Research on the vocational habilitation of the retarded: The present, the future. In: N.R. Ellis (Ed.), *International Review of Research in Mental Retardation*. New York: Academic Press Vol. 6, pp. 97-147.

23. GOLD, M. W. (1975). Vocational training. In: J. Wortis (ed.), *Mental Retardation and Developmental Disabilities*. Vol. VII, New York: Brunner/Mazel. pp. 254-264.

24. GOODMAN, J. F. (1977). Aging and intelligence in young retarded adults: a cross-sectional study of fluid abilities in three samples. *Psychol. Rep., 41*, 255-263.

25. GOODMAN, J. F. (1977). IQ decline in mentally retarded adults: a matter of fact or methodological flaw. *J. Ment. Defic. Res., 21*, 199-203.

26. HEAL, L. W., SIGELMAN, C. K., and SWITZKY, H. N. (1978). Research on community residential alternatives for the mentally retarded. In: N. R. Ellis (ed.). *International Review of Research in Mental Retardation*. Vol. 9. New York: Academic Press, pp. 210-249.

27. HEATON-WARD, A. (1977). Psychosis in mental handicap. *Brit. J. Psychiat., 130*, 525-533.

28. HERKERT, E. E., WALD, A., and ROMERO, O. (1972) Tuberous sclerosis and schizophrenia. *Dis. Nerv. Syst., 33*, 439-445.

29. HUGSON, E. A., and BROWN, R. I. (1975). A bus training programme for mentally retarded adults. *Brit. J. Ment. Subnorm., 21*, 79-83.

30. KLEIN, M., PALUCK, R. J., and BERESFORD, P. (1976). The modification of disruptive behaviours by a group of trainable mentally retarded adults. *J. Behav. Ther. Exp. Psychiat., 7*, 189-190.

31. KRAMER, M., PERSON, R. H., TARJAN, G., MORGAN, R., and WRIGHT, S. W. (1957). A method for determination of probabilities of stay, release and death for patients admitted to a hospital for the mentally deficient. *Amer. J. Ment. Defic., 62*, 199-203.

32. KRIGER, S. F. (1975) *Life Styles of Aging Retardates Living in Community Settings in Ohio*. Columbus, Ohio: Psychologia Metrika.

33. KRIGER, S. F (1976). Geriatrics. In J. Wortis (ed.), *Mental Retardation and Developmental Disabilities*. Vol. 8. New York: Brunner/Mazel, pp. 156-167.

34. LEFF, R. B. (1975). Teaching TMR and adults to dial the telephone. *Ment. Retard., 13*, 9-11.

35. MACFARLANE, A. C. (1962). Dental health in mental deficiency hospitals. In: Richards, B. W. (ed.), *Proceedings of the London Conference on the Scientific Study of Mental Deficiency*. Vol. 1. Dagenham: May & Baker, pp. 189-198.

36. MALAMUD, N. (1972). Neuropathology of organic brain syndromes associated with aging. In: C. M. Gaitz (ed.), *Aging and the Brain*. New York: Plenum Press. pp. 63-87.

37. MCCARVER, R. B., and CRAIG, E. M. (1974). Placement of the retarded in the community: prognosis and outcome. In: N. R. Ellis (ed.), *International Review of Research in Mental Retardation*. Vol. 7. New York: Academic Press, pp. 146-207.

38. NIHIRA, K. (1976). Dimensions of adaptive behavior in institutionalized mentally retarded children and adults: Developmental perspective. *Amer. J. Ment. Defic., 81*, 215-226.

39. NIHIRA, K. (1977). Development of adaptive behavior in the mentally retarded. In: P. Mittler (ed.), *Research to Practice in Mental Retardation*. Vol. 2. Baltimore: University Park Press, pp. 157-168.

40. NIHIRA, K., FOSTER, R., SHELLHAAS, M., and LELAND, H. (1974). *AAMD Adaptive Behavior Scale*. 1974 Revision. Washington: AAMD.

41. PENROSE, L. S. (1938). *A Clinical and Genetic Study of 1280 Cases of Mental Defect*. Medical Research Council, Special Report Series, No. 229. London: H.M.S.O.

42. PENROSE, L. S. (1963). *The Biology of Mental Defect*. 3rd Edition. London: Sidgwick & Jackson.

43. REID, A. H. (1972). Psychoses in adult mental defectives: I. Manic-depressive psychosis; II. Schizophrenic and paranoid psychoses. *Brit. J. Psychiat., 120*, 205-218.

44. REYNOLDS, W. M., and REYNOLDS, S. (1979). Prevalence of speech and hearing impairment

of noninstitutionalized mentally retarded adults. *Amer. J. Ment. Defic.*, *84*, 62-66.

45. RICHARDS, B. W. (1975). Mental retardation. In: J. G. Howells (ed.), *Modern Perspectives in the Psychiatry of Old Age*. New York: Brunner/Mazel. pp. 363-378.

46. ROSEN, M., CLARK, G. R., and KIVITZ, M. S. (1977). *Habilitation of the Handicapped: New Dimensions in Programs for the Developmentally Disabled*. Baltimore: University Park Press.

47. SCALLY, B. G. (1974). Marriage and mental handicap: Some observations in Northern Ireland. In: F. F. de la Cruz and G. D. La Veck (eds.), *Human Sexuality and the Mentally Retarded*. Baltimore: Penguin Books, pp. 186-194.

48. SCHROEDER, S. R., and HENES, C. (1978). Assessment of progress of institutionalized and deinstitutionalized retarded adults: A matched-control comparison. *Ment. Retard.*, *16*, 147-148.

49. SMITH, G. F., and BERG, J. M. (1976). *Down's Anomaly*. 2nd edition. Edinburgh: Churchill Livingstone.

50. SYLVESTER, P. E. (1974). Aortic and pulmonary valve fenestrations as ageing indices in Down's syndrome. *J. Ment. Defic. Res.*, *18*, 367-376.

51. TSUANG, M. T. (1974). Sex chromatin anomaly in Chinese females: psychiatric characteristics of XXX. *Brit. J. Psychiat.*, *124*, 299-305.

52. WHELAN, E. (1977). Basic work-skills training and vocational counselling of the mentally handicapped. In: P. Mittler (ed.), *Research to Practice in Mental Retardation*. Vol. 2. Baltimore: University Park Press. pp. 377-386.

NAME INDEX

SUBJECT INDEX

411